Emergency Radiology

Ajay Singh

Editor

Emergency Radiology

Imaging of Acute Pathologies

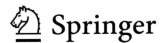 Springer

Editor
Ajay Singh, MD
Department of Radiology
Massachusetts General Hospital
Harvard Medical School
Boston, MA
USA

ISBN 978-1-4419-9591-9   ISBN 978-1-4419-9592-6   (eBook)
DOI 10.1007/978-1-4419-9592-6
Springer New York Heidelberg Dordrecht London

Library of Congress Control Number: 2013938161

Printed on acid-free paper

Springer is part of Springer Science+Business Media (www.springer.com)

Preface

The practice of emergency radiology has evolved rapidly over the last two decades, playing an important part in the triage of emergency room patients. Plain radiography and CT imaging are the most commonly used imaging modalities in managing emergency conditions in the more than 115,000 patients visiting the emergency room. Ultrasound, MR, and nuclear medicine imaging, although less often used, play crucial roles in managing specific conditions.

This textbook of emergency radiology represents the state-of-the-art radiology practice in the management of emergency room patients by leading experts in the field. The chapters are based on different organ systems, with few chapters being imaging modality based.

I would like to take this opportunity to thank the publishers for the privilege of editing this textbook and their staff for professional production of this issue. I must thank the authors of the book chapters for sharing their expertise and case material in preparing the manuscript.

Boston, MA, USA   Ajay Singh, MD

Contents

Contributors

Laura Avery, MD Department of Radiology, Massachusetts General Hospital, Boston, MA, USA

Brett W. Carter, MD Department of Radiology, Baylor University Medical Center, Dallas, TX, USA

Harigovinda R. Challa, MD Division of Pediatric Radiology, University of Kentucky, Lexington, KY, USA

Andrew Chen, MD Department of Radiology, University of Massachusetts, Worcester, MA, USA

Jeanette Chun, MD Department of Radiology, University of Massachusetts Memorial Medical Center, Worcester, MA, USA

Dennis Coughlin, MD Department of Radiology, University of Massachusetts Memorial Medical Center, Worcester, MA, USA

Terry S. Desser, MD Department of Radiology, Stanford University School of Medicine, Stanford, CA, USA

Johanne E. Dillon, MD Division of Pediatric Radiology, University of Kentucky, Lexington, KY, USA

Sathish Kumar Dundamadappa, MD Department of Radiology, University of Massachusetts, Worcester, MA, USA

Melanie Ehinger, MD Department of Radiology, University of Massachusetts, Worcester, MA, USA

Joseph Ferucci, MD Department of Radiology, University of Massachusetts Memorial Medical Center, Worcester, MA, USA

Dale E. Hansen III, MD Department of Radiology, University of Tennessee, Memphis, TN, USA

Chris Heinis, MD Department of Emergency Radiology, University of Massachusetts Memorial Medical Center, Worcester, MA, USA

Paul F. von Herrmann, MD Department of Radiology, University of Kentucky, Lexington, KY, USA

Mai-Lan Ho, MD Department of Radiology, Beth Israel Deaconess Medical Center, Boston, MA, USA

Paul Jaffray, MD Department of Radiology, University of Massachusetts Memorial Medical Center, Worcester, MA, USA

Rathachai Kaewlai, MD Department of Radiology, Ramathibodi Hospital and Mahidol University, Ratchatewi, Bangkok, Thailand

Majid Khan, MD Department of Radiology, Oakland University, William Beaumont School of Medicine, William Beaumont Hospital, Royal Oak, MI, USA

Amisha Khicha, MD Department of Radiology, Wesley Medical Center, University of Kansas School of Medicine, Wichita, KS, USA

John J. Krol, MD Department of Radiology, University of Kentucky, Lexington, KY, USA

Joshua Leeman, MD Department of Radiology, Shady Side Hospital, Pittsburgh, PA, USA

Jonathan E. Leeman, MD Department of Radiology, Shady Side Hospital, Pittsburgh, PA, USA

Robin Levenson, MD Department of Radiology, Beth Israel Deaconess Medical Center, Boston, MA, USA

Chris Malcom, MD Department of Radiology, William Beaumont Hospital, Royal Oak, MI, USA

Caterina Missiroli, MD Department of Diagnostic Imaging, Azienda Ospedaliera della Provincia di Lecco – Presidio Ospedaliero A. Manzoni, Lecco, Italy

Victorine V. Muse, MD Department of Radiology, Massachusetts General Hospital, Harvard Medical School, Boston, MA, USA

David J. Nickels, MD, MBA Department of Radiology, Division of Emergency Radiology, University of Kentucky, Lexington, KY, USA

Robert A. Novelline, MD Department of Radiology, Massachusetts General Hospital, Harvard Medical School, Boston, MA, USA

M. Elizabeth Oates, MD Department of Radiology, University of Kentucky, Lexington, KY, USA

Neil Patel, MD Department of Radiology, University of Tennessee, Memphis, TN, USA

Sneha Patel, MD Department of Diagnostic Radiology, William Beaumont Hospital, Royal Oak, MI, USA

Parul Penkar, MD Department of Radiology, Massachusetts General Hospital, Boston, MA, USA

Sridhar Shankar, MD, MBA Department of Radiology, University of Tennessee, Memphis, TN, USA

Ajay Singh, MD Department of Radiology, Massachusetts General Hospital, Harvard Medical School, Boston, MA, USA

Benjamin Yeh, MD Department of Radiology, University of California San Francisco, San Francisco, CA, USA

Jeanette Chun and Ajay Singh

Introduction

Acute aortic conditions include, but are not limited to, aortic rupture, aortic dissection, intramural hematoma, and penetrating aortic ulcer. Prompt diagnosis of these conditions is essential for managing these conditions. Because these conditions often have similar symptoms, namely, chest and abdominal pain, the imaging characteristics are key to prompt and accurate diagnosis.

Abdominal Aortic Aneurysm and Aortic Rupture

Abdominal aortic aneurysm (AAA) is seen in 5–10 % of elderly male smokers. Most AAAs are true aneurysms and involve all three layers of the aortic wall. The two most common etiologies of AAA are degenerative and inflammatory (Table 1.1).

Other less frequent etiologies of AAA include mycotic aneurysm, which constitutes 1–3 % of aortic aneurysms. However, mycotic aneurysm is known to more commonly involve aorta than any other artery. Staphylococcus and Streptococcus species are the most common pathogens of mycotic aneurysm. The cases of mycotic aneurysm due to Salmonella species are more common in East Asia and demonstrate an early tendency to rupture.

The most significant complication of AAA is aortic rupture. The mortality rate for ruptured AAA is 50 %; thus, an accurate diagnosis is essential for prompt surgical

Table 1.1 Causes of abdominal aortic aneurysm

Degenerative (most common)
Inflammatory (5–10 % of all)
Mycotic
Syndromes: Marfan's syndrome, Ehlers-Danlos syndrome
Vasculitis: Takayasu's disease, Behcet's disease
Traumatic

intervention. The risk of rupture is proportional to the maximum cross-sectional diameter, with 1 %/year risk for aneurysms measuring 5–5.9 cm. The risk of rupture increases up to 20 %/year for an aneurysm measuring greater than 7 cm in diameter. Although AAAs are less common in females (M:F = 4:1), they are more likely to rupture when compared to males.

Ultrasound is the most commonly used imaging modality to screen for AAA and has been shown to reduce mortality. The imaging criteria to diagnose AAA include aortic caliber of more than 3 cm and an aortic caliber of more than 1.5 times the expected diameter of the abdominal aorta (Fig. 1.1). The aortic caliber is measured perpendicular to the long axis of the aorta, from outer wall to outer wall. Although ultrasound is highly sensitive in making the diagnosis of abdominal aortic aneurysm, it is not as reliable as CT in diagnosing aortic rupture. However, the demonstration of normal caliber of abdominal aorta by ultrasound makes aortic rupture an unlikely possibility.

Most aortic aneurysms rupture involves the middle third of the aneurysm, through the posterolateral wall and into the retroperitoneum (Fig. 1.2a). However, intraperitoneal rupture and rupture into the bowel (usually the duodenum) and very rarely into the IVC may occur (Fig. 1.2b, c).

Risk Factors for Aortic Rupture

Progressive aneurysmal dilatation of the aorta with increased wall tension is directly related to the risk of rupture. The

J. Chun, MD
Department of Radiology,
University of Massachusetts Memorial Medical Center,
Worcester, MA, USA

A. Singh, MD (✉)
Department of Radiology,
Massachusetts General Hospital, Harvard Medical School,
10 Museum Way, # 524, Boston, MA 02141, USA
e-mail: asingh1@partners.org

A. Singh (ed.), *Emergency Radiology*,
DOI 10.1007/978-1-4419-9592-6_1, © Springer Science+Business Media New York 2013

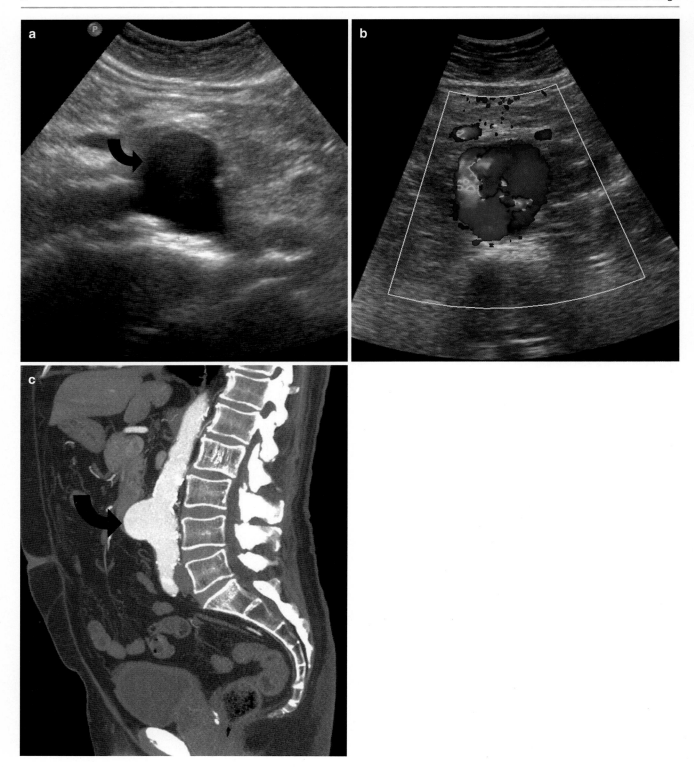

Fig. 1.1 Saccular abdominal aortic aneurysm. (**a** and **b**) US demonstrate a saccular infrarenal aortic aneurysm (*curved arrow*) with yin-yang sign on color Doppler imaging. (**c**) Sagittal reformation demonstrates the saccular infrarenal abdominal aortic aneurysm (*curved arrow*)

decreased proportion of thrombus to lumen ratio is also thought to play a part, as a larger thrombus better protects against rupture by providing protection against the high aortic pressures [1]. In addition, the amount of thrombus calcification, which is thought to be related to the amount of thrombus present, is also an indirect measure [2].

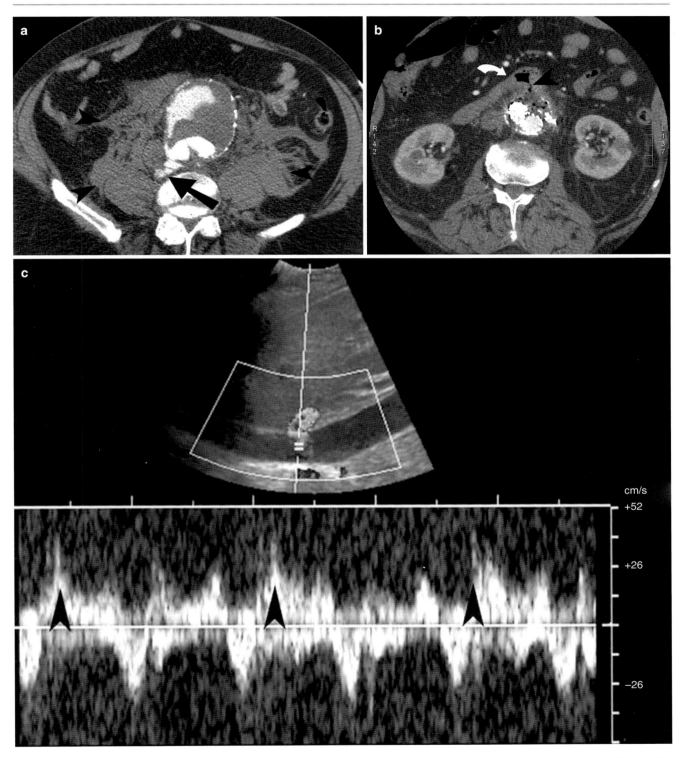

Fig. 1.2 Abdominal aortic aneurysm rupture, aorto-enteric and aorto-caval fistula. (**a**) Contrast-enhanced CT scan study of the lower abdomen demonstrates active extravasation of contrast (*arrow*) from infrarenal abdominal aortic aneurysm. There is retroperitoneal hemorrhage (*arrowheads*) identified around the aortic aneurysm. (**b**) Aorto-enteric fistula. Contrast-enhanced CT scan study demonstrates communication (*arrowhead*) of the third portion of the duodenum (*arrow*) with the infrarenal abdominal aortic aneurysm sac. The patient had recently undergone endovascular stent placement. (**c**) Aortocaval fistula. Doppler US shows the combination of arterial and venous spectral waveform in the inferior vena cava lumen, in a patient with aortocaval fistula

Table 1.2 CT findings of aortic rupture

1. Active extravasation of contrast
2. Retroperitoneal hematoma around the aortic aneurysm
3. Periaortic stranding
4. Draped aorta sign
5. Hyperdense crescent sign
6. Tangential calcium sign
7. Discontinuity of intimal calcification

Imaging

The imaging modality of choice is a contrast-enhanced multidetector CT (MDCT). The CT can demonstrate an AAA with surrounding retroperitoneal hemorrhage into psoas compartment, pararenal space, and perirenal space. A contrast-enhanced CT provides additional information about the aortic size, presence or absence of active extravasation, and anatomic relationships (Table 1.2). A hyperdense crescent sign and draped aorta sign are indicators of contained aortic leak or impending rupture. Focal discontinuity of intimal calcification is also a secondary sign of aortic rupture.

Hyperdense Crescent Sign

Hyperdense crescent sign is seen as a well-defined peripheral, high-density, crescent configuration within a thrombus where there is internal dissection of hemorrhage into the thrombus and ultimately reaching the aortic wall. It is a sign of acute or impending rupture (Fig. 1.3a) [1].

Draped Aorta Sign

Draped aorta sign indicates a contained aortic rupture and shows posterior aortic wall not identifiable as a separate structure and draping over the adjacent vertebral bodies (Fig. 1.3b, c). If rupture should occur, the most common sign of aneurysmal rupture is a retroperitoneal hematoma adjacent to the aneurysm.

Tangential Calcium Sign

The intimal calcification in the aorta points away from the circumference of the aneurysm (Fig. 1.3d).

The typical imaging features of mycotic aneurysm (Fig. 1.3e) include rapidly increasing caliber of a saccular aortic aneurysm with wall irregularity, periaortic edema and soft tissue mass, and the presence of gas. Periaortic soft tissue stranding and soft tissue mass are the most common features seen on imaging of mycotic aneurysm. Calcifications and thrombus are uncommon in a mycotic aneurysm. The lack of calcification in the aortic wall is due to the nonatherosclerotic origin of the aneurysm.

Aortic Dissection

Aortic dissection is the most common acute presentation involving the aorta [3]. It usually originates with a tear in the intima, which causes high-pressure blood to enter and dissect the aortic wall (Table 1.3).

The most commonly used classification for aortic dissection is the Stanford classification system.

1. *Type A aortic dissection:* Regardless of origin and extent of dissection, a Type A aortic dissection involves the ascending aorta (Fig. 1.4) [4]. The potential for complications with Type A dissection necessitates urgent surgical intervention [4]. The complications include dissection into the pericardium resulting in cardiac tamponade, dissection into the coronary arteries resulting in occlusion, and aortic insufficiency with involvement of the valve [4].
2. *Type B aortic dissection:* The aortic dissection originates past the left subclavian artery [5]. Unlike Type A dissection, the Type B dissections are usually medically treated.

Imaging

The imaging modality of choice to evaluate aortic dissection is MDCT. It allows accurate assessment of the extent of the disease, including the origin of the dissection, involvement of the visceral branches, and presence of a false lumen [3, 4]. The most characteristic findings of aortic dissection include an intimal flap and two distinct lumens. Secondary findings include intimal displacement of calcified wall, delayed enhancement of false lumen, pericardial or mediastinal hematoma, and ischemia or infarction of distal organs supplied by the false lumen [4].

True Versus False Lumen

Once the recognition of an aortic dissection is made, it is important to distinguish between the true and false lumen for treatment purposes, especially endovascular repair. Lepage et al. evaluated signs to distinguish between the true and false lumen and determined two consistent signs: beak sign and larger cross-sectional area of false lumen as the best indicators. The beak sign is present in the false lumen and consists of an acute angle between the dissection flap and the aortic wall [5]. The larger caliber lumen is generally the false lumen and is most commonly present anteriorly, to the right side in the ascending aorta (Figs. 1.4, 1.5, and 1.6). In the descending thoracic aorta, the false lumen is most

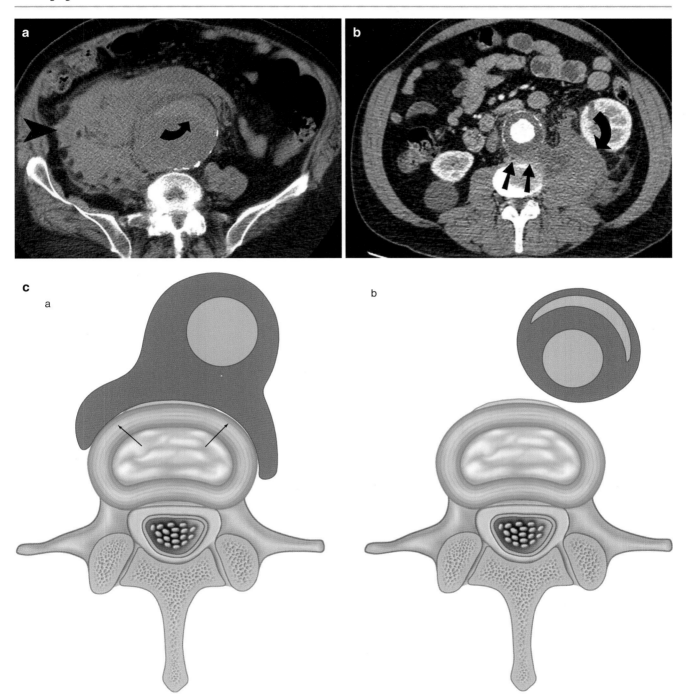

Fig. 1.3 CT features of abdominal aortic aneurysm rupture. (**a**) Hyperdense crescent sign. Noncontrast CT demonstrates large retroperitoneal hematoma (*arrowhead*) from the ruptured aortic aneurysm. A hyperdense crescent (*curved arrow*) is present in the anterior wall of the infrarenal abdominal aortic aneurysm. (**b**) Draped aorta sign. Contrast-enhanced CT demonstrates draping of the posterior wall of the aorta (*straight arrows*) on the anterior aspect of the lumbar spine. There is large retroperitoneal hematoma (*curved arrow*) identified in the psoas compartment and left posterior pararenal space. (**c**) Schematic representation of the *draped aorta sign* (*a*) and *hyperdense crescent sign* (*b*).

Draped aorta sign is characterized by draping of deficient aortic wall on the anterior aspect of the vertebral body. Hyperdense crescent sign is characterized by the presence of a high-density sickle-shaped blood clot in the aortic wall. (**d**) Tangential calcium sign in a patient with contained aortic leak. Noncontrast CT demonstrates intimal calcifications (*arrowheads*) displaced from their expected location and pointing away from the aortic circumference. (**e**) Rupture of mycotic aneurysm. Noncontrast CT demonstrates air in the wall of the aortic aneurysm, secondary to clostridial infection. Breech in the aortic wall is indicated by the presence of air (*arrowheads*) outside the aortic adventitia

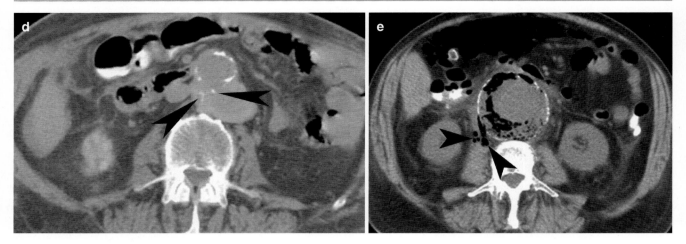

Fig. 1.3 (continued)

Table 1.3 Factors predisposing to aortic dissection

| Hypertension (most common) |
| Syndromes |
| Marfan's syndrome |
| Turner syndrome |
| Noonan syndrome |
| Ehlers-Danlos syndrome |
| Coarctation, bicuspid aortic valve |
| Cocaine use |
| Pregnancy |
| Trauma |

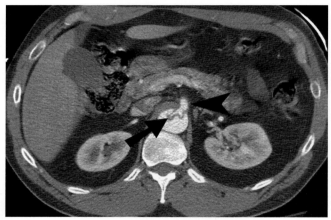

Fig. 1.5 Aortic dissection involving the abdominal aorta. Contrast-enhanced CT scan study demonstrates small caliber of the true lumen (*arrow*) supplying the superior mesenteric artery (*arrowhead*)

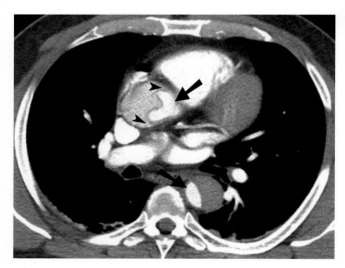

Fig. 1.4 Type A aortic dissection. Contrast-enhanced CT scan study of the chest demonstrates aortic dissection involving the ascending as well as the descending thoracic aorta. The true lumen can be identified by the smaller caliber (*arrows*) and higher density. The beak sign (*arrowheads*) is identified in the false lumen

often seen posteriorly and to the left. Cobwebs are seen in the false lumen while aortic wall calcifications are usually seen around true lumen.

Intramural Hematoma

Intramural hematoma is a hematoma that has dissected through the media without an originating intimal tear (Figs. 1.7 and 1.8). The intramural hematoma may represent hemorrhage of the vasa vasorum (nutrient vessels for the vessel wall) that has dissected through the media [6]. It can be seen in hypertensive and can also be seen after blunt trauma. It can progress to rupture of the aortic wall or aortic dissection.

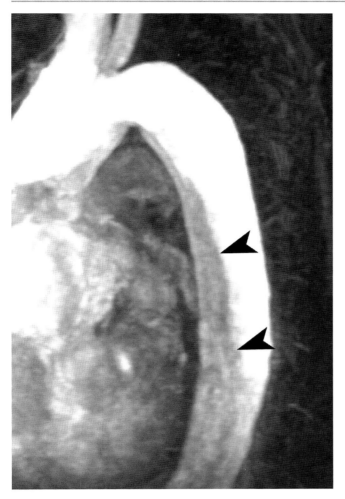

Fig. 1.6 Type B aortic dissection on MR angiogram. Gadolinium-enhanced MR angiogram demonstrates the dissection flap (*arrowheads*) present in the descending thoracic aorta

Unlike mural thrombus, intramural hematoma is deep to the intimal calcification and does not demonstrate the continuous flow seen with aortic dissection. Intramural hematoma can be diagnosed on CT, transesophageal echocardiography, and MRI. Since there is no intimal disruption, it cannot be diagnosed on conventional aortography. The treatment of intramural hematoma is similar to aortic dissection.

Penetrating Ulcer

Penetrating ulcer is characterized by atherosclerotic ulceration that has penetrated through the elastic lamina and formed a hematoma in the media. On CT scan, it is seen as an ulcer with focal hematoma and adjacent arterial wall thickening (Fig. 1.9) [7, 8]. Unlike penetrating ulcer, an atherosclerotic plaque with ulceration does not extend beyond the intima and is not associated with intramural hematoma.

Penetrating ulcer and aortic dissection are characterized by disruption of the intima, while aortic rupture is characterized by disruption of the aortic wall.

CT is the key diagnostic modality in the emergency room evaluation of acute aortic syndromes and allows different pathologies to be diagnosed for proper triage as well as treatment.

Teaching Points

- There is increased risk of rupture with increasing caliber of the aneurysm and reduced thrombus to lumen ratio.
- Hyperdense crescent sign and draped aorta sign are indicators of contained aortic leak or impending rupture.
- Type A aortic dissection involves the ascending aorta and is surgically managed.
- Type B aortic dissection originates past the left subclavian artery and is usually medically managed.
- Intramural hematoma represents hemorrhage of the vasa vasorum and is not associated with intimal discontinuity (unlike penetrating ulcer).

Penetrating ulcer   Intramural hematoma

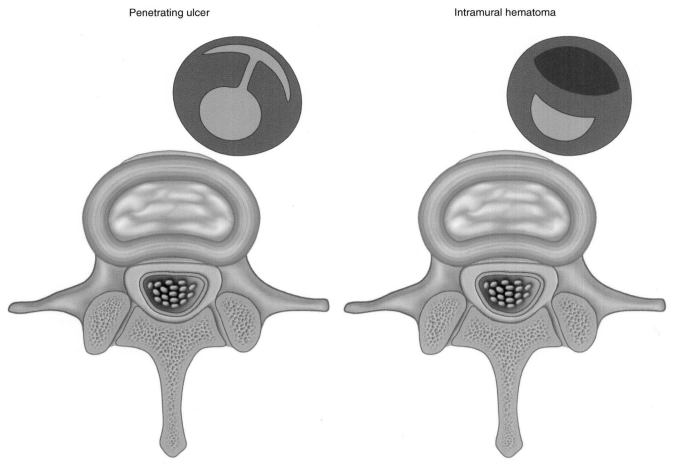

Fig. 1.7 Schematic representation of penetrating ulcer and intramural hematoma. Penetrating ulcer is characterized by communication of the arterial lumen with the hematoma located in the media. Intramural hematoma is characterized by lack of direct communication of the arterial lumen with the hematoma in the media

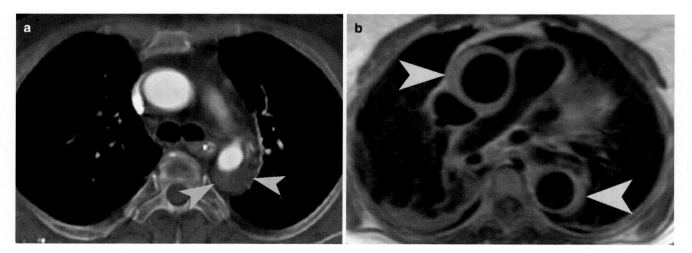

Fig. 1.8 Intramural hematoma. (**a**) Contrast-enhanced CT demonstrates asymmetric aortic wall thickening, consistent with intramural hematoma (*arrowheads*) in the descending thoracic aorta. (**b**) Noncontrast axial T1-weighted MR shows intramural hematoma (*arrowheads*) causing asymmetric aortic wall thickening in the ascending and descending thoracic aorta

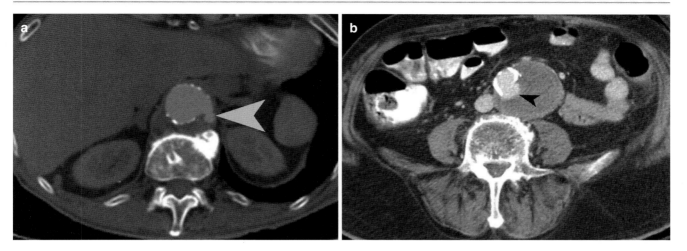

Fig. 1.9 Aortic ulcer. (**a** and **b**) Contrast-enhanced CT scan study of the abdomen demonstrates abdominal aortic aneurysm with an aortic ulcer (*arrowheads*) along with intramural hemorrhage

References

1. Rakita D, Newatia A, Hines JJ, Siegel DN, Friedman B. Spectrum of CT findings in rupture and impending rupture of abdominal aortic aneurysms. Radiographics. 2007;27:497–507.
2. Schwartz SA, Taljanovic MS, Smyth S, O'Brien MJ, Rogers LF. CT findings of rupture, impending rupture, and contained rupture of aortic abdominal aneurysm. AJR Am J Roentgenol. 2007;188:W57–62.
3. Petasnick JP. Radiologic evaluation of aortic dissection. Radiology. 1991;180:297–305.
4. Fisher ER, Stern E, Godwin II JD, Otto C, Johnson JA. Acute aortic dissection: typical and atypical imaging. Radiographics. 1994;14:1263–71.
5. Lepage MA, Quint LE, Sonnad SS, Deeb M, Williams DM. Aortic dissection: CT features that distinguish true lumen from false lumen. AJR Am J Roentgenol. 2001;177:207–11.
6. Sawhney NS, DeMaria AN, Blanchard DG. Aortic intramural hematoma: an increasingly recognized and potentially fatal entity. Chest. 2001;120:1340–6.
7. Hayashi H, Matsuoka Y, Sakamoto I, Sueyoshi E, Okimoto T, Hayashi K, et al. Penetrating atherosclerotic ulcer of the aorta: imaging features and disease concept. Radiographics. 2000;20:995–1005.
8. Sebastià C, Pallisa E, Quiroga S, Alvarez-Castells A, Dominguez R, Evangelista A. Aortic dissection: diagnosis and follow-up with helical CT. Radiographics. 1999;19:45–60.

Caterina Missiroli and Ajay Singh

Gallbladder is seen as an anechoic structure with wall thickness of less than 3 mm on ultrasound imaging. The normal common bile duct caliber is up to 5 mm in young adults, and it progressively increases with age, at the rate of 1 mm for each decade above 40 years. The intrahepatic ducts should not be more than 2 mm in diameter (not more than 40 % of the caliber of the accompanying portal vein branch).

Gallstones are seen in up to 10 % of the population, most commonly in middle-aged and elderly females. While majority of gallstones have cholesterol as the main component, a minority of stones are constituted by calcium bilirubinate and are called pigment stones. Ten to twenty percent of the gallstones contain enough calcium to be visible on plain radiograph (Fig. 2.1a). The stones are most commonly multiple and sometimes faceted. A triradiate collection of nitrogen gas within the fissures inside the gallstone produces Mercedes-Benz sign (Fig. 2.1b and c).

Typically, gallstones are seen as echogenic foci with clean distal acoustic shadowing (Fig. 2.1d). *Wall echo shadow sign* refers to the parallel echogenic lines produced by a combination of the gallbladder wall, echogenic stone, and associated distal acoustic shadowing (Fig. 2.1e). The hypoechoic line seen between the two echogenic lines represents interposed bile. This sign is seen in gallbladder filled with either a single large gallstone or multiple small gallstones. Ultrasound has higher sensitivity than CT in diagnosing gallstones and is therefore the screening modality of choice. Although ultrasound remains the exam of choice for suspected cholecystitis,

there are ever more cases of acute cholecystitis being detected today with CT in the evaluation of abdominal pain than in the past.

Majority of the patients with gallstones are asymptomatic. Sometimes the gallstone can cause transient gallbladder outflow obstruction, leading to biliary colic. Biliary colic patients present with transient pain for 1–3 h with nausea and vomiting. The symptoms subside when the gallstone falls back into the gallbladder or passes distally into the biliary tree.

Acute Cholecystitis

Acute cholecystitis usually is caused by the gallstone obstruction of the cystic duct or the gallbladder neck (one-third of cases). Acute cholecystitis without stones (5–10 % of cases) can be seen in patients with adenomyomatosis, gallbladder polyp, and malignant neoplasm [1, 2]. The predisposing factors for acute acalculous cholecystitis include history of trauma, mechanical ventilation, hyperalimentation, postoperative/postpartum state, diabetes mellitus, vascular insufficiency, prolonged fasting, and burns [2].

The clinical presentation includes right upper quadrant pain for more than 6 h (vs. biliary colic), nausea, vomiting, and fever in a patient with history of gallstones. No clinical or lab finding provides high enough positive predictive value in making the diagnosis of acute cholecystitis.

Imaging

Ultrasound is the first-line imaging modality in diagnosing acute cholecystitis because of wide availability, ability to detect gallstones as well as biliary ducts, and accuracy in diagnosing acute cholecystitis. The ultrasound findings of acute cholecystitis include gallbladder wall thickening (>3 mm), gallbladder distension (>5 cm transverse dimension), and positive Murphy's sign (Fig. 2.2) [1, 3]. Sonographic Murphy's sign by itself does not have a high

C. Missiroli, MD
Department of Diagnostic Imaging,
Azienda Ospedaliera della Provincia di
Lecco – Presidio Ospedaliero A. Manzoni, Lecco, Italy

A. Singh, MD (✉)
Department of Radiology,
Massachusetts General Hospital, Harvard Medical School,
10 Museum Way, # 524, Boston, MA 02141, USA
e-mail: asingh1@partners.org

A. Singh (ed.), *Emergency Radiology*,
DOI 10.1007/978-1-4419-9592-6_2, © Springer Science+Business Media New York 2013

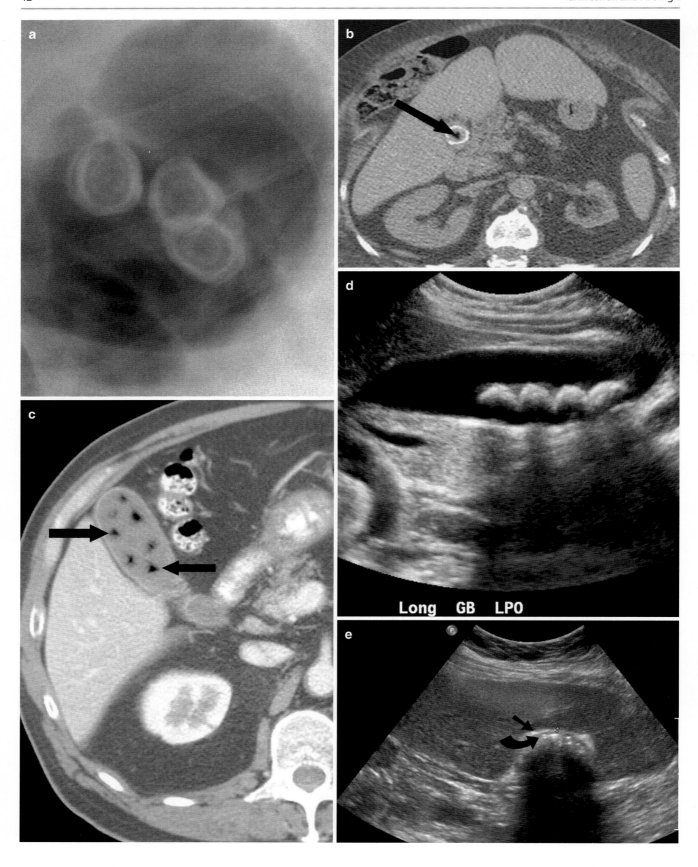

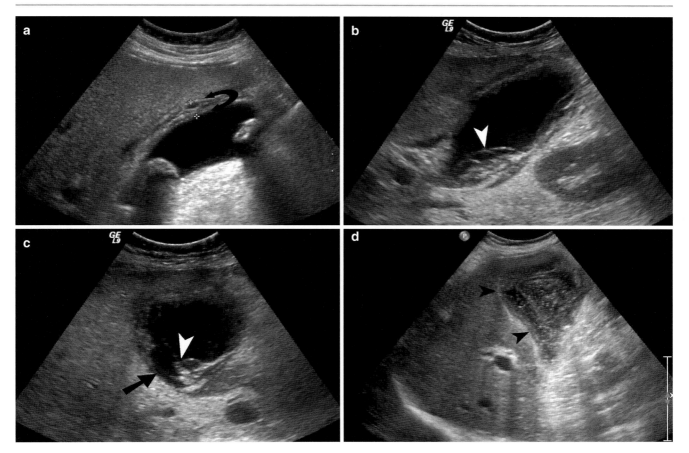

Fig. 2.2 Ultrasound imaging of acute cholecystitis. (**a**) Ultrasound in a patient with acute cholecystitis demonstrates multiple gallstones and striated thickening of the gallbladder wall (*arrow*). (**b** and **c**) Ultrasound in a patient with gangrenous cholecystitis demonstrates striated thickening of the gallbladder wall, intraluminal sludge, and sloughed mucosa (*arrowhead*). Focal thinning of the necrotic gallbladder is indicated by the *straight arrow* and appears to represent the donor site for the sloughed-off mucosa. (**d**) Ultrasound in a patient with acute cholecystitis shows gallbladder wall thickening (*arrowheads*) and complex fluid, which represented pus during cholecystostomy tube placement

positive predictive value and can be falsely negative in patients who have received analgesic medication. Another imaging finding of acute cholecystitis is the presence of a pericholecystic fluid collection, sometimes extending to the perihepatic space [2, 4].

Gallbladder wall thickening is a finding of acute cholecystitis which can also be seen in other conditions such as hypoproteinemia, ascites, pancreatitis, right heart failure, renal failure, liver failure, and hepatitis. Striated gallbladder wall thickening is no more specific for acute cholecystitis than the observation of gallbladder wall thickening from other causes. In the clinical setting of acute cholecystitis, the presence of striated gallbladder wall thickening suggests gangrenous cholecystitis.

Cholescintigraphy (HIDA scan) is considered second-line imaging modality which can be used after equivocal ultrasound study. Cholescintigraphy has a sensitivity and specificity which is superior to ultrasound. Although it may take more than 2 h to complete the study, the use of morphine (0.04 mg/kg) allows cholescintigraphy to be completed in 1.5 h. The classic findings on cholescintigraphy include nonvisualization of the gallbladder 30 min after morphine injection and presence of a curvilinear area of increased

Fig. 2.1 Imaging appearance of gallstones on plain radiograph and ultrasound. (**a**) Plain radiograph demonstrates laminated radiopaque gallstones in the *right upper quadrant*. Up to a fifth of the gallstones can be seen on plain radiograph of the abdomen. (**b** and **c**) Noncontrast CT of the gallbladder shows gallstones with Mercedes-Benz sign (*arrows*). Mercedes-Benz sign is due to nitrogen collection in triradiate configuration, within fissures of a gallstone. (**d**) Ultrasound shows multiple echogenic gallstones with distal acoustic shadowing, within the gallbladder lumen. (**e**) Ultrasound shows wall echo shadow sign in a patient with multiple gallstones and chronic cholecystitis. The outer echogenic line (*straight arrow*) represents the gallbladder wall, while the inner echogenic line (*curved arrow*) represents the outer edge of gallstones

Fig. 2.3 Gangrenous cholecystitis on cholescintigraphy. Cholescintigraphy study (HIDA scan) demonstrates nonvisualization of the gallbladder and a curvilinear area of increased radiotracer activity (*rim sign*) in the pericholecystitic liver parenchyma (*arrowheads*)

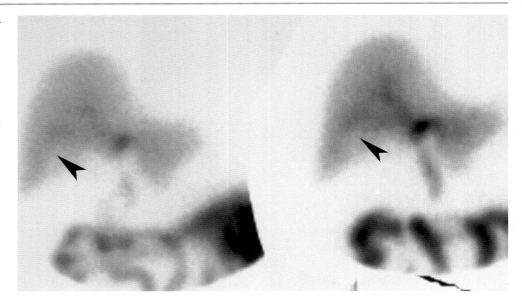

radiotracer activity (rim sign) in the liver adjacent to the gallbladder (Fig. 2.3). Rim sign is most commonly seen in patients with gangrenous cholecystitis and is due to extension of inflammation beyond the gallbladder.

If ultrasound and/or cholescintigraphy show no evidence of acute cholecystitis or any other cause for the right upper quadrant pain, a contrast-enhanced CT is considered the next most appropriate imaging modality. The CT findings include gallstones, gallbladder wall thickening, gallbladder wall enhancement, increased bile attenuation (possibly indicative to empyema), distended gallbladder, and pericholecystic fluid collection (Table 2.1; Fig. 2.4) [5]. CT has lower sensitivity than US in detecting gallstones and can miss noncalcified gallstones.

Table 2.1 CT findings of acute cholecystitis

Thickening of the gallbladder wall (normal wall thickness is up to 3–4 mm)
Gallstones
Gallbladder distention (>5 cm in transverse dimension)
Pericholecystic fluid
Indistinct interface between the gallbladder wall and the liver
Pericholecystic inflammatory changes
Transient focal attenuation difference
Increased density bile

MR imaging is not a frontline imaging modality for acute cholecystitis and can be used after equivocal US study. The advantage of MR over CT is its ability to reliably study

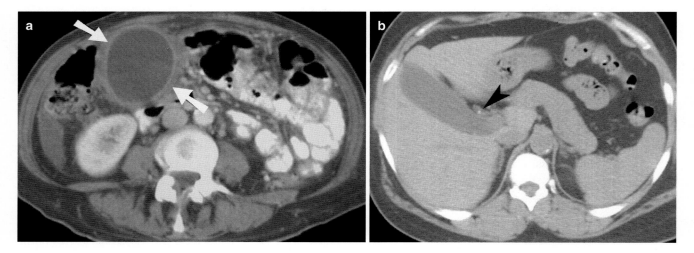

Fig. 2.4 CT findings of acute cholecystitis. (**a**) Contrast-enhanced CT shows distended gallbladder with wall thickening (*arrows*) and pericholecystic inflammatory changes. (**b**) Contrast-enhanced CT shows small calculus (*arrowhead*) causing cystic duct obstruction

common bile duct and the lack of ionizing radiation which is especially important in pregnant population. Although, gadolinium is useful in making the diagnosis of acute cholecystitis, it should not be used in pregnant population. The important findings of cholecystitis on MR imaging are described in Table 2.2 (Fig. 2.5).

The complications of acute cholecystitis include gallbladder empyema, gangrenous cholecystitis, emphysematous cholecystitis, gallbladder perforation, Mirizzi syndrome, and gallstone ileus.

Mirizzi Syndrome

The obstruction of the common bile duct or common hepatic duct by calculus impacted in the Hartmann's pouch or cystic duct constitutes Mirizzi syndrome (Fig. 2.6). Mirizzi syndrome or choledocholithiases should be suspected when-

Table 2.2 MR findings of acute cholecystitis

Gallbladder empyema	Low-signal intensity on T2 and high-signal intensity on T1 WI
Gallstones	Signal void on MRCP and low signal on T1–T2 WI
Gallbladder wall thickening	Enhancing wall and high signal on T1 and low to high on T2 WI
Gas within the gallbladder wall	Signal void in the wall
Pericholecystic inflammation	High intensity on T1 and T2 WI
Hemorrhage	High intensity on T1 and T2 WI
Fluid collection	High intensity on T1 and T2 WI

ever there is elevated bilirubin level along with clinical symptoms of acute cholecystitis.

Empyema

It is also called suppurative cholecystitis and occurs typically in diabetic patients, when the bile becomes infected and pus fills the distended gallbladder [1]. On imaging, gallbladder empyema is manifested as gallbladder distension, wall thickening, pericholecystic fluid accumulation, intraluminal sludge/pus, and intraluminal air (Fig. 2.7).

Gangrenous Cholecystitis

It is an advanced form of acute cholecystitis, most frequently seen in elderly men. It is characterized by increased intraluminal pressure, gallbladder distension, gallbladder wall necrosis, intramural hemorrhage, and abscess formation (Fig. 2.8) [1, 2]. There is an increased association of gangrenous cholecystitis with cardiovascular disease and leukocytosis of more than 17,000 WBC/mL. Although CT is highly specific (>90 %) in identifying patients with acute gangrenous cholecystitis, it is not very sensitive (Table 2.3).

Once gangrenous cholecystitis is suspected, the patients require emergency cholecystectomy or cholecystostomy to avoid life-threatening complications. These patients frequently require an open surgical procedure rather than laparoscopic cholecystectomy.

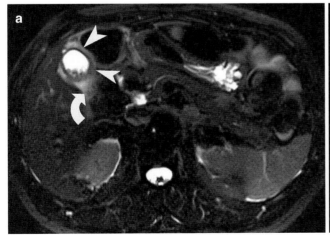
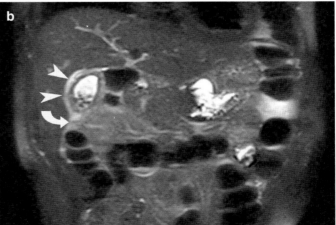

Fig. 2.5 MR findings of acute cholecystitis. (**a** and **b**) HASTE sequence shows gallbladder wall thickening (*arrowheads*), increased signal intensity (*curved arrows*), and multiple small gallstones. HASTE is a high-speed, heavily T2-weighted sequence with partial Fourier technique which has high sensitivity for fluid and a fast acquisition time (<1 s/slice)

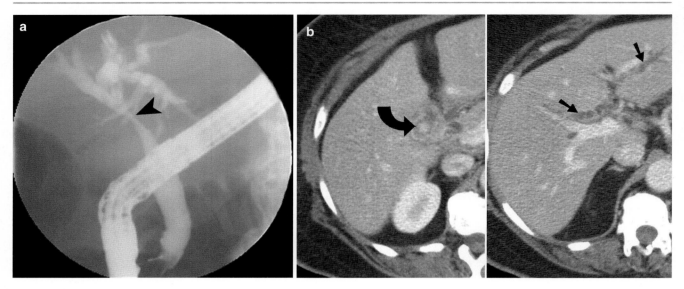

Fig. 2.6 Mirizzi syndrome. (**a**) ERCP demonstrates narrowing of the proximal CBD (*arrowhead*) due to extrinsic impression produced by calculus in the gallbladder neck. (**b**) Contrast-enhanced CT shows the calculus (*curved arrow*) in the gallbladder neck with secondary inflammation causing intrahepatic biliary ductal dilatation (*arrows*)

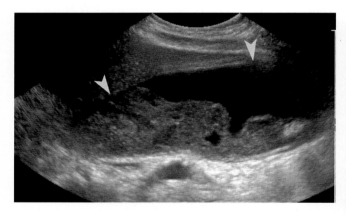

Fig. 2.7 Gallbladder empyema. Ultrasound shows marked distention (*arrowheads*) of the gallbladder lumen and intraluminal debris in a patient with gallbladder empyema

Table 2.3 CT findings of gangrenous cholecystitis

Gas in the gallbladder wall or lumen
Intraluminal membranes
Irregularity of wall
Pericholecystic abscess
Lack of mural enhancement
Greater degree of gallbladder distention and wall thickening

Emphysematous Cholecystitis

This is a rare life-threatening complication of acute cholecystitis and is characterized by gas within the gallbladder wall and/or lumen due to gas-forming bacteria. It has high mortality, especially when the diagnosis is missed. On ultrasound, gas can be recognized by the presence of dirty distal

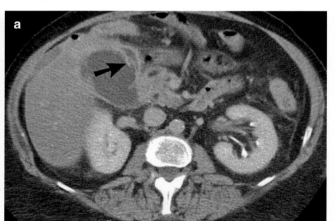

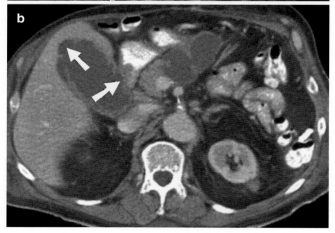

Fig. 2.8 Gangrenous cholecystitis. (**a** and **b**) Contrast-enhanced CT scan in two patients with gangrenous cholecystitis shows irregularity (*arrows*) of the gallbladder wall, gallbladder wall thickening, and pericholecystic inflammation

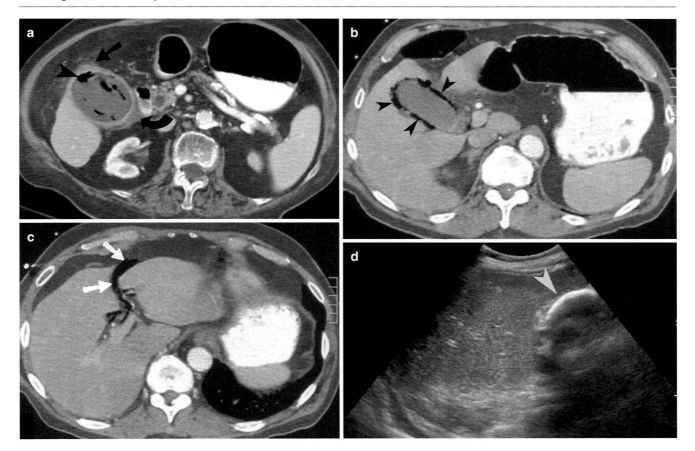

Fig. 2.9 Emphysematous cholecystitis. (**a**) Contrast-enhanced CT scan shows pericholecystic inflammation (*straight arrow*), pericholecystic fluid (*curved arrow*), and air within the gallbladder lumen (*arrowhead*). There was no air seen in the gallbladder on a previous CT study. (**b** and **c**) Contrast-enhanced CT shows air (*arrowheads*) in the wall of the gallbladder. Air is also seen to track along the ligamentum teres (*straight arrows*), indicating the presence of concomitant perforation. (**d**) Ultrasound demonstrates echogenic air (*arrowhead*) with dirty distal acoustic shadowing in the gallbladder lumen

acoustic shadowing. CT reliably allows distinction of gallbladder wall gas from porcelain gallbladder (Fig. 2.9).

Perforation

This is usually a complication of acute gangrenous cholecystitis and is associated with a high mortality of 19–24 % [1, 2]. It can be associated with generalized peritonitis, pericholecystic abscess, and cholecystoenteric fistula (chronic perforation).

The most common site of the gallbladder perforation is the fundus. These patients can develop pericholecystic or intrahepatic abscesses, cholecystoenteric fistulas, or biliary peritonitis. The CT findings of gallbladder perforation include gallbladder wall defect/bulge, streaky densities in the omentum or mesentery, pericholecystic fluid collection, and striated appearance of the gallbladder wall (Fig. 2.10).

The definitive treatment for gallbladder perforation is cholecystectomy (surgical or laparoscopic).

Gallbladder Torsion

It is characterized by acalculous cholecystitis and is most commonly seen in elderly women. A long or absent mesentery leading to abnormal mobility of the gallbladder predisposes to rotation of the gallbladder along its axis. If the torsion of gallbladder is partial (<180°), it leads to cystic duct obstruction. If the gallbladder torsion is complete (>180°), it leads to interruption of blood flow, leading to ischemia and gangrene.

On US, there is enlargement of the gallbladder which is abnormally oriented, with thickened wall and intramural or intraluminal gas due to gangrene [2].

Biliary Ductal Obstruction

Jaundice secondary to biliary obstruction is associated with pain, nausea, and vomiting. CT is the first-line imaging modality whenever malignancy is suspected as the cause of

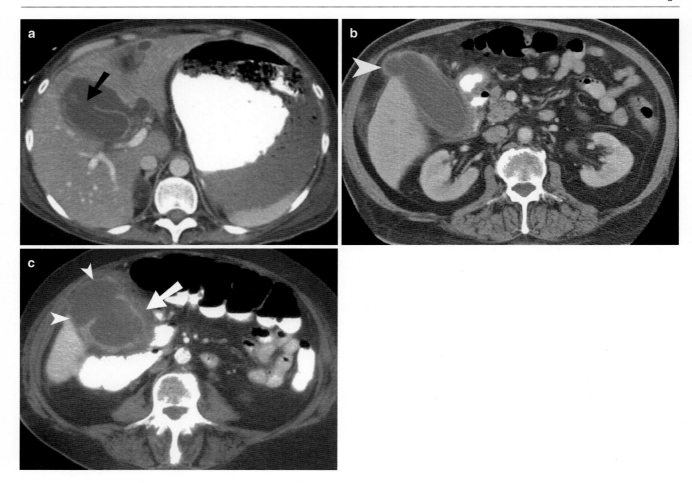

Fig. 2.10 Gallbladder perforation. (**a**) Axial contrast-enhanced CT image shows discontinuity of the gallbladder wall (*arrow*) and pericholecystic fluid. (**b**) Contrast-enhanced CT performed 3 months after cholecystostomy for acalculous cholecystitis shows CT findings of acute cholecystitis with focal perforation at the fundus (*arrowhead*). The fundal perforation was present at the site of entry of a previously placed cholecystostomy tube. (**c**) Contrast-enhanced CT demonstrates gallbladder wall perforation with intense pericholecystic inflammatory changes (*arrow*) and gallbladder wall edema. A contained perforation with bile collection (*arrowheads*) is seen anterior to the gallbladder

biliary obstruction. The most sensitive noninvasive imaging test in diagnosing choledocholithiasis is MRCP (Fig. 2.11). Therefore, it is the first-line imaging modality whenever choledocholithiasis is suspected to be the cause of biliary obstruction. Ultrasound is less effective than CT or ERCP in determining the site or cause of biliary obstruction.

Although ERCP is more expensive than other modalities, it is the first-line procedure for symptomatic choledocholithiases. The complication as well as diagnostic success rate of ERCP is lower than PTC. In patients with suspected malignant biliary obstruction and negative CT, ERCP with endoscopic ultrasound can provide cytologic diagnosis. Since ERCP has a 3 % complication rate and 0.4 % mortality rate, the use of MRCP can decrease the use of indiscriminate ERCP. ERCP is preferred when there is high likelihood of finding choledocholithiases, which requires therapeutic interventions. Percutaneous transhepatic cholangiography is useful when the obstruction is present proximally in the biliary tree. In clinical practice, PTC is most commonly performed after failed ERCP.

Percutaneous biliary decompression by catheter provides the decompression of the bile duct enlargement in patients with unresectable pancreatic head neoplasm, multifocal biliary strictures, and diffuse ductal strictures [6].

Cholangitis

Bacterial cholangitis is secondary to bile stasis, biliary ductal obstruction, and increased biliary pressure, followed by colonization by bacteria. Besides choledocholithiases, other causes of cholangitis include malignancy, sclerosing cholangitis, and biliary instrumentation.

The causes of cholangitis include bacteria, parasites, and viruses (AIDS patients). AIDS cholangiopathy is an acquired sclerosing cholangitis and is seen in patients

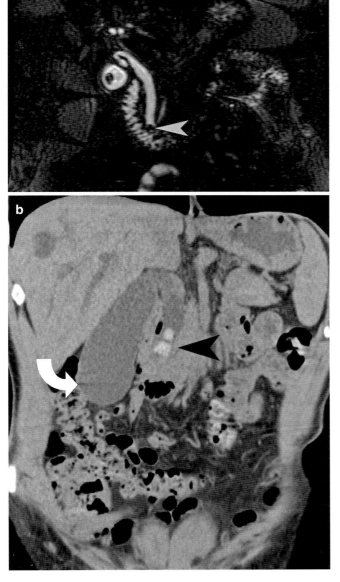

Fig. 2.11 Choledocholithiases. (**a**) MRCP shows dilatation of the CBD with choledocholithiases (*arrowhead*) at its lower end. (**b**) Coronal CT reformation shows two calculi (*arrowhead*) causing biliary obstruction at the lower end of the CBD. The gallbladder (*curved arrow*) is distended secondary to the biliary obstruction

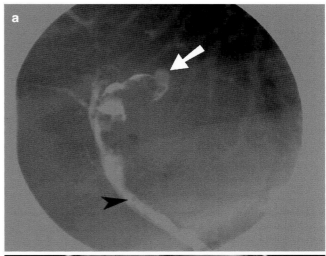

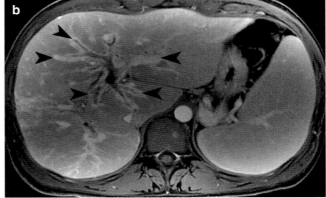

Fig. 2.12 Pyogenic cholangitis (**a**) ERCP shows irregularity of the biliary ducts, choledocholithiases (*arrowhead*), intraductal debris, and intrahepatic abscess (*arrow*). (**b**) T1-weighted gadolinium-enhanced MR shows biliary ductal dilatation and intense enhancement (*arrowheads*) of the biliary ductal wall

where CD4 count is less than 100/mm³. In posttransplant patients, bacteria (Mycobacterium avium complex), viruses (adenovirus, Cytomegalovirus, and Cryptosporidium parvum), and fungi (Candida, Microsporidium) may be the cause of cholangitis [7, 8].

The classic clinical presentation (Charcot's triad) includes fever, pain, and jaundice. In immunocompromised patients the symptoms are less typical than in immunocompetent patients.

Ultrasound is the first-line imaging tool in patients with suspected cholangitis and demonstrates biliary duct enlargement, biliary duct wall thickening, fluid collection, and abscess. The MR findings include increased T2 signal intensity in a wedge-shaped configuration or in the parenchyma surrounding the infected biliary ducts. Wedge-shaped, peribiliary, or patchy contrast enhancement is seen most often in the arterial phase. Patchy hepatic enhancement and bulging as well as enhancing papilla are most often associated with pyogenic cholangitis. Biliary ductal wall enhancement is a common finding and best seen on delayed postgadolinium T1-weighted images (Fig. 2.12).

The imaging findings in HIV patients are often similar to sclerosing cholangitis (Fig. 2.13). The imaging findings include intra- and extrahepatic biliary dilatation, saccular dilatations, biliary strictures, pruning, irregular thickening of the extrahepatic biliary tree wall, papillary stenosis, and cholecystitis [7].

The complications of bacterial cholangitis include sepsis, hepatic abscesses, portal vein thrombosis, biliary peritonitis,

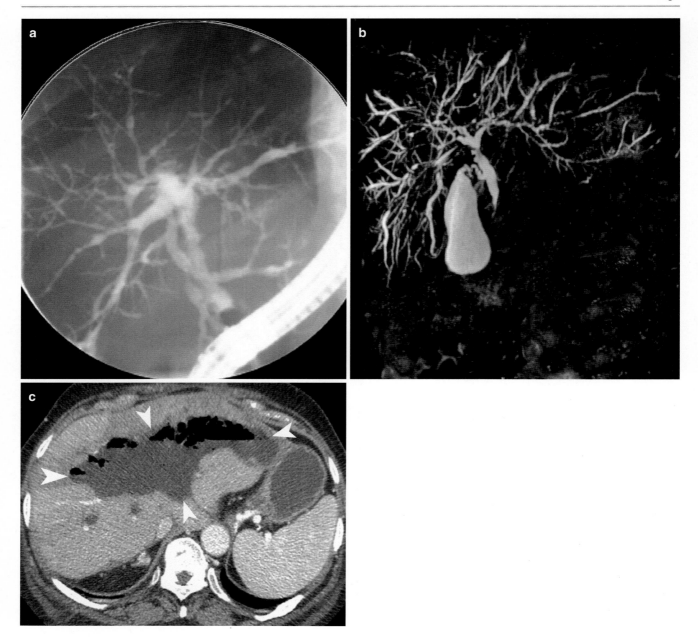

Fig. 2.13 Other biliary pathologies, including sclerosing cholangitis and biliary necrosis. (**a**) Sclerosing cholangitis. ERCP shows multiple areas of biliary dilatation, strictures, and pruning in the right as well as the left hepatic ducts. (**b**) Sclerosing cholangitis. MRCP demonstrates multiple intrahepatic biliary ductal narrowing and dilatation. (**c**) Contrast-enhanced CT in a patient with hepatic artery occlusion after liver transplant demonstrates biliary necrosis. The biliary ducts (*arrowheads*) are dilated secondary to sloughed-off ductal walls

recurrent pyogenic cholangitis, sclerosing cholangitis, and suppurative cholangitis.

Hemobilia

Hemobilia is characterized by upper gastrointestinal bleeding which originates in the biliary tree. Clinically, the classic presentation is known as Quincke's triad and is characterized by right upper quadrant pain, upper gastrointestinal bleeding, and jaundice.

The most common cause of hemobilia is blunt and penetrating abdominal trauma. The other causes include malignancy, rupture of an aneurysm, hemorrhagic cholecystitis, and blood dyscrasias (Fig. 2.14).

The imaging findings indicative of hemobilia include blood clots, appearing as filling defects in the gallbladder lumen and hemorrhagic bile, seen as altered density/signal

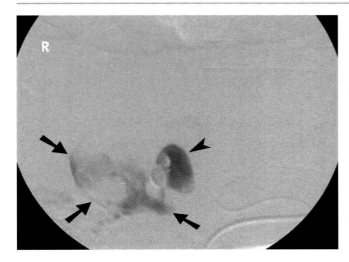

Fig. 2.14 Hemobilia. Conventional angiogram demonstrates a post-traumatic pseudoaneurysm (*arrowhead*) with active extravasation (*arrow*) of contrast. The pseudoaneurysm was subsequently embolized using endovascular coils

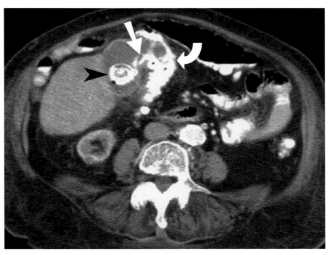

Fig. 2.15 Cholecystocolonic fistula. Axial contrast-enhanced CT image shows reflux of contrast (*straight arrow*) from the transverse colon (*curved arrow*) into the gallbladder lumen through the cholecystocolonic fistula. The gallbladder contains a gallstone (*arrowhead*) which is abutting the colonic contrast

intensity on unenhanced CT or MR imaging (increased signal on T1-weighted and decreased signal on T2-weighted images). The other findings include fluid-fluid level within the gallbladder, pseudoaneurysm, and extravasation of contrast on contrast-enhanced CT. The diagnosis can be confirmed on endoscopy or conventional angiography.

The management of hemobilia can be conservative (most common), intra-arterial embolization or surgery.

Gallstone Ileus

Gallstone ileus is the result of recurrent gallstone cholecystitis leading to a cholecystoenteric fistula formation. Gallstone ileus is most often seen in elderly females (70–75 years old; M:F 1:5) with history of gallstones [8, 9]. Although gallstone ileus overall accounts for less than 1 % of small bowel obstructions, in elderly population it may account for up to 20 % of the cases of small bowel obstruction [9, 10].

Since gallbladder is in anatomical contact with the duodenum and transverse colon, gallbladder perforation may create fistulous communication with these structures. The cholecystoduodenal fistula is the most common gallbladder fistula and allows passage of gallstone into the bowel. Although most stones will pass through the bowel without causing obstruction (85 %), the larger stones may cause small bowel obstruction (15 %) (Fig. 2.15). The most frequent site of small bowel obstruction is in the ileum because it represents the narrowest segment of the small bowel (Table 2.4). Gastric outlet or duodenal obstruction by a gallstone is rare and constitutes the Bouveret's syndrome [11].

The plain radiograph of patients with gallstone ileus may show pneumobilia (one-third of cases) and multiple air-fluid

Table 2.4 Sites of bowel obstruction in patients with gallstone ileus

1.	Terminal ileum (60 %)
2.	Proximal ileum (30 %)
3.	Distal jejunum (5–10 %)
4.	Colon or rectum (2–4 %)
5.	Duodenum (1–3 %)

levels in small bowel loops (Fig. 2.16a). The presence of gas within the gallbladder is not always recognized on plain radiograph, and this contributes to the delay in diagnosis [12]. On ultrasound, it may be difficult to identify the gallbladder, because of the presence of air and gallbladder contraction (chronic inflammation). Ultrasound may also show bowel dilatation and rarely find the site of the bowel obstruction. However, CT better demonstrates all findings necessary to make the diagnosis. Contrast-enhanced CT in patients with gallstone ileus can show the Rigler's triad of distended small bowel loops, pneumobilia, and ectopic calcified gallstone (Fig. 2.16b–d).

Bouveret's syndrome (duodenal or pylorus obstruction) is an uncommon type of gallstone ileus most commonly seen in elderly women where the gallstone is lodged in the duodenum or stomach (Fig. 2.16e) [13]. Pneumobilia may be present in about 30–50 % of patients with intestinal obstruction from gallstones [14]. The diagnosis of Bouveret's syndrome can be made by endoscopy (60 %), upper GI series (45 %), or abdominal radiograph (23 %). The mortality rate is approximately 12 % in recent years [13].

Intestinal obstruction in gallstone ileus typically occurs when stones larger than 2.5 cm migrate through the bowel [15]. It is recommended to obtain an early abdominal CT scan for the investigation of bowel obstruction in the elderly,

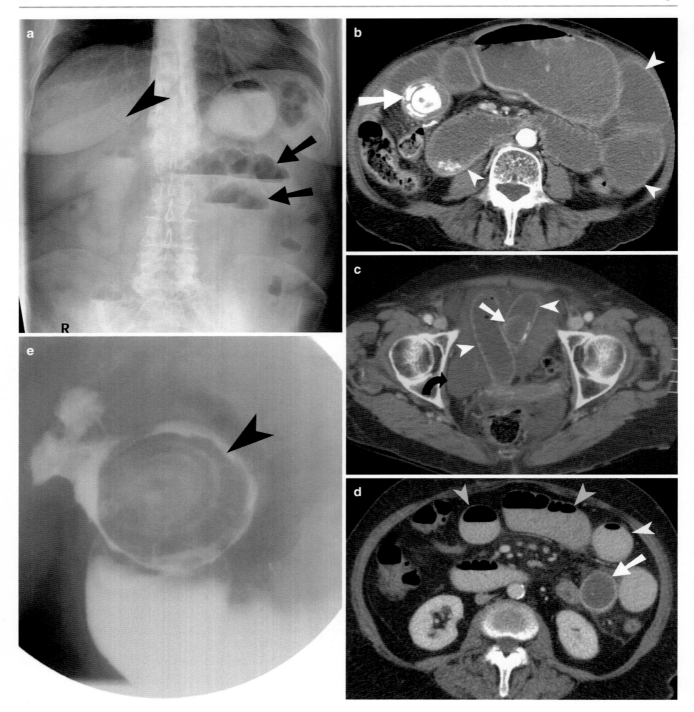

Fig. 2.16 Gallstone ileus. (**a**) Plain radiograph of a patient with gall-stone ileus demonstrates pneumobilia (*arrowhead*) and multiple air-fluid levels in dilated small bowel loops (*arrows*). (**b–d**) Contrast-enhanced CT scan in three different patients with gallstone ileus demonstrates the obstructing gallstone (*arrows*) causing dilatation of small bowel loops (*arrowheads*). Free fluid (*curved arrow*) in the pelvis is identified in one of the patients. (**e**) Upper GI study in a patient with Bouveret's syndrome demonstrates a 6.8 cm gallstone (*arrowhead*) in the duodenal bulb with gastric outlet obstruction

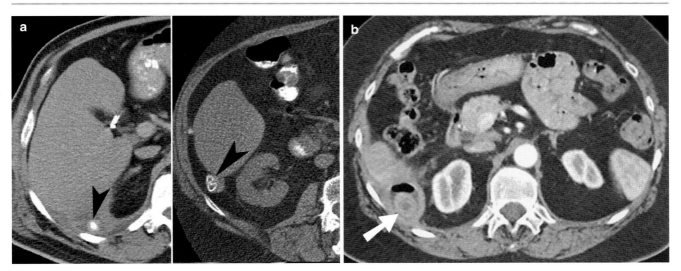

Fig. 2.17 Dropped gallstones. (**a**) Contrast-enhanced CT demonstrates dropped gallstones (*arrowheads*) incidentally detected adjacent to the caudal edge of the liver in two patients with remote history of cholecystectomy. (**b**) Contrast-enhanced CT demonstrates an abscess develop-ing around a dropped gallstone (*arrow*) in the Morrison's pouch, in a patient where the gallstone was lost during laparoscopic cholecystectomy

as gallstone ileus is a disproportionately more common cause than in younger population [16].

Complications After Biliary Surgery

Each year, approximately 1.5 million of patients undergo cholecystectomy, and 80,000 patients undergo biliary tract surgery for various causes (obstructive jaundice or pancreaticobiliary disorders) in the USA. The complication rate of these surgeries is 14.3 % and mortality rate is 0.52 % [17].

Intraperitoneal gallstone loss is not uncommon and can occur in up to 40 % of cholecystectomies. Dropped gallstones can lead to abscess (perihepatic, pelvic, or abdominal wall) and biliary-enteric fistula formation (Fig. 2.17) [18].

On CT and ultrasonography, bilomas are invariably well demarcated, but most do not have an identifiable capsule (Fig. 2.18). Communication with ducts of Luschka (ducts that drain a portion of the right lobe of the liver) or cystic duct stump can lead to accumulation of bile in the subhepatic area after cholecystectomy (Fig. 2.19). Ducts of Luschka or subvesical ducts are small biliary ducts which originate from the right hepatic lobe and course along the gallbladder fossa bed. Injuries to the ducts of Luschka are the second most frequent cause of postcholecystectomy bile leaks.

Postcholecystectomy bilomas are usually well drained by image-guided percutaneous catheter placement. ERCP, PTC, and CT are the usual modalities in making the diagnosis of biliary leak. ERCP allows diagnosis as well as treatment (stenting and nasobiliary drainage) of patients with postcholecystectomy bile leak.

The other complications after cholecystectomy include biliary perforation, biliary stricture, retained surgical sponge, biliary peritonitis, and hemorrhage (Fig. 2.20).

Teaching Points

- The first-line imaging modality for the diagnosis of acute cholecystitis is ultrasound and cholescintigraphy.
- Ultrasound is preferred over cholescintigraphy because of wider availability, shorter duration of the investigation, and ability to diagnose gallstones as well as choledocholithiases.
- Although the sensitivities of ultrasound and cholescintigraphy are both high, ultrasound has relatively lower sensitivity and specificity compared to cholescintigraphy.
- CT and MR are second-line imaging modalities, most appropriately used when ultrasound results are equivocal.
- CT is especially useful in diagnosing complications of acute cholecystitis and extrabiliary disorders.

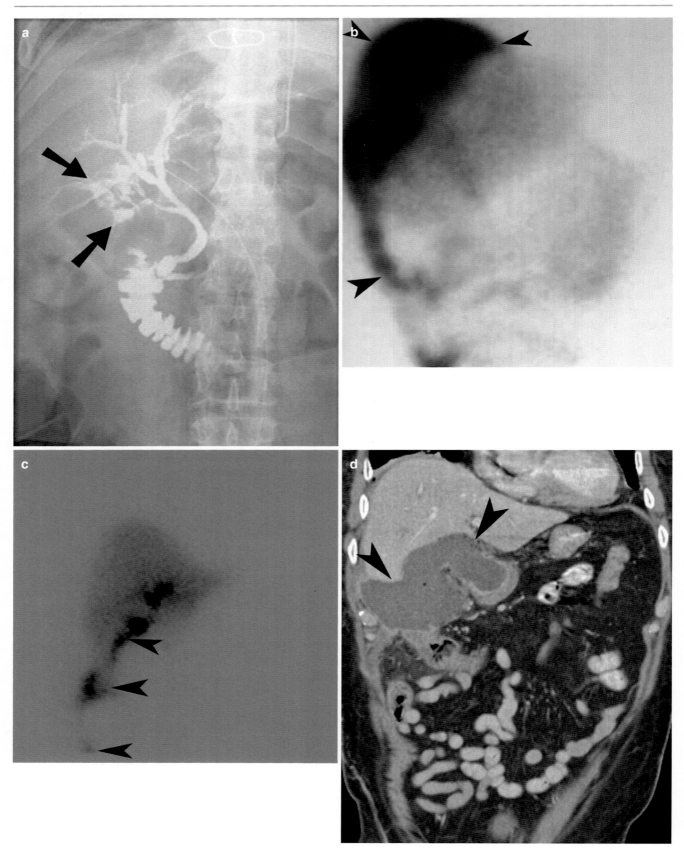

Fig. 2.18 Postcholecystectomy bile leaks. (**a**) Percutaneous transhepatic cholangiogram demonstrates leakage of contrast from the cystic duct stump in a patient with recent cholecystectomy and dehiscence of cystic duct stump. (**b** and **c**) Cholescintigraphy demonstrates accumulation of radiotracer outside the biliary system, into the peritoneal cavity (*arrowheads*). (**d**) Coronal CT reformation demonstrates biloma (*arrowheads*) in the right subhepatic location

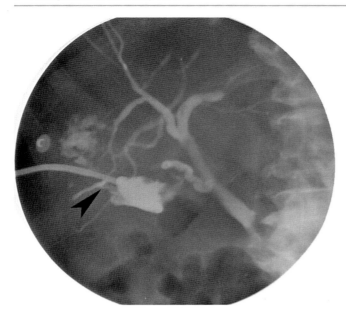

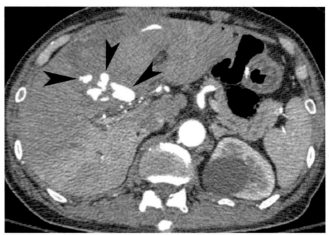

Fig. 2.20 Postcholecystectomy hemorrhage. Postcholecystectomy CT angiogram of the abdomen demonstrates active extravasation of contrast (*arrowheads*) into the gallbladder fossa

Fig. 2.19 Postcholecystectomy biloma communicating with ducts of Luschka. Pigtail catheter injection after image-guided pigtail catheter drainage of a biloma demonstrates communication of the biloma with ducts of Luschka (*arrowhead*)

References

1. Watanabe Y, Nagayama M, Okumura A, Amoh Y, Katsube T, Suga T, et al. MR imaging of acute biliary disorders. Radiographics. 2007;27:477–95.
2. Hanbidge AE, Buckler PM, O'Malley ME, Wilson SR. From the RSNA refresher courses: imaging evaluation for acute pain in the right upper quadrant. Radiographics. 2004;24:1117–35.
3. Bortoff GA, Chen MYM, Ott DJ, Wolfman NT, Routh WD. Gallbladder stones: imaging and intervention. Radiographics. 2000;20:751–66.
4. Leopold GR. The acute abdomen: ultrasonography. Radiographics. 1985;5:273–83.
5. Teefey SA, Baron RL, Bigler SA. Sonography of the gallbladder: significance of striated (layered) thickening of the gallbladder wall. AJR Am J Roentgenol. 1991;156:945–7.
6. May GP, James EM, Bender CE, Williams Jr HJ, Adson MA. Diagnosis and treatment of jaundice. Radiographics. 1986;6: 847–90.
7. Catalano OA, Sahani DV, Forcione DG, Czermak B, Liu CH, Soricelli A, et al. Biliary infections: spectrum of imaging findings and management. Radiographics. 2009;29:2059–80.

8. Murthy GD. Bouveret's syndrome. Am J Gastroenterol. 1995;90(4): 638–9.
9. Delabrousse E, Bartholomot B, Sohm O, Wallerand H, Kastler B. Gallstone ileus: CT findings. Eur Radiol. 2000;10(6):938–40.
10. Madrid A. Image of the month-diagnosis. Gallstone ileus. Arch Surg. 2003;138(7):808.
11. Tuney D, Cimsit C. Bouveret's syndrome: CT findings. Eur Radiol. 2000;10(11):1711–2.
12. Swift SE, Spencer JA. Gallstone ileus: CT findings. Clin Radiol. 1998;53(6):451–4.
13. Frattaroli FM, Reggio D, Guadalaxara A, Illomei G, Lomanto D, Pappalardo G. Bouveret's syndrome: case report and review of the literature. Hepatogastroenterology. 1997;44(16):1019–22.
14. Herbener TE, Basile V, Nakamoto D, Butler HE, Pickering SP. Abdominal case of the day. Bouveret's Syndrome. AJR Am J Roentgenol. 1997;169:252–3.
15. Romano DR, Gonzalez EM, Romero CJ, Selas PR, Diaz MM, et al. Duodenal obstruction by gallstones (Bouveret's syndrome). Presentation of a new case and literature review. Hepatogastroenterology. 1997;44:1351–5.
16. Coulier B, Coppens JP, Broze B. Computed tomographic diagnosis of biliary ileus. J Belge Radiol. 1998;81(2):75–8.
17. Ghahremani GG, Crampton AR, Bernstein JR, Caprini JA. Iatrogenic biliary tract complications: radiologic features and clinical significance. Radiographics. 1991;11:441–56.
18. McDonald MP, Munson JL, Sanders L, Tsao J, Buyske J. Consequences of lost gallstone. Surg Endosc. 1997;11(7):774–7.

Acute Appendicitis

Ajay Singh, Benjamin Yeh, and Robert A. Novelline

Normal Anatomy

The appendix, also known as the vermiform process or processus vermiformis, is a long (2–20 cm), narrow, tubular diverticulum, which starts from the apex of the cecum and extends posteromedially (Figs. 3.1 and 3.2). The appendix is most commonly retrocecal (58 %), pelvic (22 %), or paracecal (12 %) [1].

Pathophysiology

Appendicitis is most often due to luminal obstruction followed by bacterial invasion. Appendiceal obstruction can be caused by an appendicolith, foreign body, strictures, lymphoid hyperplasia, or rarely parasitic infections (Fig. 3.3). If obstruction persists, the intraluminal pressure in the appendix may rise above that of the veins, leading to venous obstruction and appendiceal wall ischemia.

Pathological Stages of Appendicitis: Three Stages

1. Acute catarrhal appendicitis: There is early scant neutrophilic infiltrates without perforation. The inflammation of the appendix can spontaneously regress or progress to the second stage.

A. Singh, MD (✉)
Department of Radiology,
Massachusetts General Hospital, Harvard Medical School,
10 Museum Way, # 524, Boston, MA 02141, USA
e-mail: asingh1@partners.org

B. Yeh, MD
Department of Radiology, University of California San Francisco,
San Francisco, CA 94122, USA

R.A. Novelline, MD
Department of Radiology,
Massachusetts General Hospital, Harvard Medical School,
Boston, MA, USA

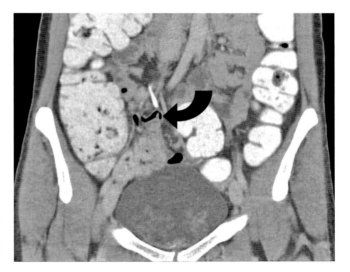

Fig. 3.1 Normal anatomy of the appendix on barium enema and CT. Coronal CT reformation of the abdomen demonstrates normal air-filled appendix (*curved arrow*) medial to the cecum. Normal appendiceal caliber is less than 7 mm

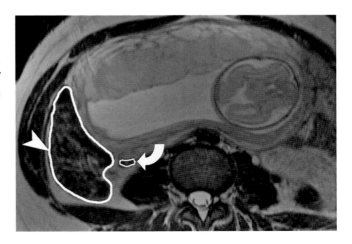

Fig. 3.2 Normal anatomy of appendix on MR imaging. Axial FSE T2-weighted sequence shows normal appendix (*arrow*) medial to the cecum (*arrowhead*). The normal appendix is low to intermediate signal intensity on T2-WI and is located between 2 and 6 o'clock position in relation to the cecum

A. Singh (ed.), *Emergency Radiology*,
DOI 10.1007/978-1-4419-9592-6_3, © Springer Science+Business Media New York 2013

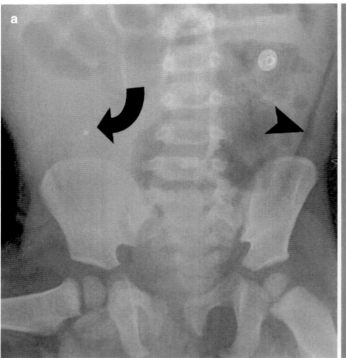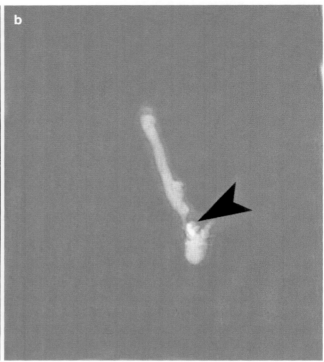

Fig. 3.3 Plain radiographic findings of acute appendicitis. (**a**) Plain x-ray of the abdomen demonstrates a small appendicolith (*curved arrow*) in the right abdomen. The properitoneal fat pad on the right is obliterated by appendiceal inflammation. The properitoneal fat pad (*arrowhead*) on the left side is well preserved. The air-containing bowel loops are displaced away from the right lower quadrant. There are changes of paralytic ileus. (**b**) Plain radiograph of the surgical specimen demonstrates an appendicolith (*arrowhead*) at the base of the appendix

2. Purulent (phlegmonous) stage: Neutrophilic infiltrate, ulceration, and necrosis are seen. Spontaneous regression is rare and there is progression to appendiceal perforation.
3. Gangrenous stage: Necrosis, ulceration, gangrene, and peritoneal inflammation are seen without the possibility of spontaneous regression.

Current Status of US, CT, and MR

- Currently, the majority of patients with clinically suspected appendicitis undergo intravenous contrast-enhanced CT with or without oral or rectal contrast before the surgery.
- Ultrasound is considered the imaging modality of choice for pediatric and pregnant patients where appendicitis is suspected.
- MR is reserved for pregnant patients where US is nondiagnostic or equivocal.

Since the first publications on the utility of CT for appendicitis in the late 1990s, there has been dramatic increase in the use of CT to evaluate right lower quadrant pain. Rao et al. found that CT performed in patients who present with suspected appendicitis improves patient care and reduces the use of hospital cost by resources $447 per patient by avoiding negative laparotomy (Table 3.1) and showed the rate of

negative laparotomy decreased from 20 % before to 7 % after the introduction of CT [4, 5].

CT Protocol

- IV contrast: 370 mg/100 cc at 3.5 mL/s, followed by scanning after 150 s delay.
- 120 kV; 150 mA; slice thickness – 2.5 mm.
- Targeted CT may be used with scanning from L3 to the symphysis pubis.
- Reformation (3 mm) in sagittal and coronal planes. The use of coronal reformations improves the confidence of the radiologist in visualizing the appendix and making the diagnosis of acute appendicitis [6].
- Oral (2 % barium suspension) vs. rectal (1 L 3 % barium suspension). The use of oral or rectal contrast is considered appropriate by ACR appropriateness criteria in the evaluation of right lower quadrant pain.

The usage of rectal as opposed to oral contrast offers the advantage of reducing the time between ordering of the scan by the physician and the time when it is performed. There is also higher likelihood of opacifying cecum and appendix with contrast. The disadvantages of rectal contrast include increased patient discomfort and the theoretical

Table 3.1 Advantages and disadvantages of US and CT

Ultrasound	CT
1. Relatively inexpensive (technical cost = $50.28)	1. Higher cost (technical cost = $112.32) [2]
2. Wide availability	2. More restricted availability
3. Can better evaluate pelvic disease in females	3. Better identifies normal appendix (>85 % in adult and 69 % in children), phlegmon, and abscess [3]
4. No ionizing radiation (preferred in children and pregnancy)	4. Ionizing radiation (10 mSv)
5. Lower sensitivity compared to CT (sensitivity 75–85 %)	5. More accurate for appendicitis (sensitivity 90–100 %)
6. Operator dependence and technically inadequate studies due to gas	6. No operator dependence

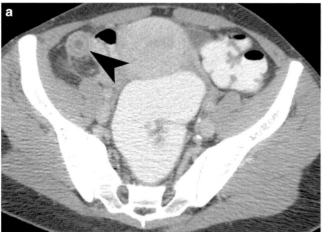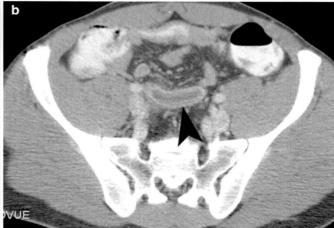

Fig. 3.4 Appendiceal wall changes in acute appendicitis. (**a** and **b**) Contrast-enhanced CT in a patient with acute appendicitis shows stratified appendiceal wall thickening (*arrowhead*). The inner hyper- dense ring indicates mucosal enhancement, while the outer hyperdense ring indicates serosal enhancement

risk of rupturing the appendix from increased intraluminal pressure in the cecum. In the adult population, the appendix is seen in more than 85 % cases, while in children the visualization rate is lower (69 %) because of the paucity of intra-abdominal fat.

Imaging Findings on CT

1. *Appendiceal caliber:* 7 mm or more in width. This criterion alone does not have high positive predictive value because up to 42 % of normal population can have an appendiceal caliber of more than 7 mm.
2. *Appendiceal wall thickness of more than 3 mm.*
3. *Appendiceal mural enhancement, homogeneous or stratified appearance of the appendiceal wall* (Fig. 3.4).
4. *Lack of intraluminal contrast in the appendix.*
5. *Periappendiceal inflammation.*
6. *Appendicoliths* (Fig. 3.5): It is seen in 10 % cases on plain radiograph and 30 % on CT study. The detection of an isolated appendicolith on CT is not sufficiently specific to be the sole basis for the diagnosis of acute appendicitis [7]. The use of bone window setting can increase the detection rate of appendicolith [8].
7. *Arrowhead sign*: Arrow-shaped configuration of the cecum due to funneling of intraluminal contrast into the

spastic cecum (Fig. 3.6). It is an indicator of extension of inflammation from the appendix to the cecum.
8. *Cecal bar sign:* It is characterized by edema and bar-like thickening of the cecum at the base of the appendix (Fig. 3.7).
9. *Hyperdense appendix:* Hyperdense appendix is seen as high-attenuation appendix on noncontrast CT and is seen in 33 % of patients with acute appendicitis [9].
10. Maximum depth of intraluminal appendiceal fluid of more th*an 2.6 mm:* This can be useful in diagnosis of appendicitis when no periappendiceal inflammation is present [10].

Complications

Appendiceal perforation, abscess, and sepsis are the dreaded complications of acute appendicitis. The frequency of appendiceal perforation is 20–25 %, with the highest frequency in the very young and old (40–70 %). The extension of inflammation outside the appendix can lead to the formation of phlegmon and abscess. The inflammatory adhesions from appendicitis can lead to small bowel obstruction. Acute appendicitis should be in the differential diagnosis whenever there is small bowel obstruction in a patient who has no history of abdominal surgery.

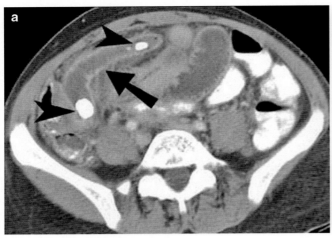 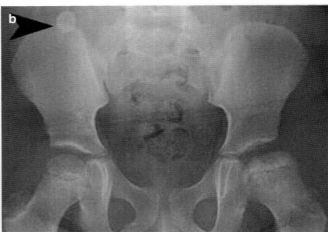

Fig. 3.5 Appendicoliths on CT and plain radiography. (**a**) Axial contrast-enhanced CT demonstrates grossly dilated appendix (*straight arrow*), containing multiple appendicoliths (*arrowheads*). The adjacent pelvic small bowel shows changes of ileus. (**b**) Plain radiograph of the abdomen demonstrates laminated appendicolith (*arrowhead*) in the right lower quadrant. Appendicoliths are seen in 10 % cases of appendicitis on plain x-ray of the abdomen

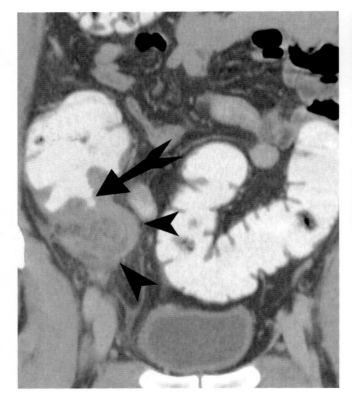

Fig. 3.6 Arrowhead sign. Contrast-enhanced CT demonstrates funneling (*straight arrow*) of contrast in the cecum with the tip pointing towards the base of the inflamed appendix (*arrowheads*) in an *arrowhead* configuration. The presence of the arrowhead sign indicates extension of inflammation from the base of the appendix into the cecal wall

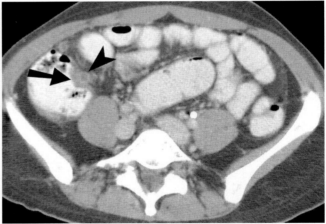

Fig. 3.7 Cecal bar sign. Contrast-enhanced CT demonstrates plaque-like thickening of the cecal wall (*straight arrow*) adjacent to the base of the inflamed appendix (*arrowhead*)

3. Abscess
4. Phlegmon
5. Defect in the enhancing appendiceal wall (sensitivity, 64 %)

Ultrasound Imaging

Graded-compression ultrasound with curvilinear probes is often performed with a 3.5-MHz transducer in larger patients and 5 MHz in thinner patients. Graded-compression ultrasound is performed in the transverse plane from the tip of liver to the pelvic brim, followed by scanning in sagittal and oblique planes. The ultrasound scanning uses uniform pressure to displace gas-filled bowel from the field of view. The

The five specific CT findings of perforated appendicitis are [11] (Figs. 3.8, 3.9, and 3.10):
1. Extraluminal air
2. Extraluminal appendicolith

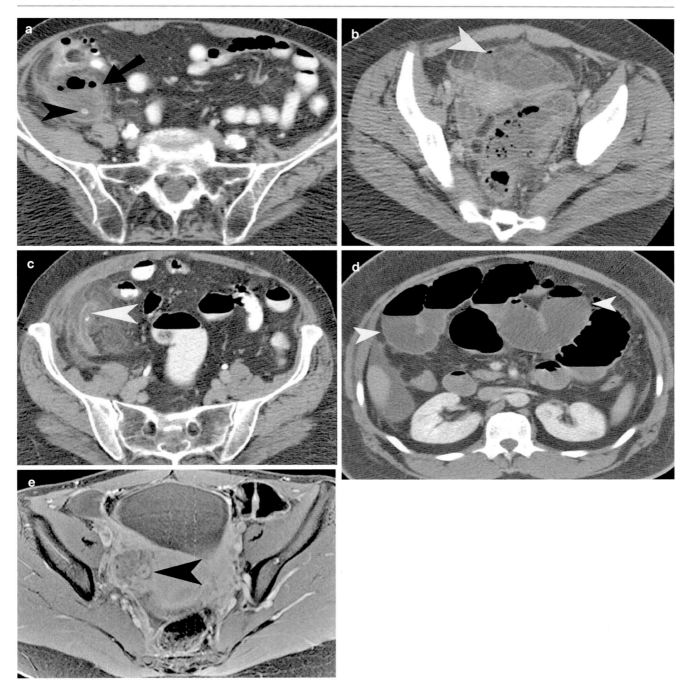

Fig. 3.8 Perforated appendicitis. (**a**) Contrast-enhanced CT demonstrates abscess (*straight arrow*) formation in the right lower quadrant from perforated appendicitis. There is an appendicolith (*arrowhead*) measuring 7 mm in diameter seen within the abscess cavity. (**b**) Contrast-enhanced CT demonstrates appendiceal perforation by the presence of tiny foci of extraluminal air (*arrowhead*) in the anterior pelvis. There is extensive inflammation present in the intraperitoneal fat. (**c**) Contrast-enhanced CT demonstrates appendiceal perforation by discontinuity of the appendiceal wall (*arrowhead*) on the medial aspect. There is tiny appendicolith seen in the appendix with surrounding inflammation seen in the right lower quadrant. (**d**) Contrast-enhanced CT demonstrates dilated small bowel loops (*arrowheads*) in a patient with small bowel obstruction caused secondary to acute appendicitis. (**e**) Gadolinium-enhanced T1-WI demonstrates a thickened appendiceal wall (*arrowhead*) to the right side of the uterus with surrounding inflammatory phlegmon

normal appendix can be usually seen in the majority of children but in only a minority (<10 %) of adults. The presence of appendiceal perforation, leading to decompression and collapse of the appendiceal lumen, is believed to decrease the sensitivity of ultrasound in diagnosing acute appendicitis. In general, the sensitivity of ultrasound (74.2 %) in the

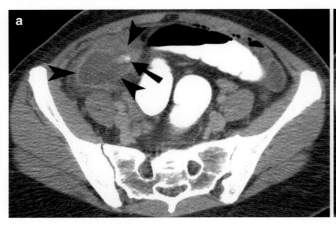 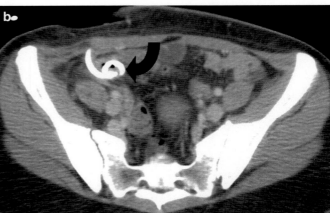

Fig. 3.9 Perforated appendicitis with abscess. (**a**) Contrast-enhanced CT scan study of the pelvis demonstrates 5-cm-diameter abscess (*arrowheads*) in the right lower quadrant, containing an appendicolith (*straight arrow*). (**b**) Axial CT image demonstrates a 10-French Dawson-Mueller pigtail drainage catheter (*curved arrow*) placed into the abscess cavity using trocar technique. Note the complete resolution of the abscess cavity following aspiration through the catheter

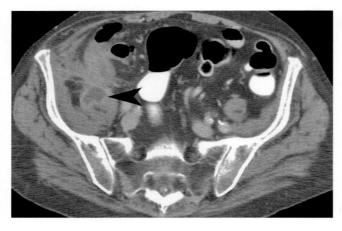

Fig. 3.10 Perforated appendicitis with psoas abscess. Contrast-enhanced CT shows ring-enhancing abscess (*arrowhead*) in the right psoas muscle, secondary to perforated appendicitis. Inflammatory phlegmon is seen in the right lower quadrant, anterior to the right psoas muscle

diagnosis of acute appendicitis is lower than the sensitivity reported with CT (100) [12]. In meta-analysis of head-to-head comparison studies performed between 1966 and 2006, the sensitivities of CT and graded-compression ultrasound studies were 91 and 78 %, respectively [13].

Ultrasound Findings of Acute Appendicitis

1. Noncompressible and aperistaltic blind-ending tubular structure (Fig. 3.11).
2. Appendiceal caliber >6 mm between outer borders of tunica muscularis.
3. Appendicolith, indicated by clean distal acoustic shadowing.
4. Inflamed fat causes "echogenic mass effect".
5. Increased blood flow in appendiceal wall, compared to normal gut on color Doppler ultrasound.

Variants of Acute Appendicitis

Tip appendicitis (Fig. 3.12) is characterized by the presence of inflammation of the appendiceal tip with normal appendiceal base. The proximal appendix is collapsed or filled with air/contrast [14]. Since the base of the appendix is not involved by the inflammation, there is no cecal bar sign or arrowhead sign. If the entire appendix is not demonstrated, the sensitivity to diagnose this condition may be reduced on ultrasound evaluation.

Stump appendicitis (Fig. 3.13) refers to acute appendicitis involving postappendectomy stump. This is a rare condition with less than 40 cases reported in the world literature. It has been reported after laparoscopic as well as open appendectomy and is due to luminal obstruction of the appendiceal stump left behind after open or laparoscopic appendectomy. The CT findings include inflammatory changes around appendiceal stump.

Acute appendicitis can occur in unusual locations and has been described in the hernia sac, the left side of abdomen, and even the thorax (Fig. 3.14). The presence of appendix in inguinal hernia sac is known as Amyand's hernia. Spontaneous resolution of acute appendicitis with conservative management has been shown to be associated with high frequency of recurrence in 38 % cases.

Acute Appendicitis in Pregnancy

Acute appendicitis is the most common cause of acute abdominal pain in pregnancy. The frequency of acute appendicitis in pregnancy is 1:800–1,500. The accuracy of diagnosis of acute appendicitis based on clinical examination is lower in pregnant patients because of the presence of nonspecific symptoms and cranial displacement of the appendix as well as omentum by the gravid uterus (Fig. 3.15a). Leukocytosis, which is present in 80 % of acute appendicitis

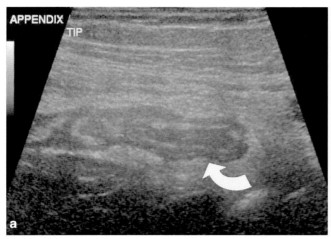
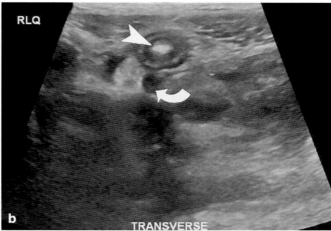

Fig. 3.11 Acute appendicitis on ultrasound imaging. (**a**) Graded-compression ultrasound image demonstrating blind-ending tubular structure measuring 12 mm in diameter with thickened wall, consistent with acute appendicitis. (**b**) Perforated appendicitis. A noncompressible tubular structure is seen in the right lower quadrant with an appendico-lith (*arrowhead*). Free fluid (*curved arrows*) is seen around the inflamed appendix

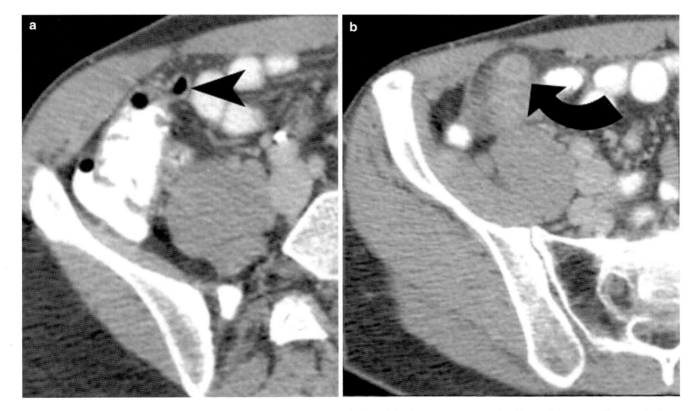

Fig. 3.12 Tip appendicitis. Contrast-enhanced axial CT scan study of the pelvis demonstrates normal caliber of the appendix near the base (*arrowhead*) (**a**). There is inflammation of the appendiceal tip (*curved arrow*) on the second image (**b**)

cases in the nonpregnant population, can be physiologically present during pregnancy, thereby reducing its usefulness.

The first-line imaging modality to diagnose acute appendicitis is graded-compression ultrasound. If ultrasound is nondiagnostic or equivocal, then noncontrast MR is indicated. Because of ionizing radiation issues, contrast-enhanced CT is considered less appropriate than ultrasound or MR in the evaluation of appendicitis.

MR Imaging

MR is the imaging modality of choice in pregnant patients when ultrasound is nondiagnostic or equivocal. We use a four-sequence protocol, which includes T2 single-shot fast spin echo (SS-FSE), T2 FSE, short tau inversion recovery, pre-gadolinium T1, and post-gadolinium T1 sequences [15]. Three-plane SS-FSE used to localize the appendix, followed by STIR and FSE T2-weighted sequences. STIR is poor at identifying the normal appendix but excellent for identifying early edema and inflammation. STIR has high sensitivities in identifying pathologies with high T1 and T2 relaxation times.

Intravenous gadolinium-based contrast material is used only if the patient is not pregnant because gadolinium is classified as class C drug and is known to cause teratogenic effects in animals. The appendix is visualized on MR in 70–100 % of patients, as opposed to 90–100 % cases on CT. The sensitivity of MR for acute appendicitis is reported to be 75–100 % [15–23].

The MR findings of acute appendicitis include dilated appendix, periappendiceal inflammation, appendiceal wall thickening, and intense enhancement of the appendix (Fig. 3.15b, c).

Postoperative Complications and Interventional Management

A retained or dropped appendicolith is a rare postsurgical complication with less than 40 cases reported in the literature. Dropped appendicolith (Fig. 3.16) can be a nidus for future intra-abdominal abscess formation and therefore needs removal. The imaging findings include abscess containing one or more high-attenuation foci, most commonly in Morison's pouch or the paracecal region. CT-guided catheter drainage has been shown to be useful in avoiding surgery in selected cases of dropped appendicolith with abscess formation. There is a single report of successful image-guided extraction of appendicolith with Witch nitinol stone basket [24].

Image-guided pigtail catheter drainage is the primary mode of management of postoperative abscess after appendectomy

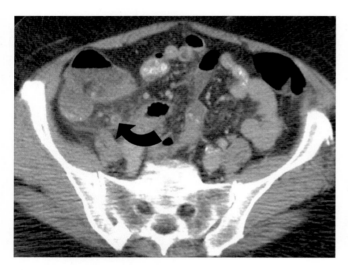

Fig. 3.13 Stump appendicitis. Contrast-enhanced axial CT scan study of the pelvis demonstrates an inflamed appendiceal stump (*curved arrow*) located posteromedial to the cecum

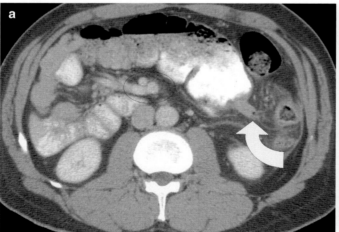
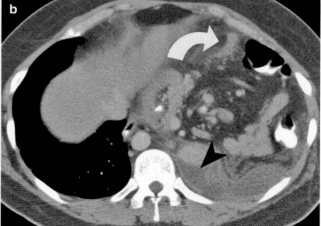

Fig. 3.14 Unusual positions of the inflamed appendix. (**a**) Contrast-enhanced CT demonstrates an inflamed left-sided appendix (*curved arrow*) in a patient with malrotation of the bowel. Note the abnormal relationship between the SMA and SMV (*oval*). (**b**) Contrast-enhanced CT shows intrathoracic location of inflamed appendix (*curved arrow*), in a patient with left diaphragmatic hernia. There is left subphrenic abscess (*arrowhead*) which required open appendectomy

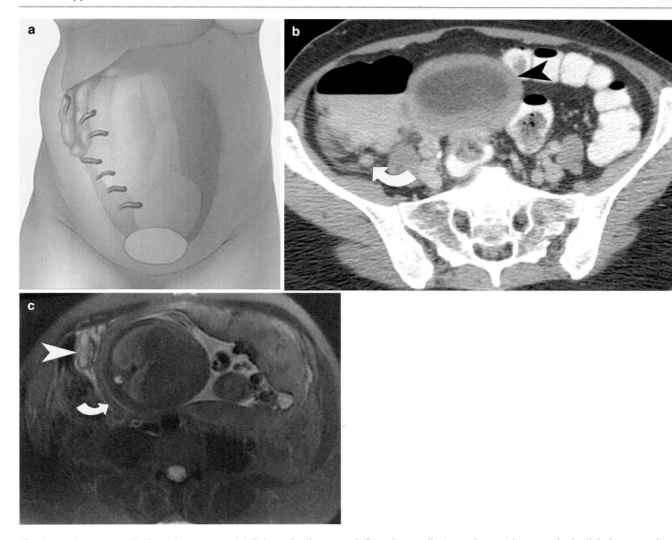

Fig. 3.15 Acute appendicitis and pregnancy. (**a**) Schematic diagram demonstrating the variable position of the appendix during pregnancy. The appendix moves out of the right lower quadrant, as the pregnancy progresses to the second trimester. (**b**) Contrast-enhanced CT demonstrates an enlarged uterus (*arrowhead*), containing gestational sac. The inflamed appendix (*curved arrow*) is present in the right lower quadrant with surrounding inflammation. (**c**) Axial T2 FSE sequence demonstrates a distended fluid containing appendix (*arrowhead*) with surrounding free fluid. Note the right midabdominal position of the appendix, secondary to the third trimester uterus (*curved arrow*)

and has been shown to have a high success rate in drainage of abdominal collections (Fig. 3.17).

The traditional treatment of retained appendicolith is open or laparoscopic surgery with abscess drainage and extraction of the calculus. Percutaneous retrieval of the retained appendicolith has been described using the Witch nitinol basket (Fig. 3.18). A trial of image-guided catheter drainage with or without percutaneous stone extraction may be beneficial in avoiding repeated surgery.

Teaching Points

1. CT is the imaging modality of choice for the evaluation of acute right lower quadrant pain.
2. Ultrasound is the first-line imaging modality in children and pregnant patients with acute right lower quadrant pain.
3. MR is second-line imaging modality for acute appendicitis, mostly used after an equivocal or nondiagnostic ultrasound in pregnant patient.

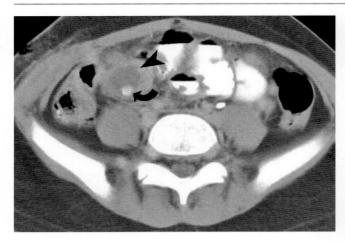

Fig. 3.16 Post appendectomy abscess and retained appendicolith. Axial contrast-enhanced CT of the lower abdomen demonstrates a well-defined abscess (*arrowhead*) in the right lower quadrant, containing an appendicolith (*curved arrow*)

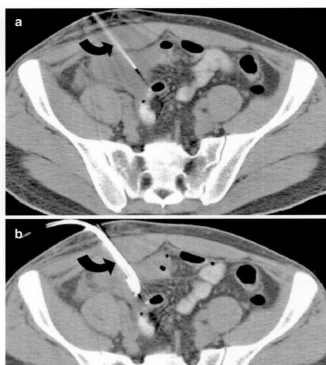

Fig. 3.17 Post appendectomy abscess drainage. (**a**) Noncontrast CT shows an 18-gauge needle (*curved arrow*) seen extending into the right lower quadrant collection at the time of the drainage procedure. (**b**) Noncontrast CT shows a 12-French pigtail catheter (*curved arrow*) placed into the collection using tandem trocar technique. Note the decrease in the size of the collection following aspiration of the catheter

Fig. 3.18 Retained appendicolith with abscess formation after appendectomy. (**a**) Noncontrast CT scan study demonstrates the abscess cavity (*arrowheads*) in the right lower quadrant, containing a subcentimeter appendicolith (*curved arrow*). (**b**) Noncontrast CT demonstrates a Witch nitinol basket (*straight arrow*) in the abscess cavity. (**c**) Witch nitinol basket (*straight arrow*) and the appendicolith (*curved arrow*) taken out during the procedure

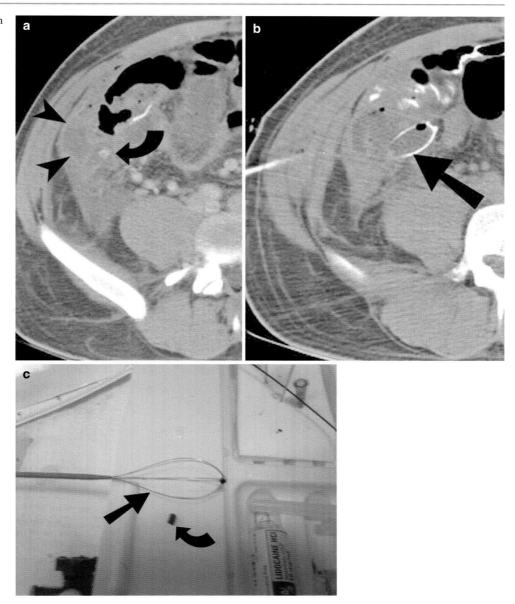

References

1. Collins DC. Acute retrocecal appendicitis: based on seven hundred and fifty-one instances. Arch Surg. 1938;36:729–43.
2. Saini S, Seltzer SE, Bramson RT, Levine LA, Kelly P, Jordan PF, et al. Technical cost of radiologic examinations: analysis across imaging modalities. Radiology. 2000;216:269–72.
3. Victoria T, Mahboubi S. Normal appendiceal diameter in children: does choice of CT oral contrast (VoLumen versus Gastrografin) make a difference? Emerg Radiol. 2010;17:397–401.
4. Rao PM, Rhea JT, Novelline RA, Mostafavi AA, McCabe CJ. Effect of computed tomography of the appendix on treatment of patients and use of hospital resources. N Engl J Med. 1998;338(3):141–6.
5. Rao PM, Rhea JT, Ratner DW, Venus LG, Novelline RA. Introduction of appendiceal CT: impact on negative appendectomy and appendiceal perforation rates. Ann Surg. 1999;229:344–9.
6. Paulson EK, Harris JP, Jaffe TA, Haugan PA, Nelson RC. Acute appendicitis: added diagnostic value of coronal reformations from isotropic voxels at multi-detector row CT. Radiology. 2005;235:879–85.
7. Lowe LH, Penney MW, Scheker LE, Perez R, Stein SM, Heller RM, et al. Appendicolith revealed on CT in children with suspected appendicitis: how specific is it in the diagnosis of appendicitis? AJR Am J Roentgenol. 2000;175:981–4.
8. Alobaidi M, Shirkhoda A. Value of bone window settings on CT for revealing appendicoliths in patients with appendicitis. AJR Am J Roentgenol. 2003;180:201–5.
9. Ng SP, Cheng SM, Yang FS, Tzen CY, Huang JK. Hyperdense appendix on unenhanced CT: a sign of acute appendicitis. Abdom Imaging. 2007;32:701–4.
10. Moteki T, Horikoshi H. New CT criterion for acute appendicitis: maximum depth of intraluminal appendiceal fluid. AJR Am J Roentgenol. 2007;188:1313–9.

11. Horrow MM, White DS, Horrow JC. Differentiation of perforated from nonperforated appendicitis at CT. Radiology. 2003;227:46–51.

12. Gaitini D, Beck-Razi N, Mor-Yosef D, Fisher D, Itzhak OB, Krausz MM, et al. Diagnosing acute appendicitis in adults: accuracy of color Doppler sonography and MDCT compared with surgery and clinical follow-up. AJR Am J Roentgenol. 2008;190:1300–6.

13. van Randen A, Bipat S, Zwinderman AH, Ubbink DT, Stoker J, Boermeester MA. Acute appendicitis: meta-analysis of diagnostic performance of CT and graded-compression ultrasound related to prevalence of disease. Radiology. 2008;249(1):97–106.

14. Rao PM, Rhea JT, Novelline RA. Distal appendicitis: CT appearance and diagnosis. Radiology. 1997;204:709–12.

15. Singh AK, Desai H, Novelline RA. Emergency MRI of acute pelvic pain: MR protocol with no oral contrast. Emerg Radiol. 2009;16(2): 133–41.

16. Oto A, Ernst RD, Shah R, Koroglu M, Chaljub G, Gei AF, et al. Right-lower-quadrant pain and suspected appendicitis in pregnant women: evaluation with MR imaging – initial experience. Radiology. 2005;234(2):445–51.

17. Birchard KR, Brown MA, Hyslop WB, Firat Z, Semelka RC. MRI of acute abdominal and pelvic pain in pregnant patients. AJR Am J Roentgenol. 2005;184(2):452–8.

18. Pedrosa I, Levine D, Eyvazzadeh AD, Siewert B, Ngo L, Rofsky NM. MR imaging evaluation of acute appendicitis in pregnancy. Radiology. 2006;238(3):891–9.

19. Oto A, Srinivasan PN, Ernst RD, Koroglu M, Cesani F, Nishino T, et al. Revisiting MRI for appendix location during pregnancy. AJR Am J Roentgenol. 2006;186(3):883–7.

20. Hormann M, Puig S, Prokesch SR, Partik B, Helbich TH. MR imaging of the normal appendix in children. Eur Radiol. 2002;12(9): 2313–6.

21. Nitta N, Takahashi M, Furukawa A, Murata K, Mori M, Fukushima M. MR imaging of the normal appendix and acute appendicitis. J Magn Reson Imaging. 2005;21(2):156–65.

22. Incesu L, Coskun A, Selcuk MB, Akan H, Sozubir S, Bernay F. Acute appendicitis: MR imaging and sonographic correlation. AJR Am J Roentgenol. 1997;168(3):669–74.

23. Hormann M, Paya K, Eibenberger K, Dorffner R, Lang S, Kreuzer S, et al. MR imaging in children with nonperforated acute appendicitis: value of unenhanced MR imaging in sonographically selected cases. AJR Am J Roentgenol. 1998;171(2):467–70.

24. Singh AK, Hahn PF, Gervais D, Vijayraghavan G, Mueller PR. Dropped appendicolith: CT findings and implications for management. AJR Am J Roentgenol. 2008;190:707–11.

Imaging of Small Bowel

4

Ajay Singh, Terry S. Desser, and Joseph Ferucci

Small Bowel of Diverticulitis

Small bowel diverticulitis is most commonly characterized by inflammation of acquired diverticula which are typically located on the mesenteric border of the bowel. Although less frequent than duodenal diverticula, jejunoileal diverticula are more prone to develop complications, including acute inflammation with perforation and abscess formation [1]. The current mode of treatment for small bowel diverticulitis is either with conservative medical management or surgical resection of the involved segment of bowel [2–4].

Small Bowel Diverticula: True Versus False Diverticula

Small bowel diverticula are most often found in the duodenum, being identified incidentally in the duodenum of 2–5 % of patients undergoing upper GI barium studies and in 12.5 % of patients undergoing ERCP (Figs. 4.1 and 4.2) [1, 5, 6]. The duodenum is the most common site of small bowel diverticula, followed by the jejunum, with ileal diverticula being least common. Jejunal diverticula are mostly multiple and are seven times more common than ileal diverticula [7, 8]. Small bowel diverticula are most commonly detected in the elderly in the sixth and seventh decade [9].

Congenital diverticula are true diverticula and are composed of all three intestinal layers and arise from the antimesenteric border of the small bowel. Meckel's diverticula, for example, are true diverticula. By contrast, pathologic acquired diverticula are "pseudodiverticula"; that is, they lack a muscular layer and result from herniation of only the mucosa and submucosa through defects in the muscular layer. It is thought that acquired diverticula tend to form at the mesenteric border where vasa recta penetrate, creating

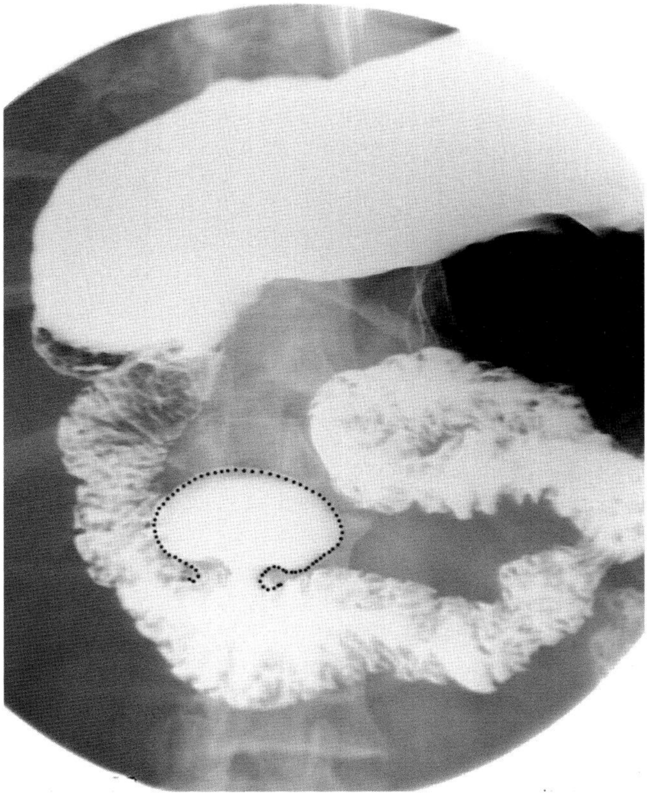

Fig. 4.1 Duodenal diverticulum. Upper GI study demonstrates an incidentally detected solitary duodenal diverticulum arising from the third portion of the duodenum

A. Singh, MD (✉)
Department of Radiology, Massachusetts General Hospital, Harvard Medical School, 10 Museum Way, # 524, Boston, MA 02114, USA
e-mail: asingh1@partners.org

T.S. Desser, MD
Department of Radiology, Stanford University School of Medicine, Stanford, CA, USA

J. Ferucci, MD
Department of Radiology, University of Massachusetts Memorial Medical Center, Worcester, MA, USA

A. Singh (ed.), *Emergency Radiology*,
DOI 10.1007/978-1-4419-9592-6_4, © Springer Science+Business Media New York 2013

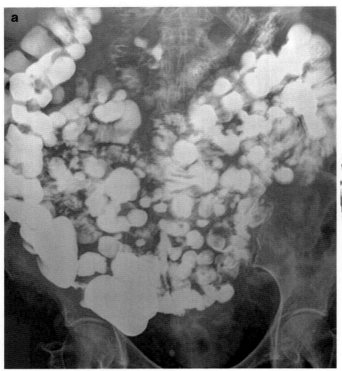

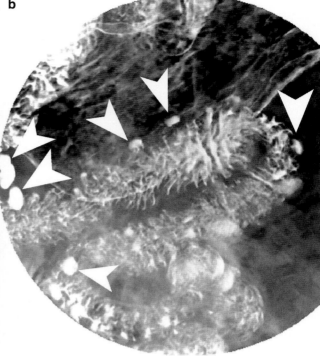

Fig. 4.2 Small bowel diverticulosis. (**a**) Small bowel follow-through examination demonstrates innumerable round collections of contrast in small bowel diverticula. (**b**) Small bowel follow-through study demonstrates multiple duodenal and jejunal diverticula (*arrowheads*) seen arising from the mesenteric border of the small bowel

areas of relative weakness [2]. Krishnamurthy et al. found histopathologic abnormalities in the wall of the jejunum of patients with jejunal diverticula, consistent with the notion that diverticula formation is associated with uncoordinated small bowel motility that results in increased intraluminal pressures [10].

Pathogenesis

Although most small bowel diverticula are of little clinical significance, approximately 10–20 % will develop complications [1]. Potential sequelae include inflammation, gangrenous change, perforation, peritonitis, bleeding, obstruction, and intestinal stasis leading to blind loop syndrome [11, 12]. Jejunoileal diverticula are more likely to have complications than duodenal diverticula [1, 13]. Of the diverticula that developed complications, jejunoileal diverticula were more likely to perforate and form abscesses, whereas duodenal diverticula were more prone to bleeding [1].

Diverticula in the small bowel are less likely to develop inflammation than those in the colon, probably due to the relative sterility of small bowel contents and the lesser degree of stasis that occurs in the larger diverticula of the small bowel [2]. Stasis of diverticular contents may be promoted by foreign bodies, enteroliths, inspissation of bowel contents, or a smaller

diverticular ostium which can reduce the outflow of intestinal fluid from the diverticulum [2, 11, 14]. Because small bowel diverticulitis is more commonly found at the mesenteric side of the bowel, the mesentery can close off the localized inflammatory process from the rest of the peritoneal cavity. As a result, peritonitis and pneumoperitoneum may not be detected clinically or radiologically unless there is rupture of the mesenteric peritoneum that had previously sealed off the abscess [11].

Clinical Presentation

Small bowel diverticulitis presents a diagnostic challenge on clinical exam and can mimic a host of more common abdominal pathologies including acute appendicitis, cholecystitis, perforated peptic ulcer disease, and colonic diverticulitis [12, 15]. A patient with small bowel diverticulitis may present with intermittent abdominal discomfort, acute abdominal pain, fever, chills, and leukocytosis [4, 9, 16–21]. Peritoneal signs may be appreciated on abdominal exam [9, 18].

Imaging

In the setting of small bowel diverticulitis, barium study may allow detection of air- or contrast-filled diverticula along the

Fig. 4.3 Acute small bowel diverticulitis in an acquired jejunal diverticulum. (**a**) A small bowel follow-through study demonstrates segmental irregularity of valvulae conniventes (*curved arrows*) in the proximal jejunum. A small collection of air due to the jejunal loop represents the inflamed jejunal diverticulum (*straight arrows*). (**b**) Coronal reformation (CT) demonstrates the inflamed jejunal diverticulum (*straight arrow*) in the left upper quadrant, with its neck (*arrowhead*) arising from the antimesenteric border of a jejunal loop. (**c**) Sagittal reformation (CT) demonstrates the inflamed true diverticulum (*straight arrow*) arising on the antimesenteric border of the jejunal loop (*curved arrow*)

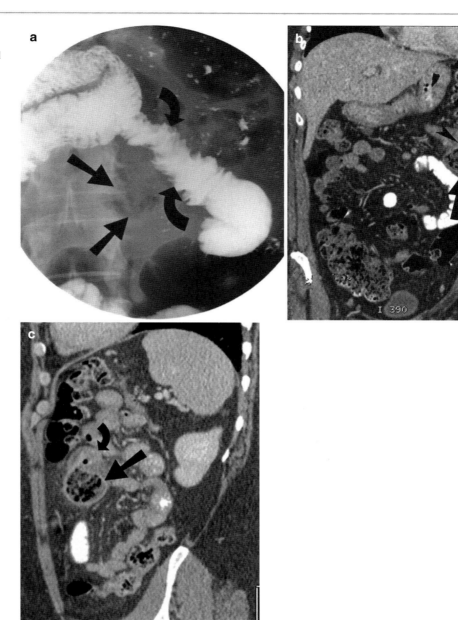

mesenteric small bowel wall, thickening of the bowel wall, bowel lumen obstruction, or extraluminal flow of contrast (Fig. 4.3) [12].

The CT findings (Table 4.1) are typically a focal inflammatory mass containing air, fluid, or an air-fluid level adjacent to asymmetrically thickened small bowel wall, with the presence of surrounding inflammation and mesenteric fat stranding [3, 9, 12]. The small bowel wall thickening is most prominent on the mesenteric side. The inflamed diverticulum may be visible along the mesenteric border of the small bowel loop (Fig. 4.4). The differential diagnosis on CT may include a perforated neoplasm, perforation secondary to a foreign body, NSAID-provoked ulceration, intramural hematoma, and local inflammatory bowel disease [3].

CT with multiplanar reconstruction can be employed to identify small bowel diverticula, with excellent visualization

Table 4.1 Findings on plain radiograph of the abdomen

Up to two air-fluid levels in the bowel
Small bowel caliber of less than 3 cm
Psoas outline (visible in 80 %)
Splenic outline (<15 cm in long axis)
Renal outlines
Gastric air

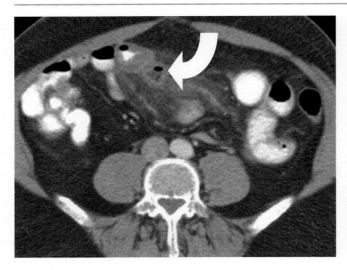

Fig. 4.4 Small bowel diverticulitis. Contrast-enhanced CT scan study of the abdomen demonstrates inflamed diverticulum (*curved arrow*) arising on the mesenteric aspect of the distal jejunal loop. There is inflammatory thickening of the adjacent small bowel wall along with inflammatory stranding in the small bowel mesentery

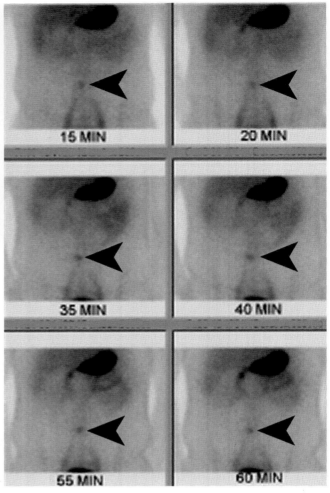

Fig. 4.5 Meckel's diverticulitis. Technetium-99m pertechnetate scan demonstrates focal increased radiotracer activity (*arrowheads*) in the lower abdomen, corresponding to the site of ectopic gastric mucosa within the inflamed Meckel's diverticulum

of the narrowed diverticular neck [2]. CT with coronal reformatting is especially useful for detecting single diverticula that are difficult to detect on axial views and can allow recognition of additional diverticula [3, 14].

CT Findings of Acute Small Bowel Diverticulitis

1. Inflamed diverticulum or focal inflammatory phlegmon along the mesenteric border of small bowel.
2. Asymmetrically thickened small bowel wall, more prominent along the mesenteric border.
3. Mesenteric fat stranding.

Meckel's Diverticulitis

Meckel's diverticulum is the most common congenital anomaly of the GI tract, seen in approximately 2 % of the population. It is a true diverticulum and is therefore present on the antimesenteric border of the distal ileum. It is most commonly located within 100 cm of the ileocecal junction [22]. It contains hypertrophic gastric mucosa (in 25–50 %) and has a lifetime complication risk of up to 4 %. Heterotropic pancreatic tissue is present in approximately 10 % of the cases.

The majority of cases of symptomatic Meckel's diverticulum are seen in the pediatric population. Hemorrhage is the most common complication and is most often painless. Bowel obstruction is the second most common complication and is

usually seen in older children and adults. The bowel obstruction can be secondary to volvulus, intussusception, or hernia.

Meckel's diverticulitis most often presents with abdominal pain and fever. It is secondary to obstruction of the mouth of the diverticulum most commonly by an enterolith, fecolith, or foreign body. Littre hernia represents Meckel's diverticulum which has herniated in a hernia sac.

Meckel's diverticulum can be seen on barium studies as a blind-ending tubular outpouching arising from the antimesenteric border of the ileum with a triradiate fold pattern at the junction of the diverticulum and ileum.

The heterotopic gastric mucosa present in a Meckel's diverticulum accumulates and secretes pertechnetate anion and is therefore detected on technetium-99m pertechnetate scan as a focal area of increased radiotracer activity (Fig. 4.5). Technetium pertechnetate scintigraphy has high sensitivity of

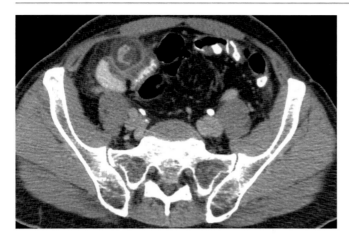

Fig. 4.6 Meckel's diverticulitis. Contrast-enhanced CT demonstrates the inflamed congenital diverticulum with thickened wall arising from the antimesenteric border of the distal ileum

more than 80 % in the pediatric population and slightly lower sensitivity of 63 % in adult population [23]. CT may show changes of small bowel diverticulitis in the right lower quadrant or may show volvulus or intussusception (Fig. 4.6).

Treatment

Laparotomy or laparoscope-assisted surgery is typically undertaken in the setting of small bowel diverticulitis associated with perforation, abscess formation, massive GI bleed, small bowel obstruction, blind loop syndrome, or refractory abdominal pain [24, 25]. Surgical approaches include both segmental resection of the involved bowel with end-to-end anastomosis and less commonly diverticulectomy [8, 24]. Conservative management consists of antibiotic therapy, IV hydration, and bowel rest [2, 3]. However, cases have been described of patients who ultimately underwent segmental bowel resection for jejunal diverticulitis, after symptoms persisted following a period of conservative management [3].

Acute Mesenteric Ischemia

Acute mesenteric ischemia is characterized by inadequate blood flow to the bowel wall, leading to ischemia. Mesenteric arterial occlusion carries a high mortality, unless the patient undergoes emergent vascular surgery.

Clinical Presentation

Clinically the patients with arterial causes of acute mesenteric ischemia are elderly and most often present with severe dull abdominal pain and vomiting. The abdominal pain is out of proportion to the tenderness elicited on palpation. Mesenteric venous thrombosis is most often seen in younger population and present with less severe symptoms which may have been present for days or sometimes weeks. Lab studies often show metabolic acidosis, elevated lactate level, and low bicarbonate level.

Pathogenesis

Superior mesenteric artery occlusion is a far more common than superior mesenteric vein occlusion as the cause of acute mesenteric ischemia. Approximately one-third of the cases are secondary to embolic occlusion and one-third secondary to thrombosis. Approximately 25 % cases are caused by nonocclusive ischemia, while the remaining cases are secondary to venous occlusion [26].

Risk Factors

The risk factor for arterial occlusion is most commonly heart diseases, such as atrial fibrillation, endocarditis, and valvular heart diseases. Atrial fibrillation is the most common cause of embolism to the superior mesenteric artery. The nonocclusive bowel ischemia may be secondary to hypotensive shock, pancreatitis, bowel obstruction, dehydration, and dialysis. Mesenteric venous thrombosis is seen with hypercoagulable states, such as protein C or S deficiency, polycythemia vera, antithrombin three deficiency, sickle-cell disease, pregnancy, and oral contraceptive use.

Imaging

The plain radiograph may show no abnormality or show paralytic ileus. Contrast-enhanced CT is the imaging modality of choice as it has sensitivity of 93.3 % and specificity of 95.9 % in a meta-analysis of 6 studies published between 1996 and 2009 [27]. Although catheter angiography has been shown to have a sensitivity of 87.5 %, the introduction of multidetector CT has obviated the need for this invasive test as the first-line imaging modality.

Biphasic CT performed 25 and 65 s after initiating contrast injection at the rate of 4 mL/s is the optimal protocol to evaluate for vascular as well as bowel wall changes. The CT angiographic phase changes management in 19 % cases by showing vascular abnormality not visible on the portal venous phase [28].

The CT imaging findings include superior mesenteric artery thrombus, small-caliber superior mesenteric vein,

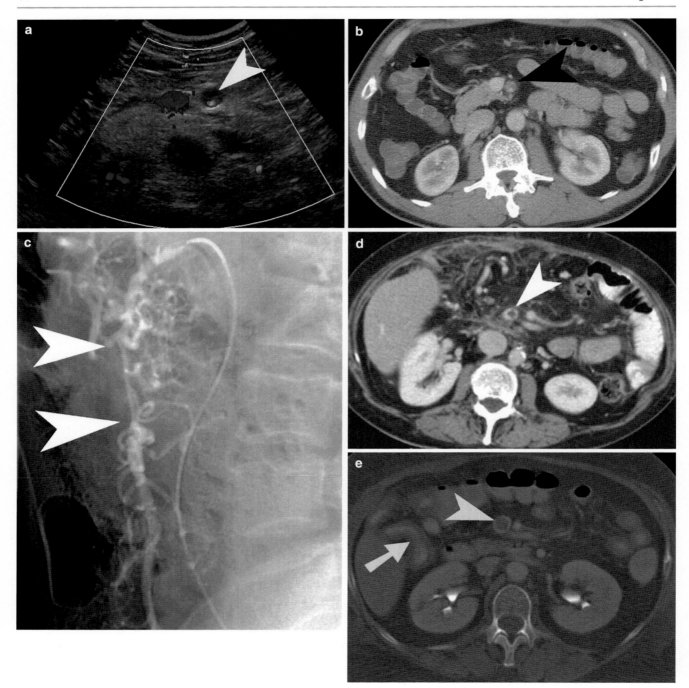

Fig. 4.7 Superior mesenteric artery and venous pathologies leading to bowel ischemia. (**a** and **b**) Color Doppler ultrasound and contrast-enhanced CT shows dissection in the superior mesenteric artery (*arrowhead*). The adjacent superior mesenteric vein is patent. (**c**) Superior mesenteric arteriogram shows narrowing (*arrowheads*) of the superior mesenteric artery lumen, secondary to nonocclusive thrombosis. (**d** and **e**) Contrast-enhanced CT shows thrombosis of the superior mesenteric vein (*arrowhead*). There are edematous changes seen in the small bowel mesentery. Ischemia in the small bowel is indicated by bowel wall edema (*arrow*)

bowel distension, and focal lack of bowel wall enhancement (Figs. 4.7 and 4.8). In the study by Kirkpatrick et al., pneumatosis intestinalis was seen in 43 % cases of acute mesenteric ischemia. Bowel wall thickening and mucosal enhancement were seen in 85 and 46 %, respectively [28]. Linear pattern of pneumatosis indicates more serious cause of pneumatosis and accounts for higher proportion of death from bowel infarction

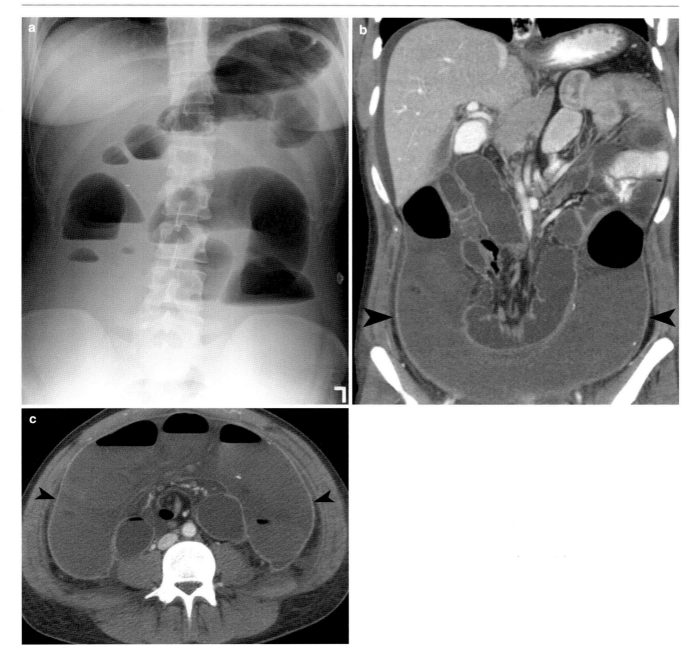

Fig. 4.8 Transmural infarction of bowel. (**a**) Plain radiograph of the abdomen demonstrates multiple air-fluid levels secondary to paralytic ileus. (**b** and **c**) Coronal CT reformation demonstrates fluid-containing, dilated small bowel loops (*arrowheads*) with no wall enhancement

than cystic pattern of intramural gas (Fig. 4.9). The presence of portomesenteric venous gas favors more serious causes of pneumatosis intestinalis, such as mesenteric ischemia, and increases mortality to 50 % (Fig. 4.10) [29]. The secondary findings seen on CT include ascites and mesenteric edema.

Colonic ischemia typically involves the inferior mesenteric artery territory, affecting splenic flexure and descending colon. The CT findings include reversible colonic wall thickening in the distribution of inferior mesenteric artery. Colonic ischemia cases usually resolve spontaneously and stricture formation is unusual.

Necrotizing enterocolitis is most commonly seen in premature neonates, developing in the first week of life. The imaging findings include pneumatosis, portal/mesenteric vein gas, pneumoperitoneum, and paralytic ileus.

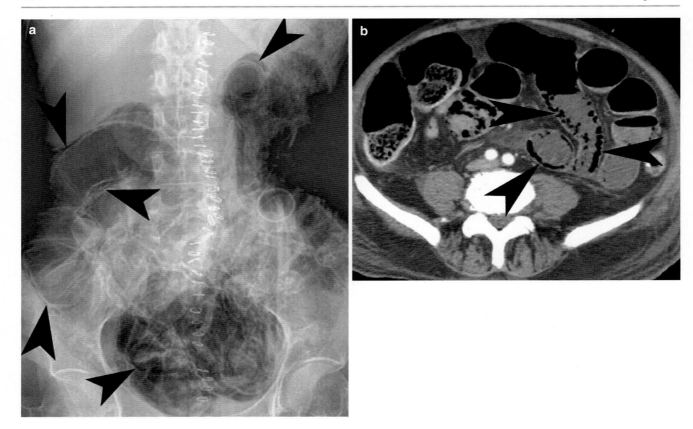

Fig. 4.9 Pneumatosis intestinalis. (**a**) Plain radiograph of the abdomen demonstrates extensive linear pneumatosis (*arrowheads*) in the small bowel wall. (**b**) Contrast-enhanced CT shows pneumatosis (*arrowheads*) in the small bowel wall, secondary to bowel wall ischemia

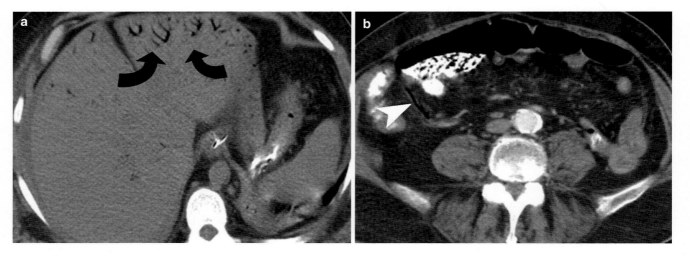

Fig. 4.10 Portal vein and superior mesenteric venous air in bowel infarction. (**a**) Noncontrast CT shows extensive air in portal vein branches (*curved arrows*). (**b**) Contrast-enhanced CT shows air in a superior mesenteric vein tributary (*arrowhead*), in a patient with bowel ischemia and portal vein gas

CT Findings of Small Bowel Ischemia

1. SMA/SMV thrombus.
2. Bowel distension, bowel wall thickening, and lack of enhancement.
3. Pneumatosis (linear pattern more ominous).
4. Portal/mesenteric vein gas.
5. Ascites.

Treatment

The treatment of acute mesenteric ischemia includes emergent laparotomy and embolectomy. Resection of infarcted bowel is performed with a second-look laparotomy often used to reassess the bowel loop viability. SMV thrombus should not be resected unless the venous thrombus is acute. Anticoagulation with heparin and broad spectrum antibiotics are utilized for mesenteric venous thrombosis.

Pneumatosis Intestinalis

Pneumatosis intestinalis is a pathological condition in which air is present submucosally or subserosally in the bowel wall. It is an imaging finding but not a clinical diagnosis, as it is associated with a multitude of causes. The causes of pneumatosis intestinalis can range from benign etiology without bowel ischemia to transmural bowel infarction, which is the most common cause (52 %) [29].

Bowel obstruction can cause pneumatosis intestinalis by causing mucosal breach secondary to increased intraluminal pressure. Pneumatosis secondary to collagen vascular disease can be secondary to abnormal peristalsis and bowel wall inflammation.

Pneumatosis cystoides intestinalis is typically characterized by colonic wall gas without bowel ischemia. Pneumatosis intestinalis with cystic appearance is more likely to be due to benign cause. Pneumatosis with linear collection of air in the bowel wall is more likely to be associated with bowel ischemia and higher mortality [29]. Unlike with bowel wall ischemia, pneumatosis cystoides intestinalis does not demonstrate gas in the portal venous system.

Benign Causes of Pneumatosis Intestinalis

1. Idiopathic.
2. Mucosal injury (including from bowel obstruction, diverticulitis, inflammatory bowel disease, corrosive ingestion, G-/J-tube placement, and recent bowel wall biopsy).
3. Steroids.
4. Emphysema.
5. Collagen vascular disease (scleroderma, SLE, PAN, polymyositis, etc.).
6. Organ transplantation.
7. AIDS.

Portal Venous Gas

Although portal venous gas is often seen in patients with transmural infarction of the bowel, it can also be seen with bowel obstruction, inflammatory bowel disease, steroid use, diverticulitis, emphysema, and organ transplantation. In patients with pneumatosis intestinalis, portal venous gas is present in 25 % cases and often indicates irreversible bowel wall infarction [29]. On CT the portal venous gas is seen as branched air lucencies present peripherally in the liver. Biliary air is typically present more centrally in the liver due to the direction of flow of bile toward the porta hepatis (Figs. 4.11 and 4.12). Mesenteric venous gas is typically seen as linear or branched lucencies present adjacent to the mesenteric border of the bowel. On ultrasound study, portal vein gas can be seen as echogenic series of gas bubbles, resembling a string of pearls.

Bowel Perforation

Free air in the abdomen is most commonly seen after surgery, G-tube placement and bowel perforation. Postoperative air progressively decreases with time and usually resolves by the seventh day. It usually takes longer time for air to resolve

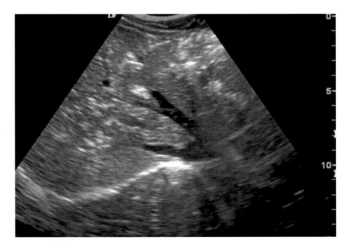

Fig. 4.11 Ultrasonographic appearance of air in the portal vein. Ultrasound shows portal venous hyperechoic foci of air seen peripherally as well as centrally in the liver

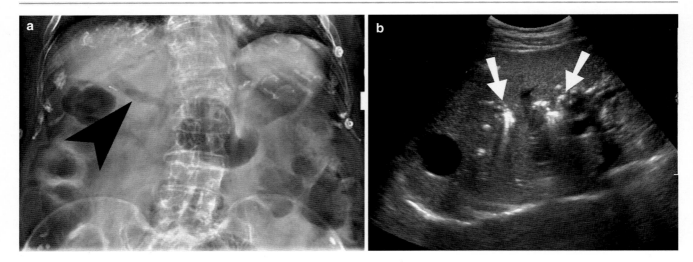

Fig. 4.12 Pneumobilia. (**a**) Plain radiograph of the abdomen shows centrally located air lucency in the common bile duct (*arrowhead*). (**b**) Ultrasound shows centrally located intrahepatic biliary ductal air (*arrows*)

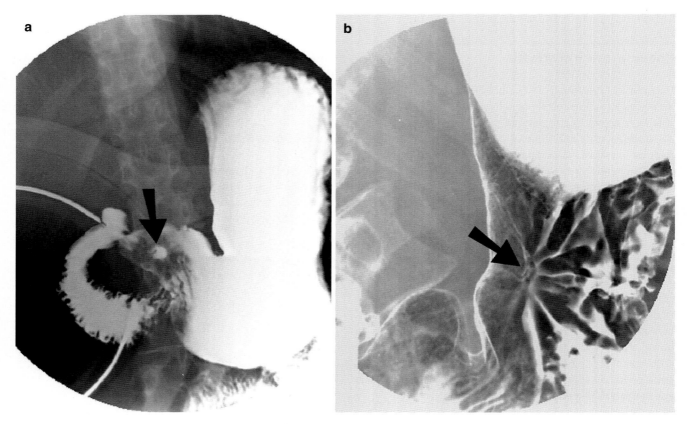

Fig. 4.13 Peptic ulcer disease. (**a**) Upper GI study demonstrates en face appearance of centrally radiopaque barium in the gastric ulcer crater (*arrow*), surrounded by a symmetric ulcer collar. (**b**) Upper GI study demonstrates smooth mucosal folds, radiating to the edge of a healing benign ulcer (*arrow*), a finding which is pathognomic of a benign peptic ulcer

in asthenic patients [30]. Free air secondary to bowel perforation is most commonly due to perforated peptic ulcer and less commonly due to perforated diverticulitis, small bowel obstruction, esophageal perforation, and appendicitis (Figs. 4.13, 4.14, and 4.15).

On upright abdominal radiographs, free air is most commonly seen under the domes of the diaphragm. On decubitus film of the abdomen, free air is seen in the nondependent abdomen, adjacent to the right hepatic margin. Supine radiograph of the abdomen has a sensitivity of 56–59 % in

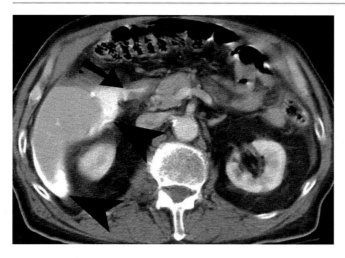

Fig. 4.14 Peptic ulcer disease with perforation. Contrast-enhanced CT shows the breech in the duodenal wall (*arrow*) with oral contrast leaking into the Morison's pouch (*arrowheads*)

patients with known free air [31, 32]. The presence of gas in the right upper quadrant constitutes a right upper quadrant gas sign and is the most common sign of free air on supine radiograph, seen in 41 % cases [32]. It is typically seen in triangular or linear configuration. On supine plain radiograph of the abdomen, the falciform ligament may be outlined by air and typically extends from right upper quadrant and pointing caudally to the left lower quadrant. This is known as ligamentum teres sign and is typically seen on supine radiograph of the abdomen. The presence of air in the fissure for ligamentum teres has been described as a new sign of intraperitoneal air [33]. The second (32 %) most commonly seen sign on the supine radiograph is the presence of air on either side of the bowel loops and constitutes the Rigler's sign, typically seen with large amount of free air (Figs. 4.16 and 4.17). The presence of a triangular configuration of air located between three loops of bowel constitutes the triangle sign.

Cupola sign refers to inverted cup-shaped lucency present under the central tendon of the diaphragm, on the supine film of the abdomen (Fig. 4.18a). When large amount of air is present on the supine radiograph of the abdomen, it can be seen as a large oval lucency (football sign) on the supine radiograph of the abdomen (Fig. 4.18b).

Visualization of medial umbilical ligaments produces inverted v-sign, which is appreciated when air is present in the nondependent part of the pelvis. It is constituted by two pairs of folds: medial umbilical folds (obliterated umbilical arteries) and lateral umbilical folds (containing inferior epigastric vessels).

"Doge's cap sign" is produced by the presence of air in the Morison's pouch. The "diaphragm muscle slip sign" is produced by air outlining the undersurface of the diaphragmatic muscles.

CT is more sensitive than plain radiograph in detecting free air, which typically accumulates in the nondependent abdomen, deep to the anterior abdominal wall. Small foci of free air can often be seen between the left lobe of the liver and the rectus abdominus.

Retroperitoneal air is often caused by duodenal or rectal perforation. Unlike free air, retroperitoneal air often outlines the kidneys and/or psoas major muscles (Fig. 4.19). Also, the retroperitoneal air is less likely to change position between supine and upright films of the abdomen than free intraperitoneal air.

Infection

Although infectious enteritis is a common cause of acute diarrheal illness in the USA, it is not usually an imaging diagnosis. Most cases of acute diarrheal illness (defined as less than 14 days in duration) in adults are due to viruses, bacteria, or less commonly protozoa. Patients are managed clinically with supportive therapy, and the illness is usually self-limited. Imaging may be indicated for chronic (>30 days' duration) diarrheal illness when inflammatory bowel disease is suspected or in the setting of acute disease in an immunocompromised patient.

Nevertheless, infectious enteritis may be present when imaging is performed for a different suspected diagnosis, such as appendicitis or diverticulitis. Findings of infectious enteritis on CT are fairly nonspecific, with diffuse bowel wall thickening and mesenteric lymphadenopathy being the most common manifestations [34]. The proximal small bowel is the typical site of infection by Giardia lamblia, the most common parasite to cause infection in the United States. Infectious enteritis affecting the distal ileum, often in combination with the cecum, can cause a confusing clinical picture, mimicking appendicitis. Frequent pathogens causing an infectious ileocolitis include Salmonella, Yersinia, Shigella, and Campylobacter [35, 36].

The clinical presentation of Campylobacter in particular may mimic that of acute appendicitis, thereby prompting CT or ultrasound imaging. The mesenteric adenitis present with this infection may be accompanied by acute inflammation of the terminal ileum, as well as an "endoappendicitis," that is, confined to the mucosal layer and visible only microscopically. Imaging manifestations include mural thickening of the terminal ileum and cecum as well as enlarged mesenteric lymph nodes (Fig. 4.20) [37].

Important causes of enteritis in patients with HIV infection include Mycobacterium avium-intracellulare (MAI), Cytomegalovirus, and Cryptosporidium. MAI more frequently affects the jejunum, causing bowel wall thickening that can be nodular. The finding of low-density, bulky mesenteric and retroperitoneal lymphadenopathy

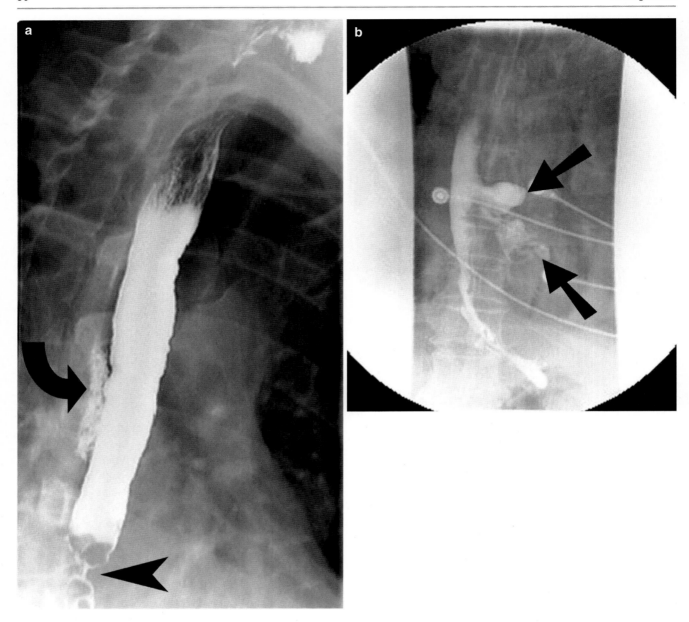

Fig. 4.15 Esophageal perforation. (**a**) Esophagram demonstrates per-foration (*curved arrow*) arising from posterior esophageal wall. There is a tight stricture (*arrowhead*) present in the distal esophagus with food residue present just proximal to it. (**b**) Esophagram demonstrates esophageal perforation (*arrows*) caused by swallowed dentures

is helpful in suggesting the diagnosis, although Whipple disease and lymphoma can have the same appearance. Cytomegalovirus enteritis is often hemorrhagic, sec-ondary to mucosal ulcerations, which can sometimes be seen on CT. Cryptosporidium infection results in bowel wall thickening, also typically involving the proximal small bowel, that can be indistinguishable from MAI and giardiasis [38].

Teaching Points

- Although less frequent than duodenal diverticula, jejunoil-eal diverticula are more prone to develop complications.
- Acquired small bowel diverticula are typically located on the mesenteric border of the bowel.
- Diverticula in the small bowel are less likely to develop inflammation than those in the colon.

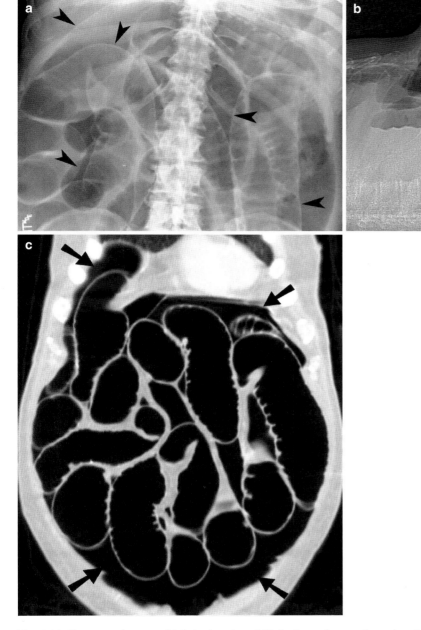

Fig. 4.16 Pneumoperitoneum: Rigler's sign. (**a** and **b**) Supine radiograph (**a**) and lateral CT scout film (**b**) demonstrate inner as well as outer wall of multiple small bowel loops (*arrowheads*). (**c**) Coronal CT reformation demonstrates large amount of free air (*arrows*) outlining the outer bowel wall margins

- CT findings include focal inflammatory mass containing air, fluid, or an air-fluid level adjacent to a segment of thickened small bowel, with the presence of surrounding inflammation and mesenteric fat stranding.

- Congenital diverticula (true diverticula) have three layers while acquired diverticula have two layers.
- Pneumatosis intestinalis with linear appearance is more likely to be secondary to bowel ischemia.

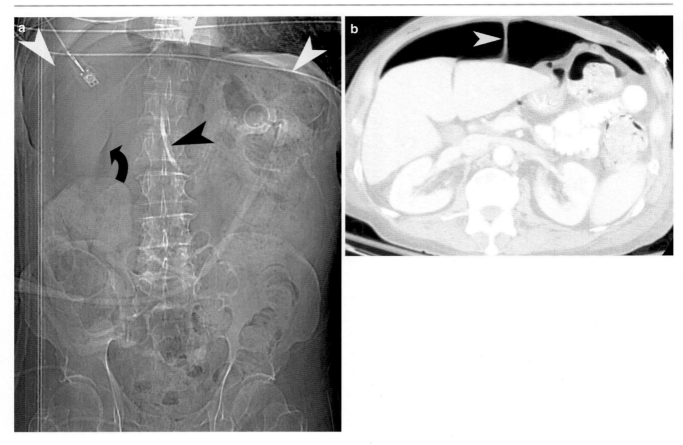

Fig. 4.17 Pneumoperitoneum: ligamentum teres sign. (**a**) Scout film of the abdomen demonstrates large amount of free air (*white arrowheads*) in the abdomen. The air is seen to outline the ligamentum teres (*black arrowhead*) as well as the undersurface (*curved arrow*) of the right lobe of the liver. (**b**) Axial CT image also demonstrates the large amount of nondependent air in the abdomen, outlining the ligamentum teres (*white arrow*)

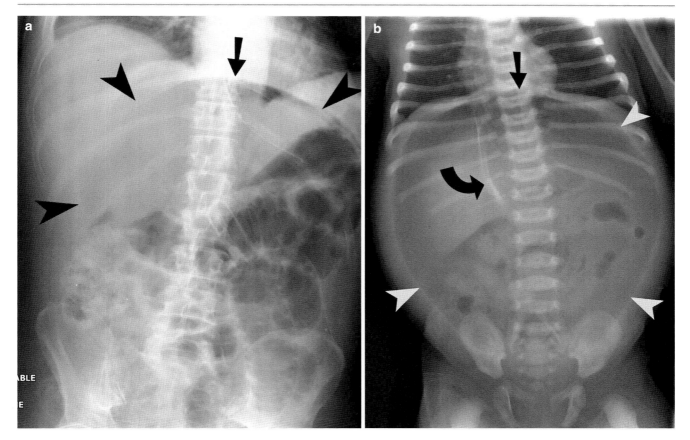

Fig. 4.18 Pneumoperitoneum: cupola sign and football sign. (**a** and **b**) Plain radiographs of the abdomen demonstrates large oval lucency (football sign, *arrowheads*) and inverted cup-shaped lucency (cupola sign, *arrow*), secondary to the free air. Ligamentum teres sign (*curved arrow*) is seen in the right upper quadrant as a sickle-shaped density outlined by air on either side

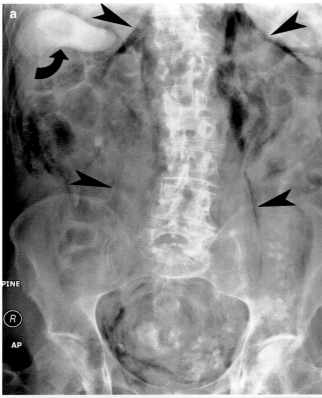

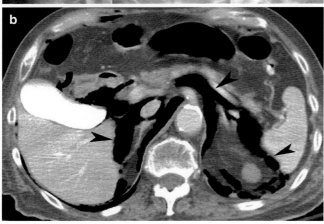

Fig. 4.19 Retroperitoneal air from perforation of the second portion of the duodenum during an ERCP study. (**a**) Plain radiograph of the abdomen demonstrates retroperitoneal air (*arrowheads*) outlining the kidneys and psoas muscles. The contrast in the gallbladder (*curved arrow*) is from the recent ERCP study. (**b**) Contrast-enhanced CT demonstrates the retroperitoneal air (*arrowheads*) and the contrast in the gallbladder (*curved arrow*)

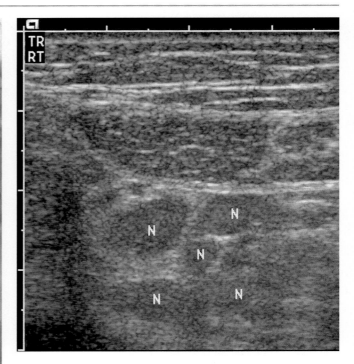

Fig. 4.20 Campylobacter ileocolitis. Ultrasound imaging demonstrates reactive mesenteric lymphadenopathy (*N*) in the right lower quadrant, in a patient with Campylobacter ileocolitis

References

1. Akhrass R, Yaffe MB, Fischer C, Ponsky J, Shuck JM. Small-bowel diverticulosis: perceptions and reality. J Am Coll Surg. 1997; 184(4):383–8.
2. Coulier B, Maldague P, Bourgeois A, Broze B. Diverticulitis of the small bowel: CT diagnosis. Abdom Imaging. 2007;32(2):228–33.
3. Macari M, Faust M, Liang H, Pachter HL. CT of jejunal diverticulitis: imaging findings, differential diagnosis, and clinical management. Clin Radiol. 2007;62(1):73–7.
4. Lempinen M, Salmela K, Kemppainen E. Jejunal diverticulosis: a potentially dangerous entity. Scand J Gastroenterol. 2004;39(9): 905–9.
5. Afridi SA, Fichtenbaum CJ, Taubin H. Review of duodenal diverticula. Am J Gastroenterol. 1991;86(8):935–8.
6. Yin WY, Chen HT, Huang SM, Lin HH, Chang TM. Clinical analysis and literature review of massive duodenal diverticular bleeding. World J Surg. 2001;25(7):848–55.
7. Maglinte DD, Chernish SM, DeWeese R, Kelvin FM, Brunelle RL. Acquired jejunoileal diverticular disease: subject review. Radiology. 1986;158(3):577–80.
8. Chendrasekhar A, Timberlake GA. Perforated jejunal diverticula: an analysis of reported cases. Am Surg. 1995;61(11):984–8.
9. Gotian A, Katz S. Jejunal diverticulitis with localized perforation and intramesenteric abscess. Am J Gastroenterol. 1998;93(7): 1173–5.
10. Krishnamurthy S, Kelly MM, Rohrmann CA, Schuffler MD. Jejunal diverticulosis. A heterogenous disorder caused by a variety of abnormalities of smooth muscle or myenteric plexus. Gastroenterology. 1983;85(3):538–47.
11. Vijayaraghavan SB, Krishnaraj B, Sarveswaran V. Sonographic features of mesenteric gas. J Ultrasound Med. 2004;23(11): 1507–10.
12. Peters R, Grust A, Gerharz CD, Dumon C, Furst G. Perforated jejunal diverticulitis as a rare cause of acute abdomen. Eur Radiol. 1999; 9(7):1426–8.
13. Tsiotos GG, Farnell MB, Ilstrup DM. Nonmeckelian jejunal or ileal diverticulosis: an analysis of 112 cases. Surgery. 1994;116(4): 726–31.
14. Pearl MS, Hill MC, Zeman RK. CT findings in duodenal diverticulitis. AJR Am J Roentgenol. 2006;187(4):W392–5.

15. Koger KE, Shatney CH, Dirbas FM, McClenathan JH. Perforated jejunal diverticula. Am Surg. 1996;62(1):26–9.

16. Williams RA, Davidson DD, Serota AI, Wilson SE. Surgical problems of diverticula of the small intestine. Surg Gynecol Obstet. 1981;152(5):621–6.

17. Kubota T. Perforated jejunal diverticulitis. Am J Surg. 2007; 193(4):486–7.

18. Novak JS, Tobias J, Barkin JS. Nonsurgical management of acute jejunal diverticulitis: a review. Am J Gastroenterol. 1997; 92(10):1929–31.

19. Prakash C, Clouse RE. Acute ileal diverticulitis. Am J Gastroenterol. 1998;93(3):452–4.

20. Franzen D, Gurtler T, Metzger U. Multiple recurrent perforated jejunal diverticulitis. Chirurg. 2002;73(12):1218–20.

21. Singh A, Raman S, Brooks C, Philips D, Desai R, Kandarpa K. Giant colonic diverticulum: percutaneous CT-guided treatment. J Comput Assist Tomogr. 2008;32(2):204–6.

22. Elsayes KM, Menias C, Harvin HJ, Francis IR. Imaging manifestations of Meckel's diverticulum. AJR Am J Roentgenol. 2007; 189:81–8.

23. Levy AD, Hobbs CM. Meckel diverticulum: radiologic features with pathologic correlation. Radiographics. 2004;24:565–87.

24. Wilcox RD, Shatney CH. Surgical implications of jejunal diverticula. South Med J. 1988;81(11):1386–91.

25. Cross MJ, Snyder SK. Laparoscopic-directed small bowel resection for jejunal diverticulitis with perforation. J Laparoendosc Surg. 1993;3(1):47–9.

26. Trompeter M, Brazda T, Remy CT, Vestring T, Reimer P. Non-occlusive mesenteric ischemia: etiology, diagnosis, and interventional therapy. Eur Radiol. 2002;12:1179–87.

27. Menke J. Diagnostic accuracy of multidetector CT in acute mesenteric ischemia: systematic review and meta-analysis. Radiology. 2010;256(1):93–101.

28. Kirkpatrick ID, Kroeker MA, Greenberg HM. Biphasic CT with mesenteric CT angiography in the evaluation of acute mesenteric ischemia: initial experience. Radiology. 2003;229(1):91–8.

29. Lassandro F, di Santo Stefano MLM, Maria Porto A, Grassi R, Rotondo A, Scaglione M. Intestinal pneumatosis in adults: diagnostic and prognostic value. Emerg Radiol. 2010;17:361–5.

30. Felson B, Wiot JF. Another look at pneumoperitoneum. Semin Roentgenol. 1973;8:437–43.

31. Menuck L, Siemens PT. Pneumoperitoneum: importance of right upper quadrant features. AJR Am J Roentgenol. 1976;127:753–6.

32. Levine MS, Scheiner JD, Rubesin SE, Laufer I, Herlinger H. Diagnosis of pneumoperitoneum on supine abdominal radiographs. AJR Am J Roentgenol. 1991;156:731–5.

33. Cho KC, Baker SR. Air in the fissure for the ligamentum teres: new sign of intraperitoneal air on plain radiographs. Radiology. 1991; 178:489–92.

34. Orchard JL, Petorak V. Abnormal abdominal CT findings in a patient with giardiasis. Resolution after treatment. Dig Dis Sci. 1995;40:346–8.

35. Puylaert JBCM, Van der Zant FM, Mutsaers JA. Infectious ileocecitis caused by Yersinia, Campylobacter, and Salmonella: clinical, radiological and US findings. Eur Radiol. 1997;7:3–9.

36. Antonopoulos P, Constantinidis F, Charalampopoulos G, Dalamarinis K, Karanicas I, Kokkini G. An emergency diagnostic dilemma: a case of Yersinia enterocolitica colitis mimicking acute appendicitis in a beta-thalassemia major patient: the role of CT and literature review. Emerg Radiol. 2008;15:123–6.

37. Puylaert JBCM, Lalisang RI, van der Werf SDJ, Doornbos L. Campylobacter ileocolitis mimicking acute appendicitis: differentiation of graded-compression ultrasound. Radiology. 1988;166:737–40.

38. Horton KM, Corl FM, Fishman EK. CT of nonneoplastic diseases of the small bowel: spectrum of disease. J Comput Assist Tomogr. 1999;23:417–28.

Ajay Singh and Joseph Ferucci

Small Bowel Obstruction

Small bowel obstruction is the most common disorder of the small bowel which requires hospital admission and surgical intervention. Small bowel obstruction leads to progressive increase in the intraluminal pressure which can exceed the venous pressure and result in bowel ischemia.

The most common cause of small bowel obstruction which accounts for 60–80 % cases is adhesions [1, 2]. These adhesions are most commonly due to prior surgery and less commonly due to peritonitis. Adhesions are characterized by demonstration of transition point without surrounding inflammation in a patient with prior history of abdominal or pelvic surgery.

The plain radiographic findings of small bowel obstruction include multiple air-fluid levels (>2) and dilated small bowel loops (>3 cm). More than two air-fluid levels greater than 3 cm in diameter or more than one air-fluid level in the same dilated small bowel loop are considered abnormal (Fig. 5.1a, b). String of pearl sign is seen on upright film of the abdomen in patients with small bowel obstruction and is characterized by nondependent small air bubbles located in valvulae conniventes. Plain radiography frequently under-diagnose or overdiagnose small bowel obstruction. Small bowel follow-through has fallen out of favor due to the accuracy of CT scan and can be used selectively when the CT findings are equivocal (Fig. 5.1c).

CT scan has higher sensitivity (90 %) than plain radiograph in making the diagnosis of small bowel obstruction and is considered the most appropriate imaging modality in diagnosing high-grade small bowel obstruction. The CT should be performed with intravenous contrast, but without oral contrast. CT enteroclysis and MR enteroclysis are both equally appropriate, first-line imaging modalities in diagnosing low-grade or intermittent small bowel obstruction.

CT study in patients with small bowel obstruction is characterized by small bowel loops more than 2.5 cm in caliber, transition point, and decompressed bowel loops beyond the transition zone. Although the adhesion band itself is rarely visible, the presence of a smooth transition zone often points to adhesions as the cause of the bowel obstruction.

Small bowel feces sign is characterized by the presence of fecal material along with air bubbles in dilated small bowel loops and is believed to be due to bacterial overgrowth and water resorption from incompletely digested food [3, 4] (Fig. 5.2). It is an indicator of the site of mechanical small bowel obstruction and points to the low-grade or subacute small bowel obstruction. It is present in longer segment of small bowel in patients with higher-grade obstruction and is useful in recognizing the transition point due to its close proximity. This sign has been reported in 7–82 % cases of small bowel obstruction and should not be mistaken for fecal material which can be normally present in terminal ileum in patients with incompetent ileocecal valve [5]. Fecal material can also be in small bowel in patients with cystic fibrosis, with bezoars, and with infectious and metabolic bowel disease.

The other findings of small bowel obstruction include mesenteric edema, ascites, mesenteric venous congestion, decreased bowel wall enhancement, and free extraluminal air (Table 5.1).

A. Singh, MD (✉)
Department of Radiology,
Massachusetts General Hospital, Harvard Medical School,
10 Museum Way, # 524, Boston, MA 02114, USA
e-mail: asingh1@partners.org

J. Ferucci, MD
Department of Radiology,
University of Massachusetts Memorial Medical Center,
Worcester, MA, USA

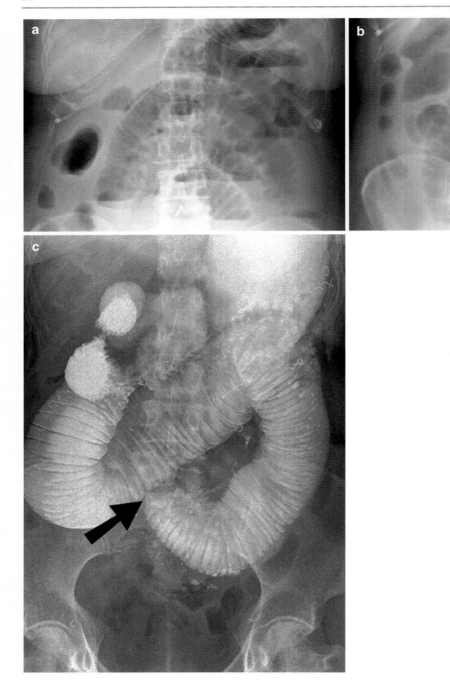

Fig. 5.1 Radiographic findings of small bowel obstruction. (**a** and **b**) Upright plain radiograph of the abdomen demonstrates dilated small bowel loops with differential air-fluid levels in a patient with high-grade obstruction. (**c**) Small bowel follow-through demonstrates dilated small bowel loops with abrupt transition in the mid-jejunum (*arrow*)

Internal Hernia

Internal hernia is characterized by herniation of small bowel through a breech in the mesentery into another compartment of the abdomen. Although paraduodenal hernia has traditionally been the most common type of internal hernia, the frequency of transmesentric internal hernia has increased with increasing popularity of gastric bypass surgeries.

The internal hernia can be paraduodenal (most common), prececal, foramen of Winslow, transmesenteric, transmesocolic, intersigmoid, and retromesenteric. The right paraduodenal hernia extends in to the Waldeyer's fossa, which is located posterior to the superior mesenteric artery and transverse colon. The left paraduodenal hernia

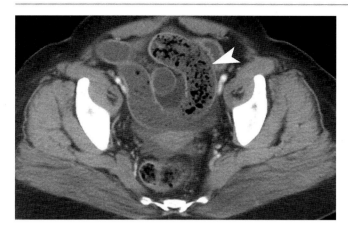

Fig. 5.2 Small bowel obstruction on CT. Contrast-enhanced CT study in a patient with small bowel obstruction demonstrates dilated small bowel loops with small bowel feces sign (*arrowhead*)

Table 5.1 Causes of small bowel obstruction

1. Adhesions (most common, 75 %)
2. Crohn's disease
3. Hernia (Fig. 5.3)
4. Neoplasia
5. Rare causes: radiation, internal hernia, intussusception, volvulus, gallstone ileus, tuberculosis, hematoma, bezoars

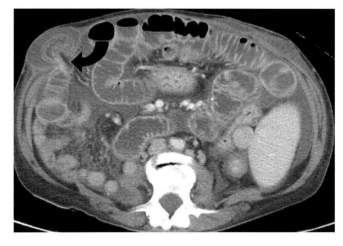

Fig. 5.3 Incarcerated hernia. Contrast-enhanced CT demonstrates small bowel obstruction secondary to bowel incarceration in hernia sac. The transition site (*curved arrow*) is located at the neck of the spigelian hernia sac

extends in to the Landzert's fossa, situated to the left of the fourth part of the duodenum.

The CT findings include saclike cluster of small bowel obstruction, anterior displacement of stomach, and crowding of mesenteric vessels [6] (Fig. 5.4). The CT findings of transmesocolic hernia, seen after gastric bypass surgery, include clustered small bowel loops cephalic to transverse mesocolon, high position of distal jejunal anastamosis, and

clustering of mesenteric vessels [7]. The right paraduodenal hernia is usually larger than left paraduodenal hernia. Transmesenteric internal hernia may also cause central displacement of colon.

Small Bowel Volvulus

Normal mesenteric attachment is broad and prevents volvulus. Anomaly in the bowel rotation and fixation, where mesenteric base is narrow, predisposes to midgut volvulus.

On barium upper gastrointestinal study, the duodenojejunal junction is located to the left of the spine and posterior to the stomach. Corkscrew configuration of the proximal small bowel is seen with midgut volvulus.

The whirl sign is characterized by twisting of the mesenteric vessels and mesenteric fat, secondary to small bowel volvulus [8]. It occurs due to twisting of afferent and efferent small bowel loops around a fixed point (Fig. 5.5). It is best appreciated when the cross-sectional imaging plane is perpendicular to the axis of rotation. Although this sign can also be seen after surgeries which involve bowel manipulation, such as hemicolectomy, it has been shown to require surgery 25 times more likely than those small bowel obstruction patients who do not have whirl sign [9].

Intussusception

Majority of small bowel obstruction seen in adults with intussusceptions has an underlying cause such as neoplasm, Meckel's diverticulum, or adhesions. The CT demonstrates a target-like appearance due to the location of intussuscepted bowel with surrounding fat-containing mesentery in the lumen of a more distal bowel (intussuscipiens) (Fig. 5.6).

Partial small bowel obstruction can be treated conservatively in majority of patients with nasogastric tube placement and gastric decompression. Surgical intervention is required in patients with closed loop obstruction and in patients with suspected strangulation.

Other Causes

Gallstone ileus causes mechanical obstruction, most commonly at the level of terminal ileum or ileocecal junction, and constitutes up to 25 % of small bowel obstruction in elderly patients (Fig. 5.7).

Duodenal hematoma is usually secondary to blunt trauma and is most often seen in children and young adults. The retroperitoneal duodenum is more prone to injury because its immobility and rich submucosal vascularity. The diagnosis can be made either with upper GI study or CT imaging (Fig. 5.8).

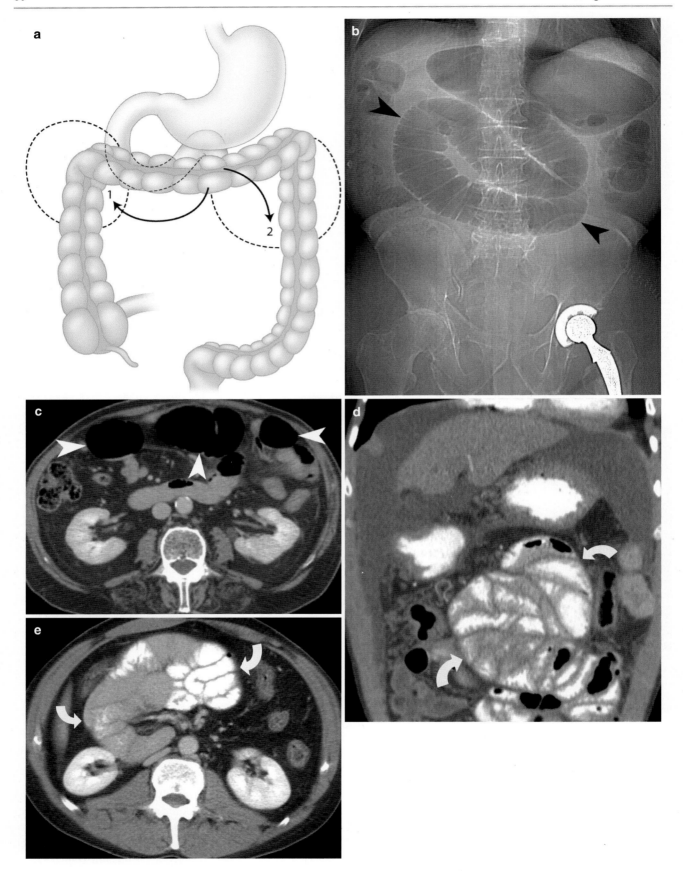

Fig. 5.4 Internal hernia. (**a**) Schematic representation of the right paraduodenal fossa (*1*) and left paraduodenal fossa (*2*). (**b**) CT scout film demonstrates dilated proximal small bowel (*arrowheads*) in the paraduodenal hernia. (**c**) Axial contrast-enhanced CT demonstrates dilated proximal small bowel loops (*arrowheads*) in paraduodenal hernia, without omental fat anterior to it. (**d**) and (**e**) Contrast-enhanced CT demonstrates clustering of small bowel loops in two different patients with paraduodenal hernia (*curved arrows*)

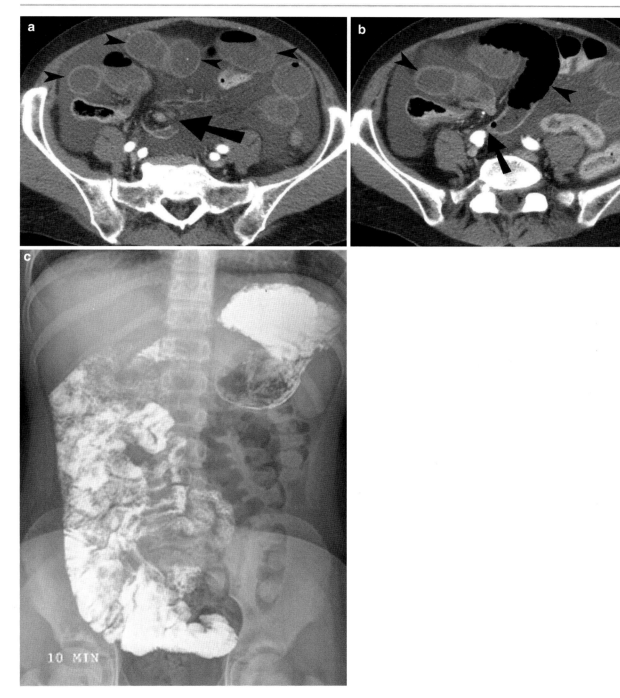

Fig. 5.5 Small bowel volvulus. (**a** and **b**) Contrast-enhanced CT demonstrates dilated small bowel loops (*arrowheads*) and whirled appearance (*arrow*) of mesentery, secondary to the volvulus. (**c**) Small bowel follow-through demonstrates the small bowel loops located to the right of midline. The air containing colonic loops can be seen to the left of midline

Closed Loop Obstruction

Closed loop obstruction is a type of mechanical obstruction with two points of obstruction present proximally as well as distally, most commonly due to adhesions. There is progressive increase in the intraluminal pressure, as the bowel cannot be decompressed with a nasogastric tube. It is the most common cause of bowel strangulation.

On cross-sectional imaging, closed loop obstruction is characterized by U-shaped configuration of dilated small bowel, radial configuration of mesenteric vessels and clustering of the abnormal bowel loop (Fig. 5.9). Small bowel strangulation is best indicated by pneumatosis intestinalis and portal venous gas.

Bowel obstruction from incarcerated hernia is characterized by dilated afferent loop extending into the hernia sac

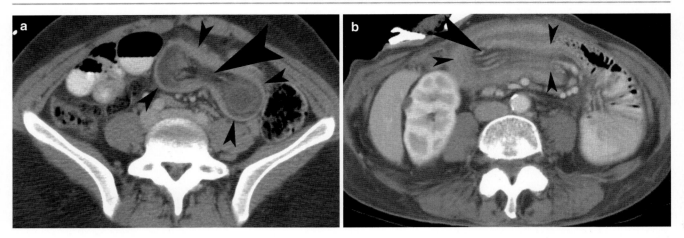

Fig. 5.6 Small bowel intussusception. (**a** and **b**) Axial contrast-enhanced CT demonstrates the mesenteric fat and mesenteric vessels in the intussusceptum (*large arrowheads*) with surrounding soft tissue density representing intussuscipiens (*small arrowheads*)

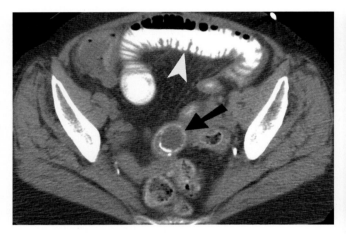

Fig. 5.7 Gallstone ileus. Contrast-enhanced CT demonstrates dilatation of small bowel (*arrowhead*) secondary to a gallstone (*arrow*) in the distal small bowel

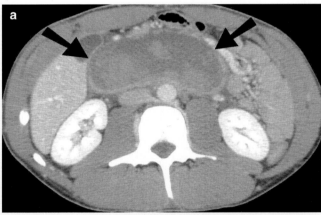

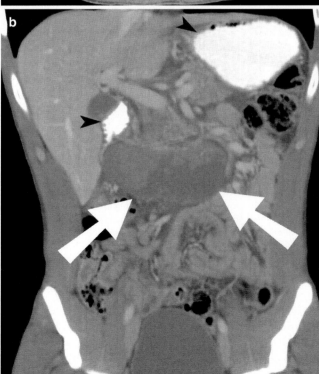

Fig. 5.8 Duodenal hematoma. (**a** and **b**) Contrast-enhanced CT demonstrates post-traumatic hematoma (*straight arrows*) in the duodenal wall, causing symptoms of proximal small bowel obstruction. (**b**) There is oral contrast (*arrowheads*) in the stomach and proximal duodenum, but not in the jejunum

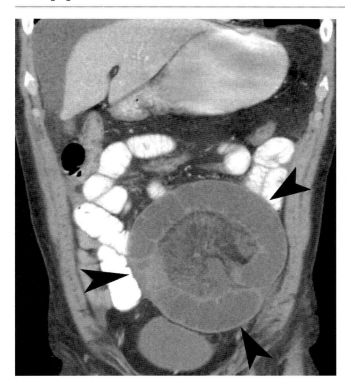

Fig. 5.9 Closed loop obstruction. Coronal CT reformation demonstrates dilated small bowel loop in circular configuration (*arrowheads*) and mesenteric vascular congestion in the left lower quadrant of the abdomen, consistent with closed loop obstruction

and decompressed efferent loop coming out of the hernia sac. Strangulating obstruction may demonstrate halo sign, mesenteric edema, mesenteric hemorrhage, lack of bowel enhancement, asymmetric wall enhancement, and pneumatosis.

Teaching Points

- Contrast-enhanced CT is considered the most appropriate imaging modality in diagnosing high-grade small bowel obstruction.

- CT enterocyclosis and MR enteroclysis are the imaging modalities of choice in diagnosing low-grade or intermittent small bowel obstruction.

- Plain radiography is not the first-line imaging modality in evaluating patients with suspected small bowel obstruction.

References

1. Balthazar EJ. CT of small-bowel obstruction. AJR Am J Roentgenol. 1994;162:255–61.
2. Miller G, Boman J, Shrier I, Gordon PH. Etiology of small bowel obstruction. Am J Surg. 2000;180(1):33–6.
3. Mayo-Smith WW, Wittenberg J, Bennett GL, Gervais DA, Gazelle GS, Mueller PR. The CT small bowel faeces sign: description and clinical relevance. Clin Radiol. 1995;50:765–7.
4. Fuchsjager MH. The small bowel feces sign. Radiology. 2002;225:378–9.
5. Lazarus DE, Slywotsky C, Bennett GL, Megibow AJ, Macari M. Frequency and relevance of the "small-bowel feces" sign on CT in patients with small-bowel obstruction. AJR Am J Roentgenol. 2004;183:1361–6.
6. Blachar A, Federle MP, Dodson SF. Internal hernia: clinical and imaging findings in 17 patients with emphasis on CT criteria. Radiology. 2001;218:68–74.
7. Reddy SA, Yang C, McGinnis LA, Seggerman RE, Garza E, Ford KL. Diagnosis of transmesocolic internal hernia as a complication of retrocolic gastric bypass: CT imaging criteria. AJR Am J Roentgenol. 2007;189:52–5.
8. Fisher JK. Computed tomographic diagnosis of volvulus in intestinal malrotation. Radiology. 1981;140:145–6.
9. Duda JB, Bhatt S, Dogra VS. Utility of CT whirl sign in guiding management of small-bowel obstruction. AJR Am J Roentgenol. 2008;191(3):743–7.

Imaging of Acute Colonic Disorders

Ajay Singh

Acute Diverticulitis

A diverticulum is a sacculation of mucosa and submucosa through the muscularis layer of the colonic wall, where the taeniae and mesentery are absent [1, 2]. The occlusion of the neck of the diverticulum may lead to inflammation, mucosal erosions, and microperforation. Although the inflamed diverticula are most commonly seen in the sigmoid and descending colon, less commonly they may be present in the transverse or ascending colon [3].

Approximately 80 % of patients with diverticulitis are more than 80 years old [2, 4]. The patients typically present with left lower quadrant pain, nausea, vomiting, fever, and leukocytosis.

Imaging

Contrast-enhanced CT is the imaging modality of choice in the evaluation of acute left lower quadrant pain. The CT can be performed with oral and/or rectal contrast and has sensitivities as high as 99 % for diagnosing acute diverticulitis. CT is not only helpful in triaging the patients into surgical and nonsurgical groups, but it is also the primary imaging modality during placement of pigtail drainage catheter in patients with abscess. The CT findings of acute diverticulitis include demonstration of inflamed, fluid-filled diverticulum with mild wall thickening and disproportionately severe surrounding inflammation (Fig. 6.1). There may be fluid in the root of sigmoid mesocolon (comma sign), engorged mesenteric vessels (centipede sign), abscesses, extraluminal air, and reactive lymphadenopathy [1–5].

A. Singh, MD
Department of Radiology,
Massachusetts General Hospital, Harvard Medical School,
10 Museum Way, # 524, Boston, MA 02141, USA
e-mail: asingh1@partners.org

Although graded compression ultrasound has been shown by some to have a sensitivity of 90 % for the diagnosis of diverticulitis, it has not gained widespread acceptance in the USA. Ultrasound is however considered the most appropriate test in the evaluation of left lower quadrant pain in women of childbearing age.

Complications

The complications of acute diverticulitis include abscess, perforation, and colovesical fistula. An uncommon complication of recurrent diverticulitis of the colon is giant colonic diverticula. A giant colonic diverticulum is more than or equal to 4 cm in diameter and is believed to result from narrowing of the diverticular neck, creating ball-valve mechanism where air can enter the diverticula but cannot escape out (Fig. 6.2).

Diverticulitis accounts for two-thirds of the vesicoenteric fistulas. Inflamed colon may adhere to the urinary bladder wall and may cause a fistula. These patients may have pneumaturia and fecaluria. The flow through the fistula predominantly occurs from the large bowel to the urinary bladder and is often indicated by the presence of air in the urinary bladder lumen (Fig. 6.3).

Treatment

The treatment of acute diverticulitis is most often conservative with antibiotic therapy. Image-guided pigtail catheter drainage is used to treat abscess and avoids the need for multistage surgery for acute diverticulitis. CT-guided catheter drainage has a 70–90 % success rate in treating a post-diverticulitis abscess. Abscess less than 3 cm in diameter may be managed conservatively, without drainage or surgery. When a collection is more than 4 cm in diameter, CT-guided catheter drainage is often preferred, followed by referral for surgical treatment (Fig. 6.4). Eventual surgical resection of the segment of colon is recommended in all patients who develop abscess.

A. Singh (ed.), *Emergency Radiology*,
DOI 10.1007/978-1-4419-9592-6_6, © Springer Science+Business Media New York 2013

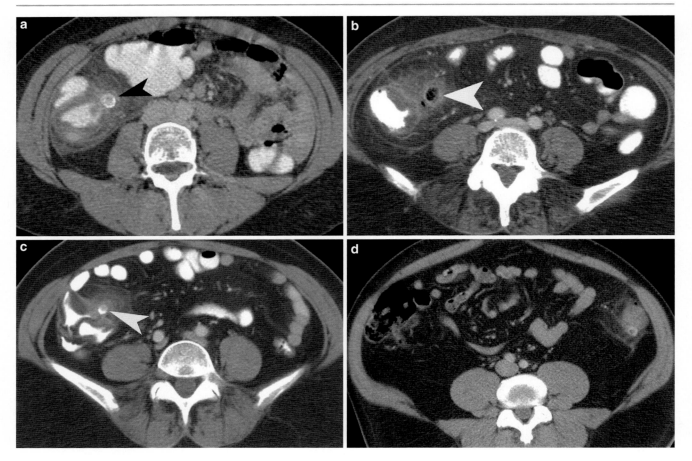

Fig. 6.1 Acute diverticulitis (**a–c**) Contrast-enhanced CT scan study of the abdomen demonstrates inflamed diverticulum (*arrowheads*) arising from the ascending colon. There are pericolonic inflammatory changes seen around the inflamed colonic diverticulum. (**d**) Contrast-enhanced CT scan study of the abdomen demonstrates inflamed diverticulum arising from the distal descending colon. There is colonic wall thickening and pericolonic inflammatory changes

Segmental Omental Infarction

Omental infarction is a rare cause of acute abdomen, which most often simulates acute appendicitis on clinical exam. It is seen in younger age group patients than acute epiploic appendagitis. Segmental omental infarction is the result of vascular compromise, either due to torsion or vascular thrombosis. It typically occurs on the right side of the omentum due to embryologic variation in the blood supply.

Omental torsion may result from conditions which cause sudden increase in intra-abdominal pressure such as coughing, sneezing, Valsalva, or heavy meal. Although most cases of segmental omental infarction is idiopathic, it can be associated with adhesions, hernias, surgery, intra-abdominal inflammation, congestive heart failure, obesity, strenuous exercise, digitalis administration, recent Whipple surgery/splenectomy surgery, and trauma.

The typical CT findings of omental infarction include a cake-like inflammatory fatty mass or whirled fatty structure, most commonly in the right lower quadrant (Fig. 6.5a, b) [6]. Unlike

acute epiploic appendagitis, omental infarction is most commonly on the right side, may or may not about the colon, and does not demonstrate ring sign around the inflamed fat. While typical acute epiploic appendagitis is less than 3.5 cm in diameter, omental infarctions are much larger (typically >5 cm) [7].

Segmental omental infarction is a self-limited condition which is best managed conservatively using Motrin. Majority of the patients are asymptomatic within 10 days of the treatment.

Acute Epiploic Appendagitis

Epiploic appendages are finger-shaped fat-containing pouches which arise off the surface of the colon and are surrounded by the visceral peritoneum. The most common location of inflammation of an epiploic appendage is adjacent the sigmoid colon and usually affects adult people in fifth to sixth decades [5]. The reason for the presence of epiploic appendagitis in the left abdomen in 80 % of cases is because of the higher number of epiploic appendages present adjacent to the sigmoid colon.

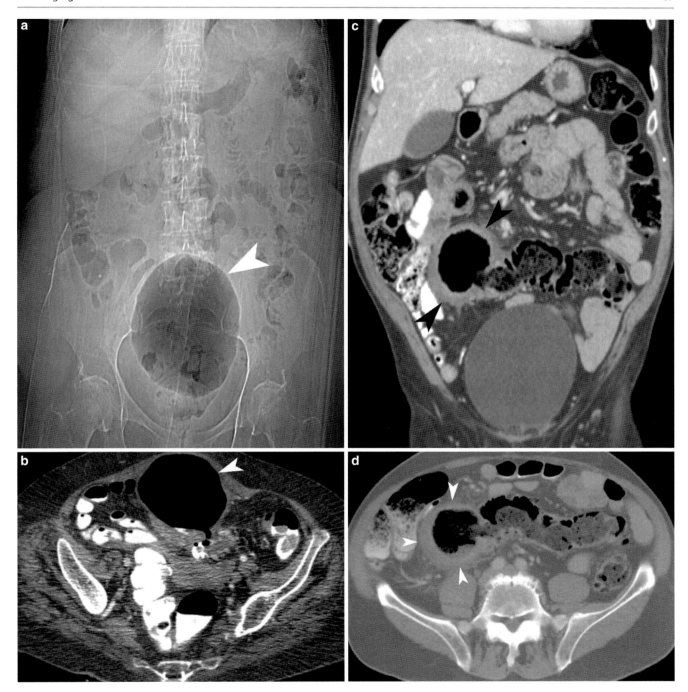

Fig. 6.2 Giant sigmoid diverticulum. (**a**) Scout film of the abdomen demonstrates a 10-cm-diameter air-containing cavity in the pelvis which corresponds to a giant sigmoid diverticulum (*arrowheads*) in a patient with recurrent episodes of diverticulitis. (**b**) Contrast-enhanced CT scan study of the pelvis demonstrates a giant sigmoid diverticulum arising from the sigmoid colon. Small amount of rectal contrast is present within the lumen of the large diverticulum. (**c, d**) Contrast-enhanced CT scan study demonstrates inflammatory thickening of the wall of a giant sigmoid diverticulum (*arrowheads*), arising from sigmoid colon

Torsion of epiploic appendages can lead to vascular occlusion and infarction. Inflamed epiploic appendage can cause bowel obstruction from adhesions and can get detached from colon to produce intraperitoneal loose body [5, 8]. It has also been rarely reported to cause intussusception and abscess formation.

Clinically, the patients may present with acute left lower quadrant pain, nausea, fever, and diarrhea or constipation [5]. When it involves the left lower quadrant, it is clinically most often mistaken for sigmoid diverticulitis. When it affects the cecum, it is clinically most often mistaken for acute

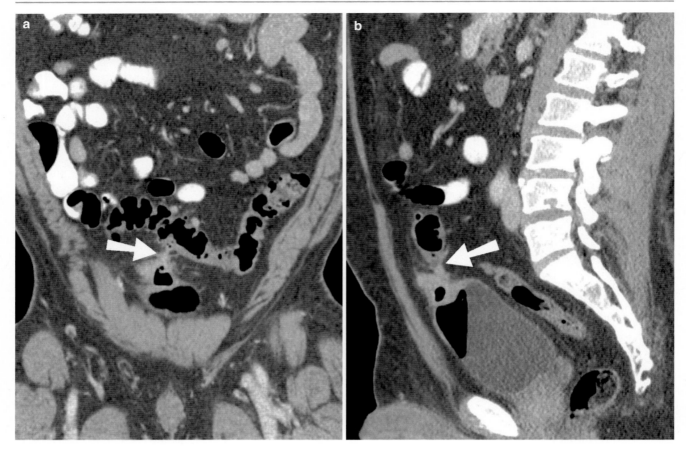

Fig. 6.3 Colovesical fistula. (**a**, **b**) Coronal and sagittal reformations of the abdomen demonstrate colovesical fistula (*arrow*) extending from the sigmoid colon to the urinary bladder dome. There is air identified within the urinary bladder lumen, secondary to the fistulous communication with the colon

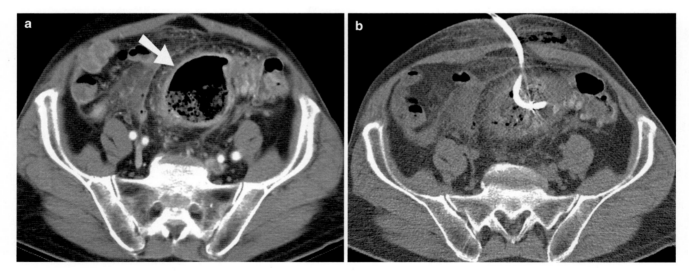

Fig. 6.4 Diverticulitis abscess. (**a**) Contrast-enhanced CT scan study of the pelvis demonstrates a well-defined abscess cavity (*arrow*) in the sigmoid mesocolon with surrounding inflammatory changes. (**b**) Contrast-enhanced CT scan study demonstrates decrease in the size of the pelvic abscess after placement of a pigtail drainage catheter

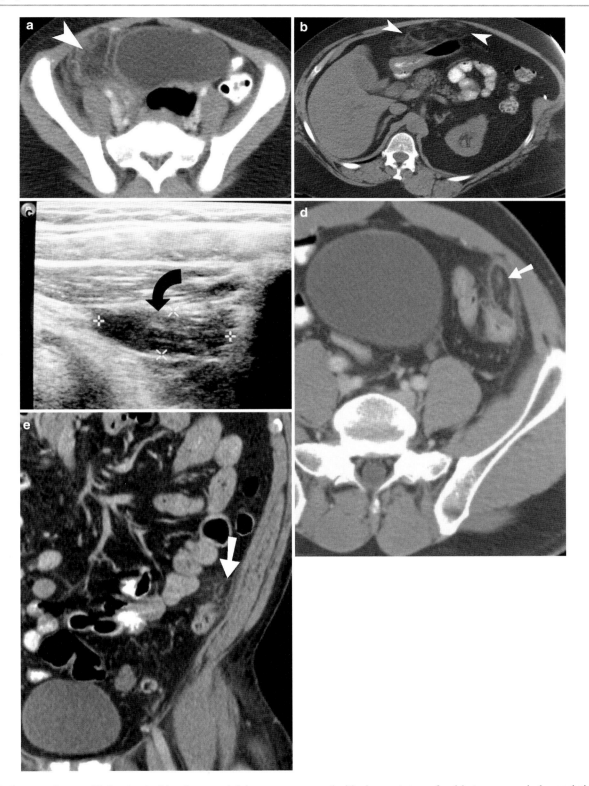

Fig. 6.5 Segmental omental infarction (**a**, **b**) and acute epiploic appendicitis (**c–e**). (**a**) Contrast-enhanced CT scan study demonstrates a 7-cm-diameter omental fat density inflammatory lesion (*arrowhead*) in the upper right lower quadrant of the abdomen of a 6-year-old patient. (**b**) Noncontrast CT of a patient with segmental omental infarction demonstrates a midline inflammatory fatty lesion anteroinferior to the left lobe of the liver. (**c**) Ultrasound of a patient with acute epiploic appendagitis demonstrates a focal heterogeneously hypoechoic lesion (*curved arrow*) located just deep to the left anterior abdominal wall musculature. (**d**, **e**) Axial and coronal contrast-enhanced CT scan study demonstrates an oval, fat density lesion (*straight arrow*) in relation to the sigmoid colonic wall with surrounding inflammatory changes. The high-density central dot corresponds to thrombosed or congested vessel within the torsed epiploic appendage. Omental infarction

appendicitis. Because of the clinical misdiagnoses, patients with primary epiploic appendagitis can get unnecessary hospitalization and treatment. The clinical management of acute appendagitis includes conservative treatment with pain medication.

Imaging

Although ultrasound has been occasionally used in diagnosing acute epiploic appendagitis, CT is the imaging tool of choice in making the diagnosis. The CT findings include a pedunculated fatty lesion, 1.5–3.5 cm in length, and associated with surrounding inflammatory stranding, hyperdense ring, high-attenuating central dot, and less commonly adjacent thickening of the colon wall (Fig. 6.5c–e) [5]. The parietal peritoneum deep to the anterior abdominal wall may be thickened. The ultrasound findings are similar to CT study and may include hypoechoic rim surrounding a hyperechoic focal lesion.

A central high-attenuation focus within the fat is a helpful finding which is believed to represent a thrombosed or congested vessel. Since it is seen in 54 % of the cases, its absence does not rule out the diagnosis of acute epiploic appendagitis. There is usually no colonic wall thickening [7]. The CT changes of acute epiploic appendagitis tend to resolve in all patients within 6 months.

The differential diagnosis of an inflammatory fat-containing lesion on CT includes acute epiploic appendagitis, mesenteric panniculitis, acute diverticulitis, trauma, omental contusion, omental metastases, and liposarcoma. Although omental infarction can have an appearance similar to that of epiploic appendagitis, it lacks the hyperdense ring that is seen in all patients with epiploic appendagitis. Majority of the cases of acute epiploic appendagitis are self-limited and can be treated with pain management using analgesics.

Inflammatory Bowel Disease

Crohn's disease is a chronic granulomatous inflammatory disease that involves the entire gastrointestinal tract with transmural and discontinuous lesions which most often affects the distal ileum and right colon [9]. The transmural inflammation is commonly associated with deep ulceration and sinus/fistula formation.

Ulcerative colitis is an idiopathic chronic inflammatory disease that most often demonstrates continuous involvement of the rectum and distal colon and rectum mucosa [10].

The common modes of presentation of inflammatory bowel disease include abdominal pain, diarrhea, weight loss, vomiting, and fever. The patients with Crohn's disease may have associated arthritis, ocular inflammatory diseases, gallstones, and skin lesions [11].

Table 6.1 Imaging findings of ulcerative colitis (Fig. 6.6)

1. Continuous involvement from rectum to colon
2. Mucosal granularity and stippling
3. Indistinctness of haustral folds
4. Collar button ulcers
5. Inflammatory pseudopolyps
6. Backlash ileitis
7. Presacral space widening (>1.5 cm)

Table 6.2 Imaging findings of Crohn's colitis (Fig. 6.7)

1. Lymphoid hyperplasia: 2 mm filling defects in the wall
2. Aphthoid ulceration: small, 1 mm diameter superficial ulcerations with radiolucent halo
3. Deep ulcerations, sinuses, and fistulas
4. Colonic wall thickening: more with Crohn's disease
5. Bowel strictures: often asymmetrical
6. Anorectal fissures, abscess, and fistulas: more commonly with Crohn's disease

Imaging

For the initial presentation of suspected Crohn's disease in patients with abdominal pain, fever, and diarrhea, CT enterography is considered the most appropriate imaging modality. The second-line imaging test for suspected Crohn's disease is small bowel follow-through study. For adult and pediatric patients with known Crohn's disease, presenting with fever, abdominal pain, and leukocytosis, routine contrast-enhanced CT is considered the imaging modality of choice. CT enterography involves the use of neutral oral contrast and imaging performed 45 s after intravenous contrast.

The CT findings include bowel wall enhancement, wall thickening, mural stratification, prominent vasa recta, and mesenteric inflammation. The mural stratification (Target or halo sign) is produced by soft tissue density mucosa, low-density submucosa (edema or fatty infiltration), and soft tissue density muscularis propria. Imaging also allows differentiation between Crohn's disease and ulcerative colitis (Tables 6.1 and 6.2).

In pediatric patients with Crohn's disease with mild symptoms, MR enterography is considered the most appropriate imaging modality because of its high sensitivity and specificity, similar to CT enterography. Ultrasound is the second-line imaging modality in similar clinical scenario and suffers from the disadvantage of operator dependence. Ultrasound may be useful in diagnosing colonic inflammatory diseases, in particular when equivocal results are obtained by other imaging techniques, because of its ability to see wall thickening (≥4 mm), target sign, sluggish peristalsis, and pericolonic extension of the disease. MR imaging may be also used, in particular when recurrent studies are needed, and allows excellent soft tissue contrast without radiation exposure [10].

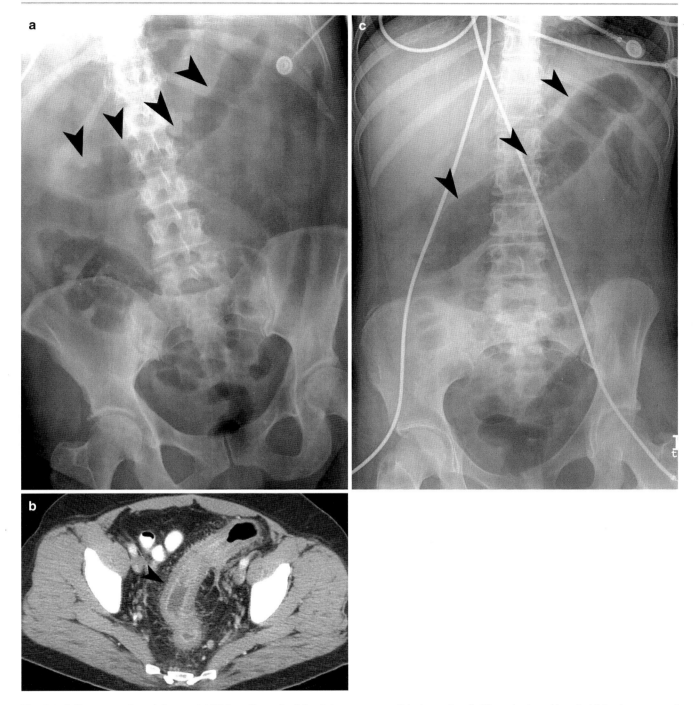

Fig. 6.6 Inflammatory bowel disease. (**a**) Plain radiograph of the abdomen demonstrates thumbprinting (*arrowheads*) involving the transverse colon in a patient with ulcerative colitis. (**b**) Contrast-enhanced CT in a patient with ulcerative colitis shows symmetrical and continuous involvement of the entire rectum and sigmoid colon by inflammatory proctocolitis (*arrowhead*). There is sigmoid wall thickening, mucosal enhancement, and pericolonic inflammatory densities. (**c**) Plain radiograph of the abdomen in a patient with Crohn's colitis demonstrates a featureless segment of the transverse colon

Complications and Treatment

The complications of inflammatory bowel disease include abscess, fistulas, and bowel obstruction [2]. Acute flare-up of Crohn's disease is usually treated with anti-inflammatory drugs and steroids. Surgery is the therapeutic tool which is reserved for nonresponsive disease, complications, and very ill patients.

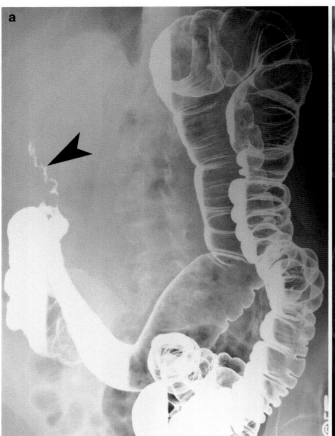

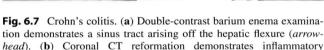

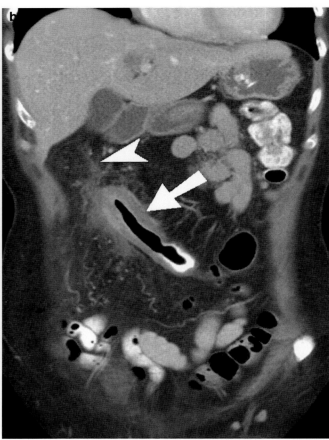

Fig. 6.7 Crohn's colitis. (**a**) Double-contrast barium enema examination demonstrates a sinus tract arising off the hepatic flexure (*arrowhead*). (**b**) Coronal CT reformation demonstrates inflammatory thickening of right transverse colon (*arrow*), secondary to Crohn's colitis. A sinus tract (*arrowhead*) is seen extending from the splenic flexure to the right subhepatic location

Pseudomembranous Colitis

Pseudomembranous colitis, also called *C. difficile* colitis, is a life-threatening condition caused by *Clostridium difficile* that produces two exotoxins and leads to colonic mucosa to generate a protein-rich membrane (pseudomembrane). Toxin A is responsible for colitis and allows Toxin B to enter the cell. The bacterium has a widespread presence in the hospitals and is the cause of up to 20 % of diarrhea associated with antibiotic therapy [12].

The disease may be asymptomatic at the beginning but then becomes clinically evident with watery diarrhea, abdominal pain and tenderness, fever, dehydration, and leukocytosis. In the life-threatening cases lethargy, tachycardia, and toxic megacolon or perforation due to necrosis may be associated. Cytoxan assay is the gold standard in detection of Toxin B and has more than 90 % sensitivity. Majority of cases in clinical practice are detected by colonoscopy and positive toxin B assay.

The CT findings include extensive mural thickening with prominent haustral folds (Fig. 6.8). In decreasing order of frequency, there is involvement of entire colon (most common), right colon, and left colon (least common). The barium enema findings include thumbprinting and small nodular or plaque-like filling defects.

While the mortality of *Clostridia difficile* infection is only 2 %, the cost of managing the patients in hospital is more than three billion dollars per year. The medical treatment involves the use of metronidazole for mild infection and vancomycin with or without metronidazole for severe infection. In resistant patients with elevated lactate levels and elevated WBC levels (>50,000/mm³), surgical intervention (partial colectomy with preservation of rectum) is needed.

Typhlitis

Typhlitis is characterized by inflammation of the cecum and ascending colon in immunocompromised patients. It is also called neutropenic colitis and is most often seen in patients with leukemia, lymphoma, aplastic anemia, AIDS, renal transplantation, or other immunocompromised conditions.

CT is considered the imaging modality of choice. The CT imaging features include cecal distension, circumferential

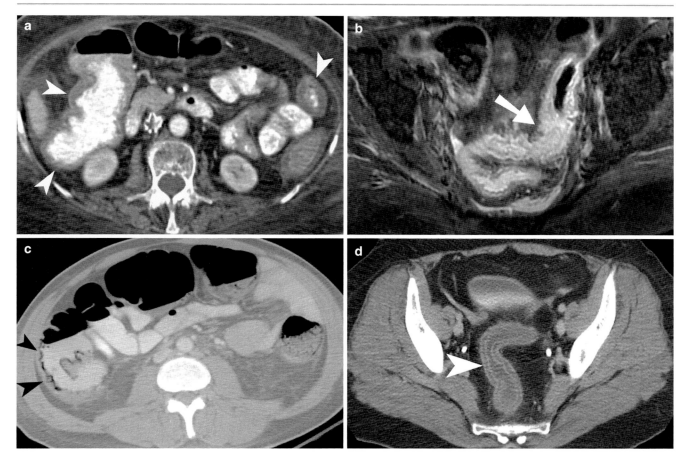

Fig. 6.8 Pseudomembranous colitis. (**a**) Contrast-enhanced CT scan study of the abdomen demonstrates diffuse thickening of the colonic wall (*arrowheads*), more prominent on the right side. (**b**) Gadolinium-enhanced T1-weighted axial image of the pelvis demonstrates enhancement and thickening of the rectal as well as sigmoid colonic wall with surrounding inflammatory changes. (**c**) Contrast-enhanced CT shows the infectious colitis affecting the right colon. There is ascending colonic wall thickening (*arrowheads*) and pneumatosis. (**d**) Contrast-enhanced CT of the pelvis shows rectosigmoidal wall thickening (*arrowhead*) from proctocolitis. The bowel wall thickening is produced by submucosal edema sandwiched between mucosal and serosal enhancements

colonic wall thickening, and pericolonic wall thickening (Fig. 6.9). The other findings include pericolonic fluid, free air, and pneumatosis.

Colonic Volvulus

Volvulus refers to torsion of a tract of free-moving bowel along its axis, usually because of a point of traction. It is more frequent in the small bowel, but may occur in the colon. Sigmoid volvulus accounts for 75 % and cecal volvulus accounts for 20 % of large bowel obstructions.

Cecal volvulus is a potentially life-threatening condition which accounts for up to 2 % of cases of bowel obstruction, 11 % of cases of intestinal volvulus, and 25–40 % of colonic volvulus [13, 14]. Cecal volvulus occurs most commonly in 20–40 years and is a misnomer as the torsion occurs in the ascending colon. The two types of cecal volvulus include the axial torsion which is characterized by 180–360° twist along the long axis of the ascending colon and cecal bascule which is characterized by cecum folding anteromedially, leading to luminal occlusion. It is often predisposed by abnormal fixation of the right colon to the retroperitoneum and abnormal motility of the right colon. Other predisposing factors include prior surgery, recent colonoscopy, recent enema, pregnancy, congenital duplication cyst, and mesenteric mass.

Transverse colonic volvulus is a rare site of colonic volvulus but most likely to be life-threatening. Sigmoid volvulus usually occurs in elderly patients (>70 years) and is the most frequent type of colonic volvulus (60–75 %). Main predisposing factors are high-fiber diet, pregnancy, hospitalization or institutionalization, and Chagas disease [14].

Imaging

Cecal volvulus demonstrates a dilated gas-filled colonic segment projecting in the left upper quadrant or mid-abdomen, single air-fluid level, and small bowel dilatation. On barium enema there is a beak-like tapering at the level of

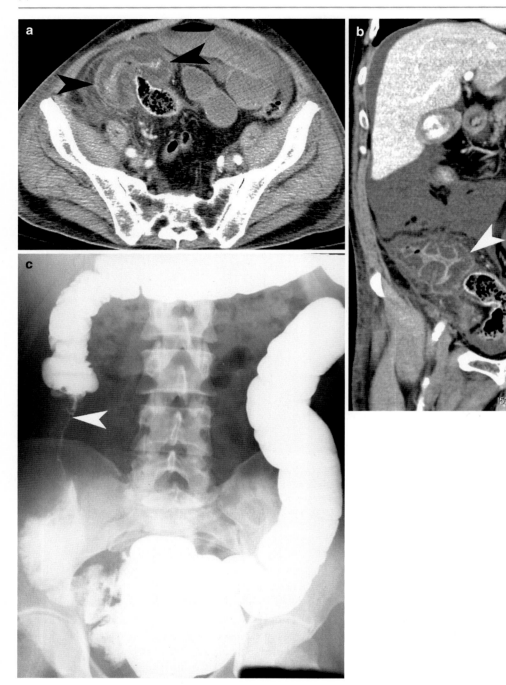

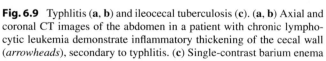

Fig. 6.9 Typhlitis (**a, b**) and ileocecal tuberculosis (**c**). (**a, b**) Axial and coronal CT images of the abdomen in a patient with chronic lymphocytic leukemia demonstrate inflammatory thickening of the cecal wall (*arrowheads*), secondary to typhlitis. (**c**) Single-contrast barium enema examination of a patient with ileocecal tuberculosis demonstrates chronic ileocecal stricture (*arrowhead*) and cranial migration of the ileocecal junction

the volvulus, adjacent to a dilated cecum. On CT, the "whirl sign" is the main finding, referring to the twisted appearance of the mesenteric vessels, afferent bowel, and efferent bowel loops (Figs. 6.10 and 6.11). The other signs include an abnormally enlarged cecum with decompressed distal colon.

For transverse colonic volvulus, conventional radiology is rarely useful. Barium enema or CT is frequently used to show the twist in the colon. On barium enema, a beak-shaped narrowing is seen at the level of the colonic twist (Fig. 6.12a, b).

On plain radiography, sigmoid volvulus is seen as a large air-filled bowel loop extending cranially from the pelvis to beyond the level of the transverse colon (northern exposure sign). Other radiological findings include the "coffee bean"

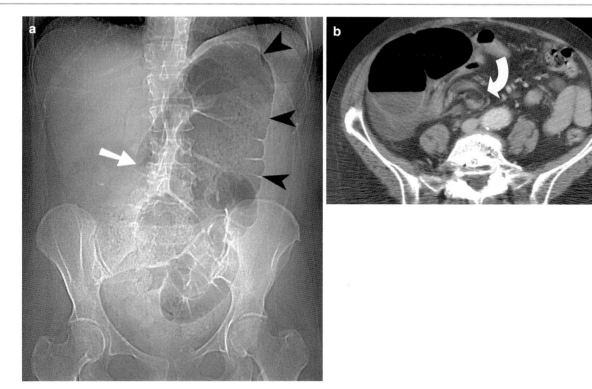

Fig. 6.10 Cecal volvulus. (**a**) Plain x-ray of the abdomen demonstrates dilatation of the cecum (*arrowheads*) which extends to the left upper quadrant. The bowel gas transition is present in the ascending colon (*arrow*). (**b**) Contrast-enhanced CT scan study of the pelvis demonstrates whirl sign in the right lower quadrant (*curved arrow*). The cecum is dilated and there is free fluid present posterior to it

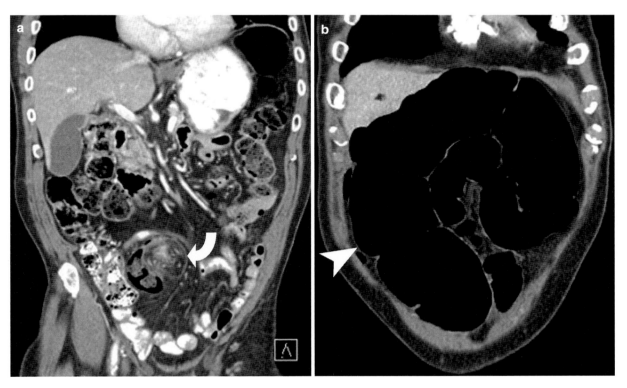

Fig. 6.11 Cecal volvulus. (**a**) Coronal CT reformation demonstrates whirled appearance of the mesentery as well as a segment of the right colon in this patient with cecal volvulus. (**b**) Coronal CT reformation demonstrates dilated sigmoid colonic loops (*arrowhead*) in this closed-loop obstruction

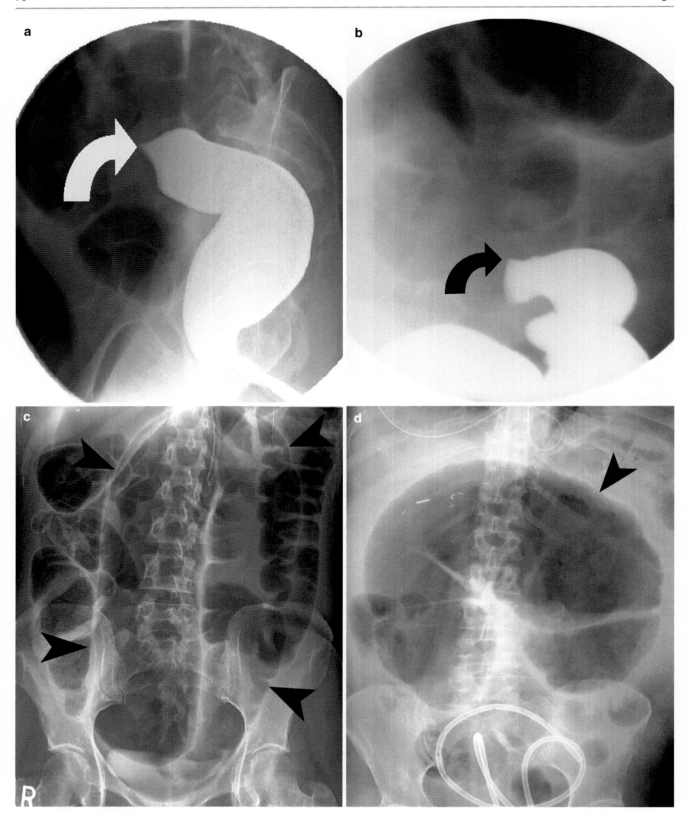

Fig. 6.12 Sigmoid volvulus. (**a**, **b**) Single-contrast barium enema examination in two patients with sigmoid volvulus demonstrates beak-like narrowing (*curved arrow*) at the rectosigmoid junction. (**c**, **d**) Plain x-ray of the abdomen demonstrates dilated loops of sigmoid colon in a coffee bean configuration (*arrowheads*) in two patients with sigmoid volvulus

sign, "closed-loop," and "three-line" or "white-stripe" signs (describing the U-shaped closed-loop appearance of the colon, between the two points of obstruction and the obliquely oriented vertical white line of the opposed walls and the space within them) (Fig. 6.12c, d) [14]. Coffee bean sign refers to a dilated C-shaped sigmoid colonic loop, extending cranial to the transverse colon and separated by a linear vertical density produced by opposing walls of sigmoid colon. CT can demonstrate the radiographic findings and few other signs (Table 6.3).

The complications of colonic volvulus include bowel wall infarction, gangrene, and perforation. Symptomatic colonic obstruction in patients with splenic volvulus is characterized by 180–720° twisting around the mesentery. Lesser degree of twisting may be asymptomatic. Although the treatment options include detorsion, cecopexy, cecostomy, and partial colectomy, if gangrenous changes are encountered, then resection of the necrotic bowel is performed.

Table 6.3 CT findings of volvulus

1. Coffee bean sign
2. Whirl sign (twisting or swirling mesenteric fat and vessels)
3. X-marks-the-spot sign (crossing transition points)
4. Split-wall sign (invagination of pericolic fat giving the impression split in twisted bowel loop)

Intussusception

Intussusception is typically seen in the pediatric age group (2 months to 6 years), accounting for up to 90 % of bowel obstruction in infants. Unlike in adults, in children majority of cases are idiopathic. Intussusception is characterized by a segment of proximal bowel and its mesentery (intussusceptum) prolapsing into a segment of contiguous distal bowel (intussuscipiens) due to peristalsis. The most frequent type of intussusception in childhood is the ileocolic intussusception and in adults is ileocolic or colocolic [15, 16]. The lead point, which is more frequent in adults than in children, can be a lipoma, adenomatous polyp, leiomyoma, or villous adenoma. Lead point is also more common in adults than in children. Majority of intussusceptions seen in small bowel on CT are transient and are idiopathic.

In plain radiograph, a crescent-shaped collection of air outlining the intussusceptum head is called "crescent sign." On barium enema, contrast trapped between intussusceptum and intussuscipiens gives a coiled spring appearance (Figs. 6.13 and 6.14). On ultrasound assessment, there is a target appearance produced by the edematous hypoechoic wall of intussuscipiens and concentric hyperechoic rings produced by layers in the wall of intussusceptum (Fig. 6.15).

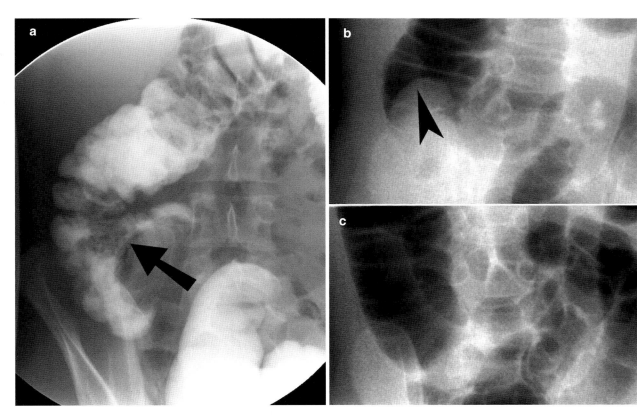

Fig. 6.13 Colonic intussusception reduction on contrast enema. (**a**) Single contrast barium enema demonstrates a large filling defect (*arrow*) in the cecal lumen due the presence of the intussusceptum. (**b**) Air enema demonstrates the tip of the intussusceptum (*arrowhead*) outlined by air introduced for reduction of intussusception. (**c**) The follow up image demonstrates resolution of the ileocolonic intussusception

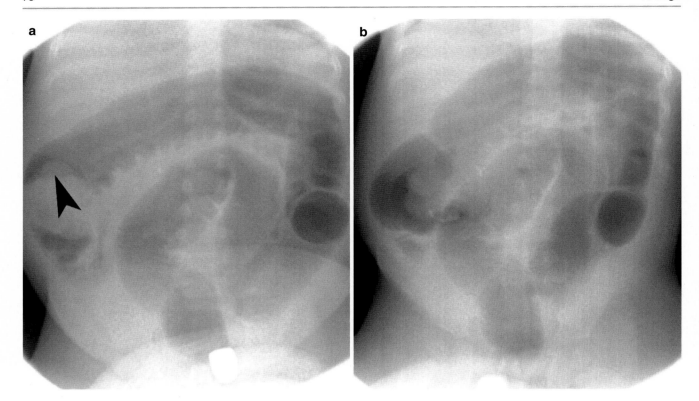

Fig. 6.14 Colonic intussusception reduction on contrast enema. (**a**, **b**) Spot images before and after contrast reduction shows the intussusceptum (*arrowhead*) outlined by air, followed by resolution of the ileocolonic intussusception

Contrast enema is used in children, more for treatment than diagnosis of intussusception. Today the main diagnostic tool is ultrasound, particularly in young patients. It allows a correct diagnosis and may find and alternative one when intussusception is not present. CT is also used in doubtful cases and in adult patients.

The CT findings include the central intussusceptum, surrounded concentrically by mesenteric fat or vessels and finally intussuscipiens (Fig. 6.16). The concentric structures may produce a target- or sausage-shaped mass. A reniform-shaped mass is seen on CT in late stages and produced by progressive wall edema and vascular compromise.

The treatment of intussusception includes radiological enema (with air, water-soluble material, or barium). The injection of liquid (water or saline) or air under US control is another technique that reduces radiation exposure of young patients. If no results are obtained or perforation is present, surgical resection is indicated [15]. Surgical treatment is the main therapy for adult intussusception, because of the high frequency of an underlying pathologic lead point.

Colonic Ischemia

Ischemic colitis is the most frequent type of ischemic disease of the gastrointestinal tract (50 %), most commonly involving the splenic flexure and the descending colon [13].

It mainly affects the elderly people and may manifest with reversible ischemia to irreversible ischemia (transmural infarction, gangrene, perforation, and stricture). The underlying cause of ischemia is insufficient vascular supply to the colonic wall which has the highest propensity to initially affect the mucosa. Although mucosal ischemia is reversible in the majority, it can also progress to transmural infarction.

The causes of bowel ischemia include thromboembolism, nonocclusive causes, colonic obstruction, tumors, vasculitis, radiation, and trauma [17]. Major vascular occlusion is seen on angiography in less than a tenth of the cases. Today the definitive diagnosis is usually made by colonoscopy. The plain radiograph may be normal or may show submucosal hemorrhage or edema (thumbprinting), ileus, transverse ridging, or ahaustral bowel pattern. Thumbprinting is most suggestive of colonic ischemia and is seen as thumb-shaped smooth projections into the colonic lumen (Fig. 6.17a). The initial diagnosis is most often suspected based on the CT imaging findings, most commonly in inferior mesenteric artery distribution (Table 6.4).

For mild cases the treatment is conservative with two-thirds of all patients recovering spontaneously within 24–48 h. In patients who do not respond to conservative treatment or those who have clinical signs of frank peritonitis or bowel perforation, surgical intervention is indicated.

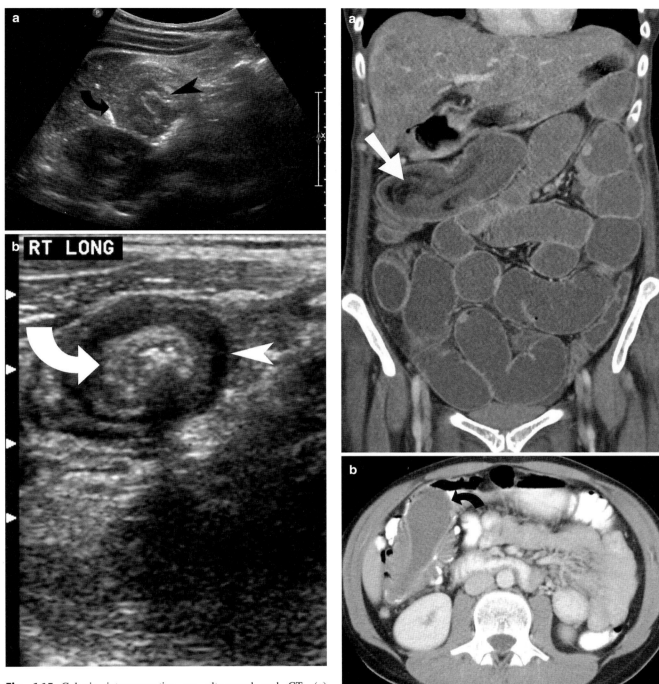

Fig. 6.15 Colonic intussusception on ultrasound and CT. (**a**) Ultrasound demonstrates concentric layers of the intussusceptum (*arrowhead*) and intussuscipiens (*curved arrow*). (**b**) Contrast-enhanced CT shows the centrally located intussusceptum (*arrowhead*), surrounded by air and intussuscipiens (*curved arrow*)

Fig. 6.16 Intussusception. (**a**) Coronal CT scan reformation demonstrates colocolonic intussusception in the hepatic flexure of the colon. The intussusceptum (*straight arrow*) is causing high-grade bowel obstruction. (**b**) Axial contrast-enhanced CT demonstrates colocolonic intussusception due to a duplication cyst (*curved arrow*)

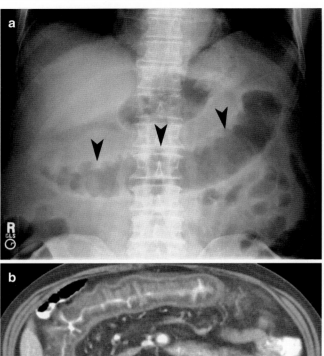

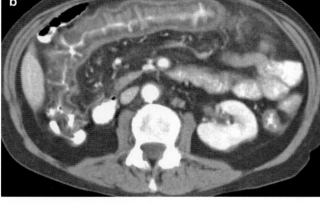

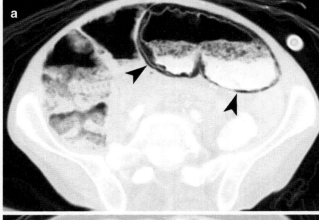

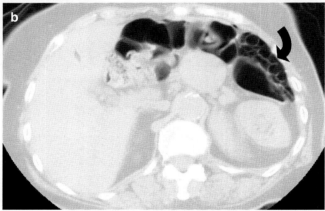

Fig. 6.18 Colonic ischemia. (**a**, **b**) CT of the abdomen (lung windows) demonstrates linear (**a**) and cystic (**b**) pneumatosis involving the transverse colon. Linear pneumatosis is believed to be associated with worse prognosis

Fig. 6.17 Ischemic colitis. (**a**) Plain x-ray of the abdomen demonstrates thumbprinting and mucosal edema (*arrowheads*) in the transverse colon of a patient with ischemic colitis. (**b**): Contrast-enhanced CT scan study of the abdomen demonstrates thickening of the transverse colonic wall with stratification, secondary to mucosal and serosal enhancement. The histopathology findings were consistent with ischemic colitis

Table 6.4 CT findings of colonic ischemia

1. Symmetric bowel wall thickening (Fig. 6.17b)
2. Most commonly involving the inferior mesenteric artery territory
3. Double halo sign due to submucosal edema
4. Colonic pneumatosis (Fig. 6.18)

GI Bleeding

Although most common site of gastrointestinal tract bleeding is from the esophagus, stomach, or duodenum, 30 % of bleeding originates from the lower gastrointestinal tract, distal to the ligament of Treitz [18]. Upper gastrointestinal bleeding accounts for two-thirds of gastrointestinal bleedings and is most commonly due to peptic ulcers and gastritis. Lower gastrointestinal bleeding is most commonly seen in older patients than upper gastrointestinal bleeding. The main causes of bleeding in the lower intestinal tract are diverticular disease (20–55 %), angiodysplasia (3–40 %), tumors (8–26 %), inflammatory diseases (6–22 %), and benign lesions of the anorectal tract (9–10 %) [18].

Clinically, lower gastrointestinal bleeding presents as hematochezia, which refers to passage of bright red blood. Small bleedings (<100 mL/day) may remain asymptomatic, but when blood loss is higher or acute (>500 mL or >15 % blood volume), the patient may suffer hypotensive shock.

In patients with lower gastrointestinal bleeding, Tc 99m-labeled RBC scan is the investigation of choice because of its ability to detect intermittent bleeding (Fig. 6.19). Unlike Tc 99m sulfur colloid, Tc 99m-labeled RBC scan allows detection of bleeding over several hours. It is less sensitive than Tc 99m sulfur colloid in detection of bleeding. Tc 99m sulfur colloid scan has extremely high sensitivity in detecting bleeding as low as 0.05–0.1 mL/min, but has the disadvantage of being sensitive only if the bleeding occurs within 20 min of radiopharmaceutical injection.

If scintigraphy demonstrates bleeding, then conventional angiography is performed for diagnostic and therapeutic reasons. If bleeding is identified on angiography, vasopressin infusion or transcatheter embolization could be performed.

Fig. 6.19 Lower gastrointestinal bleeding on Tc 99m-labeled RBC scan. Tc 99m-labeled RBC scan demonstrates progressively increasing radiotracer activity (*arrowheads*) in the cecum

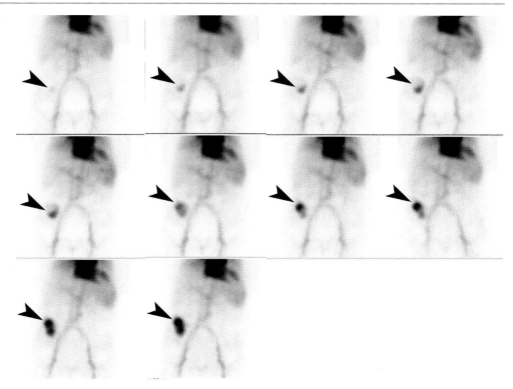

To identify bleeding on angiography, the rate of bleeding must be more than 0.5 mL/min. Colonoscopy should be performed if the hematochezia has subsided and when the diagnostic yield of angiography is low.

Acute Epiploic Appendagitis

Acute epiploic appendagitis is characterized by torsion or venous occlusion of epiploic appendages. Since epiploic appendages are more in number in the sigmoid colon, this condition most commonly affects the sigmoid colon (62 %) (Table 6.5) [7]. Unlike omental infarction, this condition is more common in older age group of fourth to fifth decades. It is clinically most often misdiagnosed as acute sigmoid diverticulitis.

On imaging, epiploic appendagitis is most often seen as a 1.5- to 3.5-cm-diameter focal fat density lesion with central high-density (54 %) and surrounding inflammation [7] (Fig. 6.20).

Acute epiploic appendagitis is medically managed with Motrin. In majority of the patients, the symptoms resolve within 10 days of symptom onset.

Acute Segmental Omental Infarction

Acute segmental infarction is a rare cause of right lower quadrant pain, often clinically misdiagnosed as acute appendicitis. The conditions predisposing to this condition include

Table 6.5 Location of acute epiploic appendagitis [7]

Location	Frequency (%)
Sigmoid colon	62
Descending colon	18
Cecum	12
Ascending colon	8
Transverse colon	0
Anterior	82
Lateral	8

obesity, trauma, overeating, laxative use, overexertion, and congestive heart failure.

The CT findings include heterogeneous fat density lesion which is usually larger than the lesion seen with acute epiploic appendagitis (Fig. 6.21). It is located in the greater omentum, most often in the right lower quadrant [6]. The importance of making the CT diagnosis of this condition is because of the medical management of this condition and its tendency to mimic a surgical abdomen.

Teaching Points

1. Contrast-enhanced CT is the imaging modality of choice in the evaluation of acute left lower quadrant pain.
2. For the initial presentation of suspected Crohn's disease in patients with abdominal pain, fever, and diarrhea, CT enterography is considered the most appropriate imaging modality.

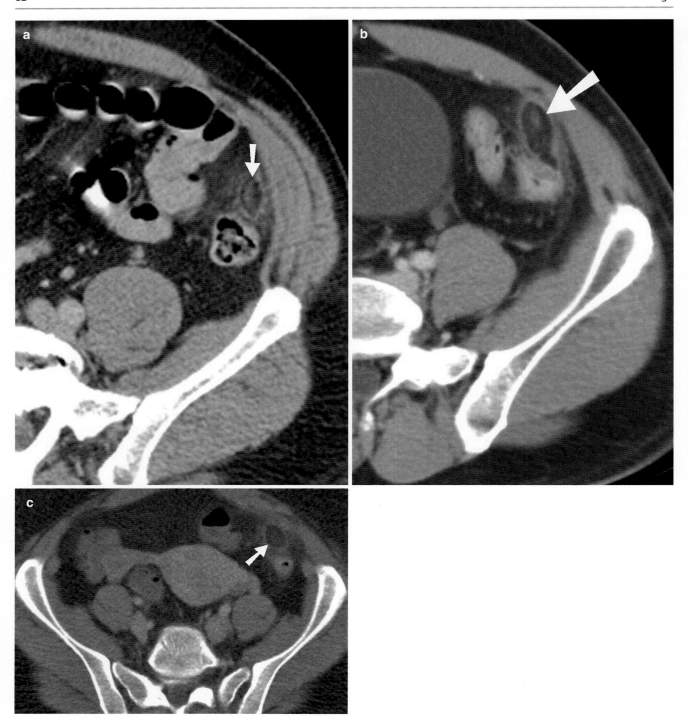

Fig. 6.20 Acute epiploic appendagitis. (**a–c**) CT study demonstrates inflamed epiploic appendage (*arrows*) in the left lower quadrant. The central high density with the fatty lesion represents thrombosed or congested vessel

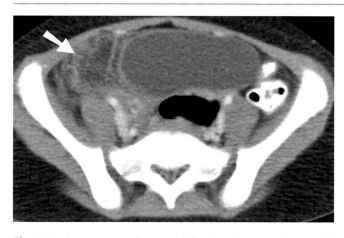

Fig. 6.21 Acute segmental omental infarction. Contrast-enhanced CT in a child shows inflammatory omental lesion (*arrow*) in the right lower quadrant. The appendix was normal and seen at a higher level

3. For adult and pediatric patients with known Crohn's disease, presenting with fever, abdominal pain, and leukocytosis, routine contrast-enhanced CT is considered the imaging modality of choice.
4. Sigmoid volvulus accounts for 75 % and cecal volvulus accounts for 20 % of large bowel obstructions.

References

1. Pereira JM, Sirlin CB, Pinto PS, Jeffrey RB, Stella DL, Casola G. Disproportionate fat stranding: a helpful CT sign in patients with acute abdominal pain. Radiographics. 2004;24:703–15.
2. Horton KM, Corl FM, Fishman EK. CT evaluation of the colon: inflammatory disease. Radiographics. 2000;20:399–418.
3. Rucker CM, Menias CO, Bhalla S. Mimics of renal colic: alternative diagnoses at unenhanced helical CT. Radiographics. 2004;24:S11–33.
4. Heverhagen JT, Klose KJ. MR Imaging for acute lower abdominal and pelvic pain. Radiographics. 2009;29:1781–96.
5. Singh AK, Gervais DA, Hahn PF, Sagar P, Mueller PR, Novelline RA. Acute epiploic appendagitis and its mimics. Radiographics. 2005;25:1521–34.
6. Singh AK, Gervais DA, Lee P, Westra S, Hahn PF, Novelline RA, et al. Omental infarct: CT imaging features. Abdom Imaging. 2006;31(5):549–54.
7. Singh AK, Gervais DA, Hahn PF, Rhea J, Mueller PR. CT appearance of acute appendagitis. AJR Am J Roentgenol. 2004;183(5):1303–7.
8. Ghahremani GG, With EM, Hoff FL, Gore RM, Miller JW, Christ M. Appendices epiploicae of the colon: radiological and pathological features. Radiographics. 1992;12:59–77.
9. Furukawa A, Saotome T, Yamasaki M, Maeda K, Nitta N, Takahashi N, et al. Cross-sectional imaging in Crohn disease. Radiographics. 2004;24:689–702.
10. Rimola J, Rodríguez S, García-Bosch O, Ricart E, Pagès M, Pellisé M, et al. Role of 3.0-T MR colonography in the evaluation of inflammatory bowel disease. Radiographics. 2009;29:701–19.
11. Gore RM, Levine MS. Textbook of Gastrointestinal Radiology (2nd ed., Volume 1). W. B. Saunders company. 2000: Chapter 41; p 726–45.
12. Kawamoto S, Horton KM, Fishman EK. Pseudomembranous colitis: spectrum of imaging findings with clinical and pathologic correlation. Radiographics. 1999;19:887–97.
13. Silva AC, Beaty SD, Hara AK, Fletcher JG, Fidler JL, Menias CO, et al. Spectrum of normal and abnormal CT appearances of the ileocecal valve and cecum with endoscopic and surgical correlation. Radiographics. 2007;27:1039–54.
14. Peterson CM, Anderson JS, Carenza JW, Menias CO. Volvulus of the gastrointestinal tract: appearances at multimodality imaging. Radiographics. 2009;29:1281–93.
15. del Pozo G, Albillos JC, Tejedor D, Calero R, Rasero M, de-la-Calle U, et al. Intussusception in children: current concepts in diagnosis and enema reduction. Radiographics. 1999;19:299–319.
16. Kim YH, Blake MA, Harisinghani MG, Archer-Arroyo K, Hahn PF, Pitman MB, et al. Adult intestinal intussusception: CT appearances and identification of a causative lead point. Radiographics. 2006;26:733–44.
17. Rha SE, Ha HK, Lee SH, Kim JH, Kim JK, Kim JH, et al. CT and MR imaging findings of bowel ischemia from various primary causes. Radiographics. 2000;20:29–42.
18. Laing CJ, Tobias T, Rosenblum DI, Banker WL, Tseng L, Tamarkin SW. Acute gastrointestinal bleeding: emerging role of multidetector CT angiography and review of current imaging techniques. Radiographics. 2007;27:1055–70.

Imaging of Genitourinary Emergencies

Robin Levenson and Mai-Lan Ho

Nontraumatic urinary tract emergencies include acute obstructive uropathy, infections which can become complicated, and acute renovascular abnormalities. Imaging plays an important role in evaluating the extent of the acute process and the location and in differentiating urinary tract emergencies from other acute conditions which may be clinical mimics.

Obstructive Uropathy

Obstructive uropathy is defined as structural or functional blockage of normal urinary outflow and may occur at any level of the urinary system. This leads to urine stasis, pressure buildup, and failure of excretion [1]. Etiologies include stones, blood clots, infection/inflammation, extrinsic compression, functional spasm, and primary or metastatic tumors. In healthy individuals, unilateral renal obstruction can be compensated for by the contralateral kidney, without measurable changes in overall excretory function. However, in patients with underlying chronic renal disease and/or bilateral obstruction, significant functional decompensation may occur. Additional complications include infection and collecting system rupture [2].

The clinical presentation of acute obstructive uropathy may include flank pain, dysuria, hematuria, oliguria, fever, and nausea/vomiting. In patients with fulminant uremia, lethargy and mental status changes may be present [2].

Imaging

Plain radiography may be used as initial screening for patients with acute abdominal/flank pain, although computed tomography is the modality of choice. Radiography has 45–60 % sensitivity and 70 % specificity for detecting renal stones (Fig. 7.1a). Findings may be falsely negative for noncalcified stones, calcified stones less than 4 mm, and patients with large body habitus. In addition, false-positive interpretations may occur with gallstones, phleboliths, and granulomatous calcifications [1]. Other causes of obstruction, including masses and blood clots, are poorly characterized. Radiography may also be used for surgical planning and follow-up.

Multidetector computed tomography (MDCT) is the gold standard for imaging patients with suspected obstructive uropathy. Stone/lesion size, location, and degree of obstruction can be quantified. Non-contrast CT (NCCT) has a sensitivity of 95–98 % and specificity of 96–100 % for detecting urinary stones [3–5]. NCCT is relatively quick, without the use of intravenous or oral contrast, making it particularly useful in the emergency setting. Most stones appear radiodense on CT. Rarely, in HIV patients who are poorly hydrated and treated with indinavir, crystalline stones develop which are radiolucent on NCCT. When findings are negative or equivocal, intravenous contrast can be administered to assess for additional renal or abdominal processes. Besides urinary stones, other etiologies of intraluminal obstruction include blood clots, which are dense but lower in attenuation than calculus; masses, which measure soft tissue attenuation and enhance following contrast administration; and ureteral spasm, strictures, or injury. Extraluminal compression may be caused by retroperitoneal masses, abscess, inflammation, or posttraumatic hematoma [4, 5].

At CT evaluation for ureteral stone, one should focus at the most common locations; narrowing of the ureter occurs naturally at the ureterovesicular junction (UVJ), the pelvic brim as the ureter crosses iliac vessels, and at the ureteropelvic junction (UPJ) (Fig. 7.1b, c) [3]. Frequently, a transition point is visible, with urinary decompression more distally. Secondary CT findings in obstructive uropathy include hydroureter, hydronephrosis, perinephric stranding, and possible enlargement of the unilateral kidney

R. Levenson, MD (✉) • M.-L. Ho, MD
Department of Radiology, Beth Israel Deaconess Medical Center,
330 Brookline Avenue, Boston, MA 02215, USA
e-mail: rlevenso@bidmc.harvard.edu

A. Singh (ed.), *Emergency Radiology*,
DOI 10.1007/978-1-4419-9592-6_7, © Springer Science+Business Media New York 2013

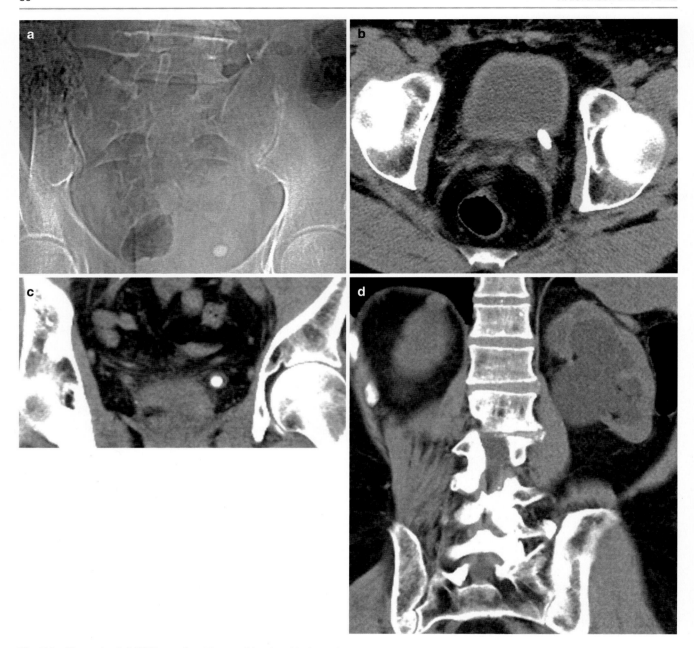

Fig. 7.1 Obstructing left UVJ stone in a 71-year-old male with elevated creatinine and hydronephrosis. (**a**) Scout view demonstrates a coarse calcification in the left pelvis corresponding to a left UVJ stone as confirmed on subsequent CT images. (**b–d**) Non-contrast-enhanced CT axial (**b**) and coronal (**c, d**) images show a 14×6×4 mm left UVJ stone (**b, c**) with soft tissue rim sign (**c**) and upstream severe left hydronephrosis (**d**)

(Fig. 7.1d) (Table 7.1). Periureteral wall thickening and perinephric/periureteral fat stranding reflect acute inflammation. The "soft tissue rim sign" is due to edema of the ureteral wall at the site of stone impaction and may help differentiate a ureteral stone from a phlebolith in an adjacent vein (Fig. 7.1c) [6]. Renal edema may be appreciated, with decrease in Hounsfield attenuation on NCCT ("pale kidney" sign). Following contrast administration, there may be delayed excretion of contrast into the collecting system/ureter or beyond the level of obstruction ("delayed nephrogram/urogram"), which may be partial or complete (Fig. 7.2). Pyelosinus or forniceal rupture manifests as a perinephric fluid (Fig. 7.3). In cases of extrinsic compression, the ureter appears abnormally deviated due to mass effect [4, 5, 7].

Ultrasonography (US) is a useful screening examination for pregnant and pediatric patients, in whom radiation exposure is a concern. The sensitivity for urinary obstruction is 60–70 %, but this is highly operator and patient dependent and involves limited ureteral assessment [8].

Table 7.1 CT findings in acute obstructive uropathy

1. Calcified stone in the GU tract (UVJ, UPJ, and pelvic brim are the most common locations)
2. Hydroureter
3. Hydronephrosis
4. Soft tissue rim sign
5. Perinephric/periureteral stranding
6. Unilateral enlarged kidney
7. Forniceal rupture
8. Pale kidney sign

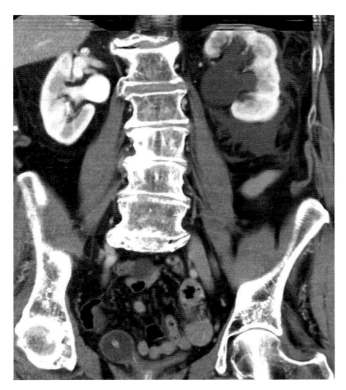

Fig. 7.2 Delayed excretion of contrast in an 87-year-old female with left abdominal pain. Contrast-enhanced coronal CT image shows left hydronephrosis and delayed excretion of contrast (delayed enhancement) from the left kidney as compared to the right in this patient with an obstructing 9 mm left UPJ stone

Renal stones are echogenic foci with or without shadowing, depending on size, composition, and technique (Fig. 7.4). Smaller stones may blend into the echogenic renal sinus and be missed. Ureteropelvic and ureterovesical junction stones, which lie superficially within good acoustic windows, may be seen. However, mid-ureteral stones are extremely difficult to detect. The finding of hydronephrosis is suggestive but may be absent in early obstruction (false negative) or present due to alternate causes such as pregnancy and reflux (false positive) (Fig. 7.5a). One must distinguish true hydronephrosis from mimics such as parapelvic cysts, extrarenal pelvis, and pelvicaliectasis. Additional signs include absent or decreased ureteral jets and a Doppler arterial resistive index greater than 0.70 (or difference between kidneys greater than 0.10). However, these findings are neither sensitive nor specific [8].

Magnetic resonance imaging (MRI) is an alternative to CT, particularly in pediatric and pregnant patients for whom radiation exposure is a concern. MRI offers superior soft tissue contrast, albeit with increased costs and longer scan times. Ultrafast scanning protocols have been developed to image the urinary system with good spatial resolution in multiple planes. Fluid-sensitive T2-weighted sequences, such as single-shot fast spin echo (SSFSE) and balanced steady-state free precession (SSFP), utilize urine as an intrinsic contrast agent [9]. Fat-suppressed sequences are also acquired to enable differentiation from intraperitoneal/retroperitoneal fat. Urinary calculi, which are proton poor, may appear as hypointense filling defects (Fig. 7.5b, c). Stones smaller than 1 cm are frequently not seen – in which case diagnosis relies on signs of urinary obstruction, such as a ureteral transition point [9]. Acute obstruction frequently presents with soft tissue wall thickening, stranding, and edema, manifesting as high T2 signal and loss of renal corticomedullary differentiation. Multiphasic gadolinium-enhanced imaging can be performed using a T1-weighted spoiled gradient echo sequence. This allows assessment of the renal parenchyma, improves urinary-calculi contrast, and quantifies collecting system transit time [9].

Complications and Treatment

In the early stages, acute obstructive uropathy is reversible with minimal renal parenchymal damage. Urinary stones smaller than 5 mm can be managed conservatively and usually pass spontaneously. Large and/or irregularly shaped stones may become impacted, predisposing to infection and collecting system rupture which can result in hematogenous dissemination of infection (urosepsis) [2].

In urgent situations, drainage procedures such as percutaneous nephrostomy, nephroureteral stenting, and suprapubic cystostomy can be performed to decompress the urinary system proximal to the site of obstruction [2].

Infections

Urinary tract infections have accounted for approximately one million emergency department visits annually in the USA [10]. Most of these are uncomplicated and only involve the urinary bladder. However, if the infection migrates proximally or is spread hematogenously, pyelonephritis may ensue.

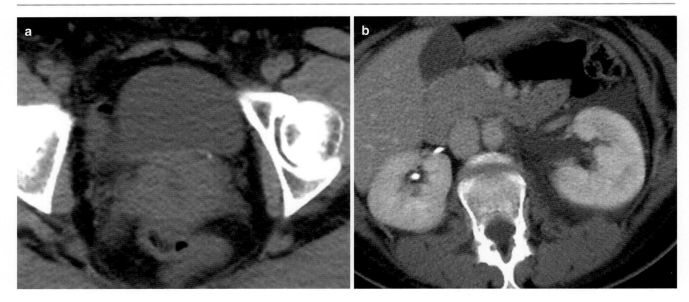

Fig. 7.3 Forniceal rupture in a 41-year-old female with left flank pain. (**a**) Non-contrast-enhanced axial CT image demonstrates 2 mm left UVJ stone. (**b**) Contrast-enhanced CT axial image demonstrates perinephric fluid consistent with forniceal rupture

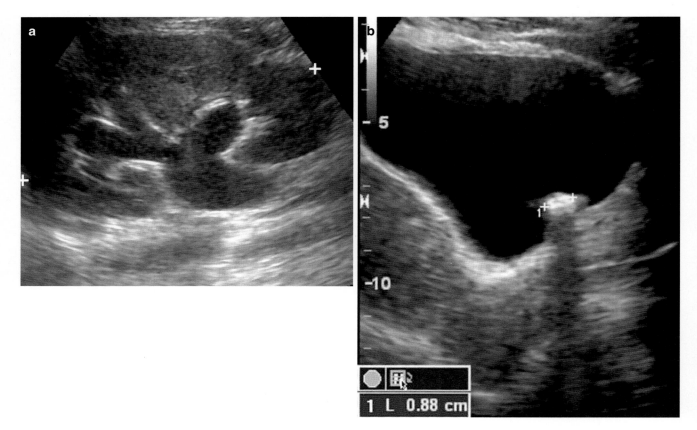

Fig. 7.4 Obstructing left UVJ stone with upstream left hydronephrosis. Ultrasound images show moderate left hydronephrosis (**a**). Shadowing echogenic focus at the left UVJ is consistent with obstructing stone (**b**)

Acute Pyelonephritis

Urinary tract infections typically begin in the urinary bladder and migrate proximally, leading to tubulointerstitial inflammation. This ascending infection often occurs in the absence of reflux due to the virulence of the bacteria, most commonly gram-negative organisms, in particular *Escherichia coli*. Pyelonephritis can also occur if the urinary infection

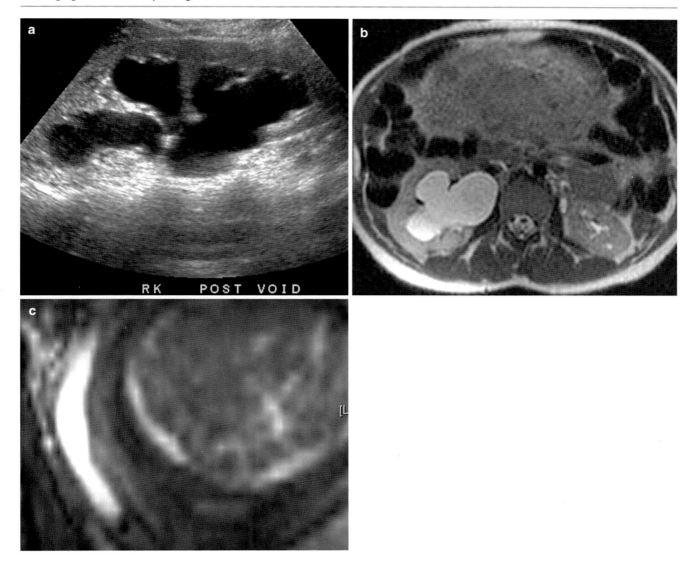

Fig. 7.5 A 27-year-old female, 34 weeks pregnant, with right abdominal pain. (**a**) Ultrasound shows moderate right hydronephrosis. Distal right ureter not visualized and etiology was unclear. (**b, c**) Subsequent MR imaging shows moderate to severe right hydronephrosis on axial SSFSE HASTE imaging (**b**) secondary to distal right ureteral stone (**c**, coronal true FISP)

is spread to the kidneys hematogenously, from skin infection or endocarditis as may be seen in intravenous drug abusers.

Patients with pyelonephritis tend to present with fever, chills, and flank pain with costovertebral angle tenderness. Symptoms often also include dysuria, urinary frequency, and urgency [10]. Additional symptoms of acute pyelonephritis may include abdominal pain, nausea, and vomiting, which overlap with many other conditions, particularly gastrointestinal. Urinalysis findings include pyuria, bacteriuria, and positive urine culture.

Imaging

The majority of patients respond well to antibiotic treatment and imaging is often not required. However, in certain circumstances, imaging can play an important role in differentiating acute pyelonephritis from other entities causing acute symptoms (particularly if the patient has failed 72 h of antibiotic treatment), detecting structural abnormalities, evaluating patients at high risk for complications, and characterizing the severity of infection and extent of possible organ damage.

MDCT is the preferred imaging modality to evaluate for acute bacterial pyelonephritis. Post-contrast imaging findings include one or more wedge-shaped hypodense areas extending from the papilla to the renal cortex, consistent with a striated nephrogram and representing decreased enhancement compared to the surrounding renal parenchyma (Fig. 7.6a). The findings result from stasis of contrast material within edematous tubules that demonstrates increasing attenuation over time The decreased enhancement or striation is due to reduced perfusion secondary to obstruction of

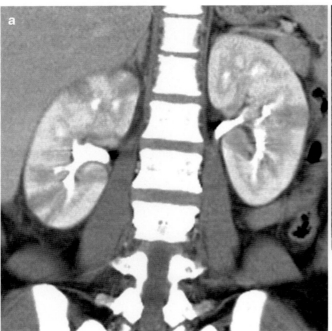

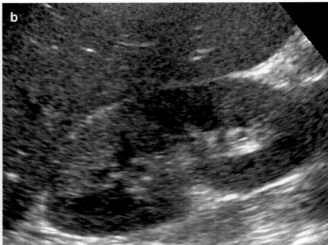

Fig. 7.6 Acute bilateral pyelonephritis in a 34-year-old female with fever, chills, and right upper quadrant pain. (**a**) Contrast-enhanced coronal CT image demonstrates bilateral, right greater than left, striated nephrograms with alternating areas of hypodensity representing decreased enhancement. No drainable fluid collection. (**b**) Ultrasound image shows wedge-shaped echogenic area in the right kidney

Table 7.2 Differential diagnosis of striated nephrogram

| 1. Acute pyelonephritis |
| 2. GU obstruction |
| 3. Renal vein thrombosis |
| 4. Contusion |

Table 7.3 Imaging of acute pyelonephritis

| 1. CT and MRI: striated nephrogram |
| 2. US: often negative but can see hypoechoic or hyperechoic areas |
| 3. Enlarged kidney |

the renal tubules by intraluminal inflammatory debris, interstitial edema, and vasospasm [10]. A "striated nephrogram" can also be seen in GU obstruction, renal vein thrombosis, and contusion [11] (Tables 7.2 and 7.3). On non-contrast-enhanced CT, affected regions of the kidney may be lower in density due to underlying edema, and there may be loss of the renal pyramids. The affected kidney may be enlarged [12]. Renal calculi may be present. Secondary findings due to inflammation in acute pyelonephritis may also include perinephric stranding, thickening of Gerota's fascia, and hydronephrosis [10, 12].

Ultrasound may be used to evaluate the urinary tract in cases of infection, in particular to assess for hydronephrosis or renal abscess. Occasionally findings of pyelonephritis may be found at ultrasound, although ultrasound is not as sensitive as CT and patients with clinically suspected pyelonephritis often have negative ultrasound results. Changes in the echotexture of the renal parenchyma may be seen and include hypoechoic areas due to edema and hyperechoic regions due to hemorrhage (Fig. 7.6b) [10]. There may be hydronephrosis, renal enlargement, and/or loss of normal corticomedullary differentiation. Regions of hypoperfusion may be seen with color Doppler. Ultrasound is limited in assessing the full extent of pyelonephritis and perinephric extension and in visualizing microabscesses [10].

The use of MRI in the evaluation of acute renal infections tends to be limited to patients who cannot undergo intravenous contrast-enhanced CT (i.e., allergy to IV contrast material), patients in who radiation is a concern, or patients with inconclusive/equivocal CT results. MRI is much more susceptible to patient motion artifact than CT is, and it can be more difficult to obtain high-quality images in sick patients. In acute pyelonephritis, similar to that seen on CT, MRI shows wedge-shaped areas of decreased enhancement of the renal parenchyma on T1 fat-saturated post-contrast images and may show areas of decreased signal on T2-weighted images (Fig. 7.7). Renal enlargement and perinephric fluid may also be seen.

Treatment and Complications

Antibiotic therapy is the mainstay of treatment in acute bacterial pyelonephritis and most patients respond well. However, complications of acute pyelonephritis can include

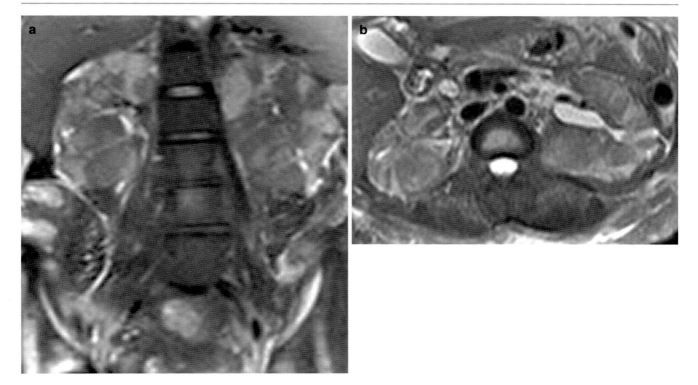

Fig. 7.7 A 62-year-old female with fever, chills, UTI, and *E. coli* bacteremia presenting with acute bacterial pyelonephritis. SSFSE (HASTE) MR coronal (**a**) and axial (**b**) images demonstrate diffuse heterogeneous signal in linear, wedge-shaped configuration in both kidneys

renal obstruction, renal or perirenal abscess, and emphysematous pyelonephritis.

Renal Abscess

Renal or perinephric abscesses typically develop from inadequately treated pyelonephritis more commonly due to ascending infection, with diabetic patients particularly prone (75 % of renal abscesses are seen in diabetic patients), and less often hematogenous spread [10]. The most common microorganisms are *E. coli* and *Proteus mirabilis*. Renal abscesses can be solitary or multiple, with multiple abscesses more commonly seen in hematogenous spread of infection [10].

Patients with renal abscess tend to have persistent symptoms of pyelonephritis despite at least 72 h treatment with antibiotics.

Imaging

CT is the preferred imaging modality to detect renal abscess in the emergent setting since some small abscesses are not seen on ultrasound. At CT, renal abscesses tend to be round and centrally hypodense, with central liquefaction, and may demonstrate significant rim enhancement at post-contrast imaging, but no internal enhancement (Fig. 7.8a). Gas may be seen within the abscess. A hypoenhancing halo may surround the abscess in the renal parenchyma during the nephrographic phase. In many cases, the entire kidney is enlarged or there may be a focal mass/bulge in the renal contour. Perinephric inflammation and thickening of Gerota's fascia are also commonly seen. A perirenal abscess tends to manifest as a fluid collection in the perinephric space and may contain gas. Extra-parenchymal collections have been found to extend into the adjacent psoas muscle [10].

On ultrasound, a renal abscess tends to be a hypoechoic thick-walled structure with increased through transmission but less so than that seen with a simple cyst of similar size. Typically, no internal vascularity is seen. Debris may be seen within the abscess (Fig. 7.8b).

Renal abscesses on MRI are centrally T2 hyperintense and T1 hypointense and tend to have a thick wall which shows variable enhancement on T1-weighted post-contrast imaging (Fig. 7.9). Perinephric inflammatory stranding may also be seen. Findings may be difficult to differentiate from cystic renal cell carcinoma; the patient's clinical symptoms and subsequent resolution on follow-up imaging help make this distinction.

Emphysematous Pyelonephritis

Emphysematous pyelonephritis is a life-threatening emergency of the kidneys, caused by gas-forming bacteria which infect the renal parenchyma, collecting system, and/or

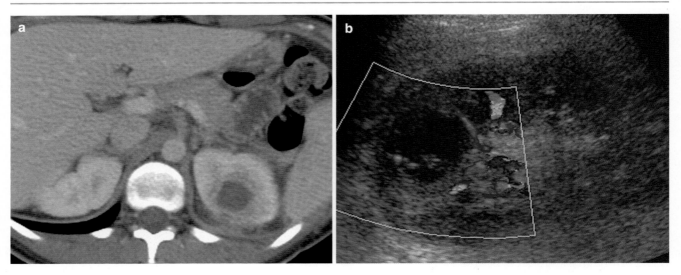

Fig. 7.8 Left renal abscess in a 26-year-old female with left flank pain and fever. (**a**) Contrast-enhanced axial CT image shows hypodense area in the left kidney with central more hypodense, necrotic core measuring 2.1×2.2 cm with adjacent perinephric fat stranding. (**b**). Ultrasound images of the left kidney show 2.3×2.1 cm hypoechoic, thick-walled structure containing echogenic internal debris and no internal vascularity

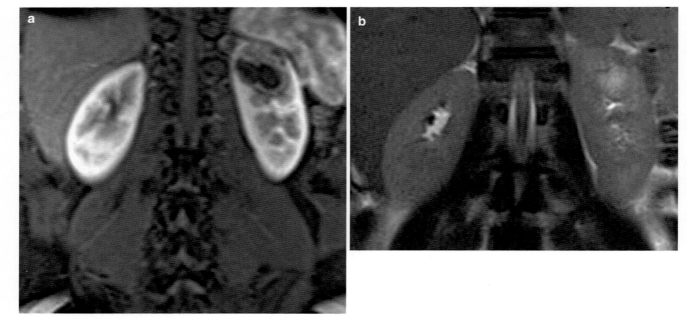

Fig. 7.9 Right renal abscess on MRI in an 18-year-old female with left upper quadrant pain and elevated WBC. (**a**) Contrast-enhanced T1-weighted coronal image demonstrates peripherally enhancing thick-walled cystic lesion. (**b**) T2-weighted coronal image shows T2 hyperintense focus in the left renal upper pole

perinephric tissue. It is highly associated with poorly controlled diabetes mellitus, present in up to 90 % of cases. Obstruction of the corresponding urinary collecting system secondary to calculus, neoplasm, and/or sloughed papilla may also be present [13, 14]. The bacteria most commonly linked to emphysematous pyelonephritis are *E. coli* (~70 %) and *Klebsiella pneumoniae* [14]. If gas is localized to the renal collecting system and does not involve the renal parenchyma, the term emphysematous pyelitis is used, which is less severe than emphysematous pyelonephritis, with lower mortality.

The presenting symptoms of emphysematous pyelonephritis include fever, flank pain, and pyuria, which are nonspecific and also seen in other urinary tract infections [14]. Patients may also present with lethargy/altered mental status, acid–base abnormalities, hyperglycemia, renal failure,

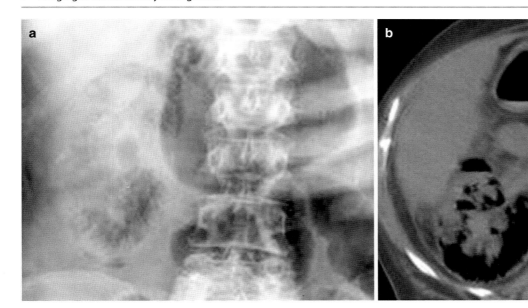

Fig. 7.10 Emphysematous pyelonephritis. (**a**) Scout image shows mottled lucencies projecting over the right renal shadow. (**b**) Non-contrast-enhanced axial CT image of the same patient demonstrates gas within the renal parenchyma (Images courtesy of Leonora Mui at Columbia University Medical Center, New York, NY)

and, in severe cases, septic shock. Emphysematous pyelonephritis is seen more often in females than in males presumably because females are more susceptible to urinary infections. On physical exam, patients may have flank pain and, rarely, crepitus may be felt over the lower back [13].

Imaging

On radiography, evidence of gas overlying the renal shadows or radially oriented gas aligning with the renal pyramids may be seen (Fig. 7.10a). In severe cases, one may see crescentic-shaped gas collection involving Gerota's fascia. Findings may also include obscuration of the ipsilateral psoas muscle shadow [13].

CT best demonstrates the extent of gas and destruction associated with emphysematous pyelonephritis. Imaging findings include foci of gas within the renal parenchyma/collecting system, renal enlargement and destruction, fluid collections with possible gas-fluid levels, and tissue necrosis (Fig. 7.10b) [10]. Two CT imaging types have been described: type 1 with streaky or mottled gas collections without fluid collections and type II with bubbly gas in the renal parenchyma/collecting system associated with renal/perirenal fluid collections [10, 13]. Mortality rates are 69 % for type 1 and 18 % in patients with type II [10, 13].

Sonographic evaluation of the kidneys in emphysematous pyelonephritis may demonstrate an enlarged kidney that contains echogenic foci with posterior dirty shadowing, indicative of gas within (Fig. 7.11). The echogenic foci representing gas may be confused with renal calculi. The true extent of emphysematous renal involvement can be underestimated on ultrasound [13].

Treatment and Complications

Initial treatment includes aggressive IV hydration, correction of electrolyte imbalances, and broad-spectrum IV antibiotics [13]. If gas is diffuse throughout the kidney, nephrectomy is often indicated. If infection is more localized and preservation of kidney is a priority, percutaneous drainage can be attempted.

Emphysematous Cystitis

Emphysematous cystitis is a rare infection of the bladder caused by gas-producing organisms, most commonly *E. coli*, *Enterobacter aerogenes*, and *Klebsiella pneumoniae* [15]. It tends to be seen in elderly patients with diabetes, with diabetes reported in over half of cases. Elderly or debilitated patients with chronic urinary retention secondary to urinary bladder outlet obstruction, neurogenic bladder, or bladder structural abnormality, as well as patients with an indwelling urinary bladder catheter, are at increased risk of developing emphysematous cystitis in part due to urinary stasis. It has been speculated that organisms within the urinary bladder cause fermentation of urinary glucose, leading to release of carbon dioxide bubbles that collect in the submucosa or lumen of the bladder [15, 16].

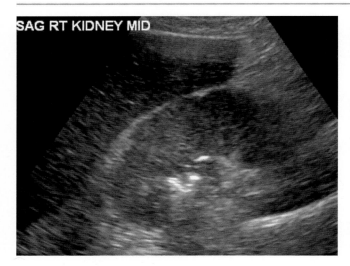

Fig. 7.11 Emphysematous pyelonephritis. Ultrasound image of the right kidney shows echogenic foci with dirty shadowing within the right kidney, consistent with gas

The presenting symptoms include dysuria, hematuria, and increased urinary frequency. The incidence of this infection is greater in females than males, 2:1 [13].

Imaging

Radiography is highly sensitive in detecting emphysematous cystitis (~97 %) [17]. On radiography, one may see curvilinear lucency, consistent with gas, outlining the bladder wall, with or without intraluminal gas (Fig. 7.12a).

In patients with emphysematous cystitis (EC), gas is seen within the wall of the urinary bladder and possibly intraluminal, particularly in the absence of recent instrumentation or fistulous communication with a hollow viscous (Fig. 7.12b). CT can detect cases of EC that are not apparent on radiography and can better depict the extent of disease. CT also helps differentiate emphysematous cystitis

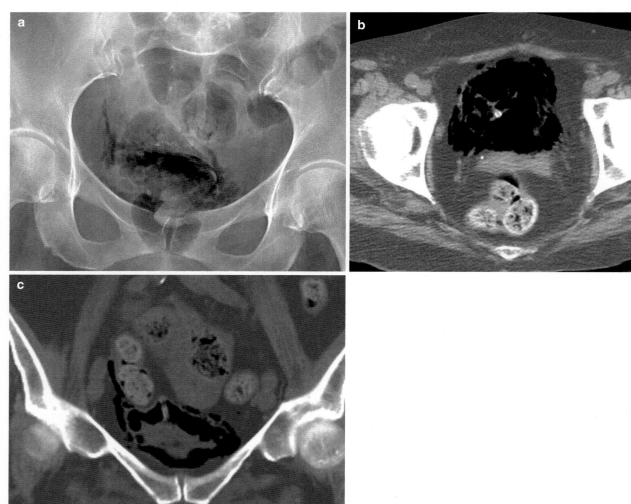

Fig. 7.12 Emphysematous cystitis in a 62-year-old female with right flank pain and UTI. (**a**) Pelvis radiograph shows pelvic lucencies consistent with bladder gas as confirmed on CT. (**b**) and (**c**) CT images demonstrate extensive gas within the lumen and wall of the urinary bladder. Coronal image depicts dissection of gas in the right space of Retzius

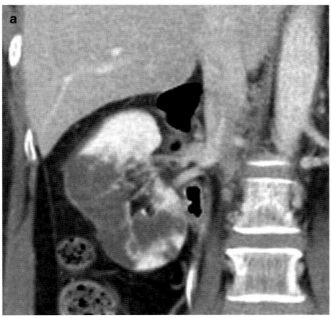
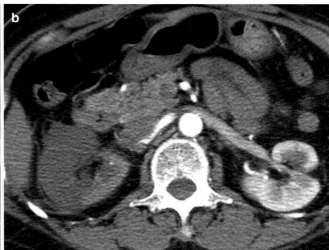

Fig. 7.13 Renal infarct in a 50-year-old female with right abdominal pain. (**a**) Contrast-enhanced coronal image of the right kidney shows wedge-shaped areas of hypodensity involving the cortex and medulla with preservation of the capsule. (**b**) Contrast-enhanced axial CT image obtained 10 days later shows lack of flow in the distal right renal artery and significantly worsened lack of right renal perfusion/enhancement

from other causes of pelvic gas, including abscess or vesicocolic fistula [13].

Treatment

Emphysematous cystitis is typically treated with early broad-spectrum antibiotics and bladder drainage with Foley catheter. If disease progresses to involve the ureters or kidney(s), surgery may be required.

Renovascular Emergencies

Acute alternations in the renal vasculature can lead to various changes in the kidney, some of which require intervention. Renovascular emergencies include renal infarct and renal vein thrombosis.

Renal Infarction

Renal infarcts may develop secondary to thrombotic disease, embolism, aortic dissection, or trauma. Sources of thrombosis include arteriosclerosis, vasculitis, and aortic or renal artery aneurysm. Renal artery embolism is most commonly cardiac in nature but can also be iatrogenic, such as following catheterization.

The presenting symptoms in patients with renal infarction tend to be flank pain with possible hematuria [12].

Imaging

CT is the imaging modality of choice in evaluating for renal infarction. The size and location of the renal infarct depends on the size of the embolus, location of arterial occlusion, and the age of the event. At contrast-enhanced CT, findings in renal infarct are one or more wedge-shaped regions demonstrating lack of enhancement that involve both the renal cortex and medulla (Fig. 7.13) [18]. Cortical rim enhancement of the kidney can be seen adjacent to a renal infarct due to collateral capsular perfusion and usually appears several days after onset of the infarct [19]. Chronic renal infarct results in scarring and loss of renal cortex.

An acute renal infarct may have a normal grayscale appearance on ultrasound. Alternatively, a wedge-shaped hypoechoic area may be present in the renal parenchyma, which may be difficult to distinguish from pyelonephritis without the use of color Doppler. With color Doppler, there will be absence of flow to a portion of or to the entire kidney.

Treatment

The mainstay of treatment for acute renal infarct is anticoagulation.

Renal Vein Thrombosis

Renal vein thrombosis is commonly due to an underlying disorder of the kidney or of the clotting system. It can also be seen in dehydration, regional neoplastic processes (involving the kidney, adrenal gland, and/or ureter) with direct extension, and trauma [18, 19].

The clinical presentation of renal vein thrombosis can vary depending on the etiology of the thrombosis. Presenting symptoms include flank pain, gross hematuria, and decrease or loss of renal function [19]. Renal vein thrombosis is more often seen on the left, which is thought to be due to the greater length of the left renal vein compared to the right. Membranous glomerulonephritis is the most common underlying disorder in adults with renal vein thrombosis [19].

Imaging

Patients suspected of having renal vein thrombosis are often first imaged with ultrasound. On ultrasound, one may see enlargement of the affected kidney and a hypoechoic renal cortex due to underlying edema. Later, the kidney decreases in size and becomes hyperechoic. On Doppler ultrasound examination, the findings include absence of venous flow, echogenic material with the renal vein lumen consistent with thrombus, reversal of arterial diastolic flow, and elevated renal artery resistive index due to high resistance.

In acute renal vein thrombosis, CT imaging demonstrates a hypoattenuating filling defect consistent with thrombus within a thickened renal vein, and the vein may be distended (Fig. 7.14). Enhancement of the thrombus suggests tumor thrombus. The kidney on the affected side may be enlarged, and there may be delay in the renal cortical nephrogram and an imaging appearance of a diminished nephrogram [18, 19]. Additionally, perinephric edema may be present. Once chronic, renal vein thrombosis leads to attenuation of the vein due retraction of the thrombus and regional collateral vessels can be seen.

Treatment and Complications

Anticoagulation is the mainstay of treatment in renal vein thrombosis. Thrombolytic therapy has been used in cases of bilateral renal vein thrombosis with acute renal failure, large clot burden with high risk of additional embolic events, and pulmonary embolism. Complications of renal vein thrombosis include acute renal failure, extension of the thrombus into the IVC, and elevated risk of pulmonary embolism.

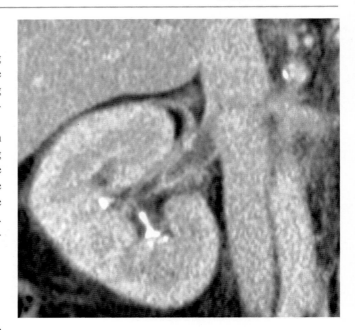

Fig. 7.14 Renal vein thrombosis in a 57-year-old female with abdominal pain and history of membranous glomerulonephritis. Contrast-enhanced coronal image shows filling defect within a distended right renal vein

Renal Transplant

With increase in renal transplantation in recent years, a greater number of renal transplant patients may present to emergency departments, and it is thus important to be aware of the potential transplant complications. In the emergent setting, evaluation of renal transplant is typically performed with ultrasound. Complications may be urologic or vascular and include peritransplant fluid collections.

Ultrasonography

Peritransplant fluid collections can be partially differentiated based on time interval since transplantation. Small hematomas are commonly seen postoperatively and usually resolve spontaneously. They are echogenic when acute, and become less echogenic over time, and may contain septations [20].

Urinomas are well-defined, simple-appearing, anechoic collections that tend occur between the urinary bladder and transplant kidney during the first 2 weeks after transplantation [20].

Lymphoceles are collections that tend to develop within 1–2 months posttransplantation, although may occur weeks to years thereafter and are usually seen between the transplant and the bladder. Sonographically, lymphoceles tend to be anechoic.

Fig. 7.15 Lack of diastolic flow. A 59-year-old female status post renal transplant with increasing creatinine. Doppler ultrasound image waveform shows lack of diastolic flow. Renal vein was patent. Differential diagnosis ATN vs. rejection

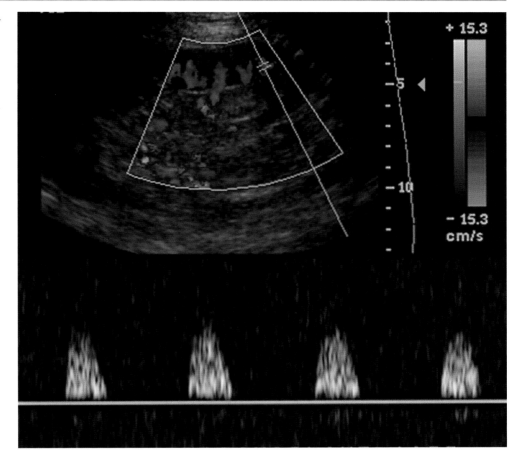

Large perinephric fluid collections can cause hydronephrosis, with lymphoceles being the most common [20]. All perinephric fluid collections can become infected and demonstrate more a complex cystic appearance with possible abscess formation. Peritransplant abscesses are rare and tend to develop during the first few weeks posttransplantation [20].

Renal transplant vascular complications include renal vein thrombosis and renal infarction, with imaging characteristics similar to that described above. Of note, in renal vein thrombosis, on color Doppler imaging, there may be lack of or reversal of diastolic flow in the intraparenchymal arteries, which may also be demonstrated in acute rejection or acute tubular necrosis (ATN). Renal vein thrombosis is differentiated from acute transplant rejection or ATN by lack of flow and thrombus in the main renal vein (Fig. 7.15).

References

1. Reddy S. State of the art trends in imaging of renal colic. Emerg Radiol. 2008;15(4):217–25.
2. Dhar M, Denstedt JD. Imaging in diagnosis, treatment, and follow-up of stone patients. Adv Chronic Kidney Dis. 2009;16(1):39–47.
3. Rucker CM, Menias CO, Bhalla S. Mimics of renal colic: alternative diagnoses at unenhanced helical CT. Radiographics. 2004;24 Suppl 1:S11–28.
4. Taourel P, Thuret R, Hoquet MD, et al. Computed tomography in the nontraumatic renal causes of acute flank pain. Semin Ultrasound CT MR. 2008;29(5):341–52.
5. Krauss T, Frauenfelder T, Strebel RT, et al. Unenhanced versus multiphase MDCT in patients with hematuria, flank pain, and a negative ultrasound. Eur J Radiol. 2012;81(3): 417–22.
6. Dyer RB, Chen MY, Zagoria RJ. Classic signs in uroradiology. Radiographics. 2004;24 Suppl 1:S247–80.
7. Cullen IM, Cafferty F, Oon SF, et al. Evaluation of suspected renal colic with noncontrast CT in the emergency department: a single institution study. J Endourol. 2008;22(11):2441–5.
8. Moş C, Holt G, Iuhasz S, et al. The sensitivity of transabdominal ultrasound in the diagnosis of ureterolithiasis. Med Ultrason. 2010;12(3):188–97.
9. Kalb B, Sharma P, Salman K, et al. Acute abdominal pain: is there a potential role for MRI in the setting of the emergency department in a patient with renal calculi? J Magn Reson Imaging. 2010;32(5):1012–23.
10. Craig WD, Wagner BJ, Travis MD. Pyelonephritis: radiologic-pathologic review. Radiographics. 2008;28(1):255–77.
11. Saunders HS, Dyer RB, Shifrin RY, Scharling ES, Bechtold RE, Zagoria RJ. The CT nephrogram: implications for evaluation of urinary tract disease. Radiographics. 1995;15(5): 1069–85.

12. Urban BA, Fishman EK. Tailored helical CT evaluation of acute abdomen. Radiographics. 2000;20(3):725–49.
13. Grayson DE, Abbott RM, Levy AD, Sherman PM. Emphysematous infections of the abdomen and pelvis: a pictorial review. Radiographics. 2002;22(3):543–61.
14. Huang JJ, Tseng CC. Emphysematous pyelonephritis: clinicoradiological classification, management, prognosis, and pathogenesis. Arch Intern Med. 2000;160(6):797–805.
15. Nemati E, Basra R, Fernandes J, Levy JB. Emphysematous cystitis. Nephrol Dial Transplant. 2005;20(3):652–3.
16. Chong SJ, Lim KB, Tan YM, Chow RK, Yip SK. Atypical presentations of emphysematous cystitis. Surgeon. 2005;3(2): 109–12.
17. Grupper M, Kratvsov A, Potasman I. Emphysematous cystitis: illustrative case report and review of the literature. Medicine. 2007; 86(1):47–53.
18. Urban BA, Ratner LE, Fishman EK. Three-dimensional volume-rendered CT angiography of the renal arteries and veins: normal anatomy, variants, and clinical applications. Radiographics. 2001; 21(2):373–86.
19. Kawashima A, Sandler CM, Ernst RD, Tamm EP, Goldman SM, Fishman EK. CT evaluation of renovascular disease. Radiographics. 2000;20(5):1321–40.
20. Akbar SA, Jafri ZH, Amendola MA, Madrazo BL, Nis KG. Complications of renal transplantation. Radiographics. 2005;25: 1335–56.

Imaging of Acute Conditions of Male Reproductive Organs

Caterina Missiroli and Ajay Singh

Hydrocele

There is normally 1–2 ml of fluid between the visceral and parietal layers of the tunica albuginea that surrounds the testis. The presence of abnormal amount of fluid in this space can be seen with hydrocele, hematocele, or pyocele (Figs. 8.1 and 8.2) [1].

Ultrasound is the imaging technique of choice in determining the type of fluid collections. While hydroceles are usually anechoic collections, hematoceles and pyoceles show complex fluid with internal echoes and variable septations and loculations.

Varicocele

Varicocele is characterized by increase in the diameter of the pampiniform plexus veins (normal range 0.5–1.5 mm), resulting in a collection of tortuous elongated veins posterior to the testicle [2].

When idiopathic, it is caused by incompetent valves in the internal spermatic vein, resulting in blood flow reversal (spermatic cord to pampiniform plexus). It is usually left-sided due to venous drainage into the renal vein rather than inferior vena cava (right vein directly drain into the inferior vena cava) [2, 3]. When acquired, it is due to increased pressure on the spermatic venous system (from hydronephrosis, hepatomegaly, and abdominal tumors). In these patients varicocele is bilateral in up to 70 % of patients and more prominent in the upright position and during valsalva maneuver [2].

Color Doppler ultrasound plays an important role in the evaluation of scrotal venous morphology and demonstrates serpentine vessels larger than 2 mm in diameter, next to the epididymis head (Fig. 8.3) [2, 4]. The blood flow is in reversed direction and typically increases during valsalva maneuver and in upright position.

Although traditionally it is surgically treated, it can also be managed with coil embolization by interventional radiologist [5].

Epididymitis and Epididymo-orchitis

Infections of testicles and epididymitis are most common in young adults and are the result of retrograde passage of organisms (*N. gonorrhoeae*, *C. trachomatis*, or *E. coli*) from the urethra, prostate, or seminal vesicles [6, 7]. Epididymitis is the most common cause of inflammatory scrotal disease. Epididymitis and epididymo-orchitis are most commonly secondary to retrograde spread of infection from urinary tract.

The main purpose of imaging in patients with presumed inflammatory disease is to distinguish inflammation from testicular torsion or other surgically treatable causes of scrotal pain, such as abscess or testicular tumor. The ultrasound finding of inflammation includes demonstration of hyperemia, which is well displayed as low-resistance hypervascularity (Fig. 8.4). The normal epididymis demonstrates no detectable flow (even at the lowest possible flow settings), so the detection of any epididymal vascularity is abnormal and indicates hyperemia [4]. Epididymis and testis are usually enlarged and edematous. The sonographic findings of epididymitis include enlarged, hypoechoic, or hyperechoic epididymis and hydrocele. In complicated cases abscess may be visualized with hypervascularity in its margins. On sonography, orchitis is seen as testicular enlargement, heterogeneous echogenicity, and hypervascularity.

C. Missiroli, MD
Diagnostic Imaging Department,
Azienda Ospedaliera della Provincia di Lecco –
Presidio Ospedaliero A. Manzoni,
Lecco, Italy

A. Singh, MD (✉)
Department of Radiology,
Massachusetts General Hospital,
Harvard Medical School,
10 Museum Way, # 524, Boston, MA 02141, USA
e-mail: asingh1@partners.org

A. Singh (ed.), *Emergency Radiology*,
DOI 10.1007/978-1-4419-9592-6_8, © Springer Science+Business Media New York 2013

Fig. 8.1 Testicular anatomy.
(**a**) Schematic diagram
demonstrates normal testicular
anatomy. (**b**) Hydrocele:
schematic diagram demonstrates
fluid between tunica albuginea
and tunica vaginalis

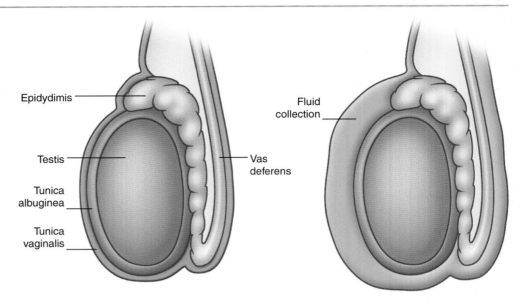

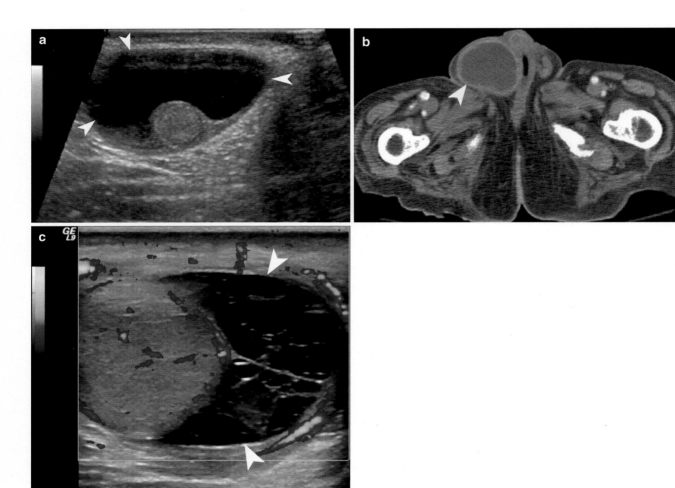

Fig. 8.2 Hydrocele and pyocele. (**a**) Hydrocele: ultrasound demonstrates anechoic fluid collection (*arrowheads*) between the parietal and visceral layers of the tunica albuginea, surrounding the testicle. (**b**) Hydrocele: contrast-enhanced axial CT imaging of the pelvis demonstrates the fluid-density hydrocele (*arrowhead*) surrounded by the parietal layer of the tunica albuginea. (**c**) Pyocele: ultrasound imaging demonstrates complex fluid collection (*arrowheads*) surrounding the testicle with multiple internal septations

Fig. 8.3 Varicocele. (**a, b**) Ultrasound demonstrates extratesticular tortuous tubular structures on grayscale imaging and color Doppler imaging

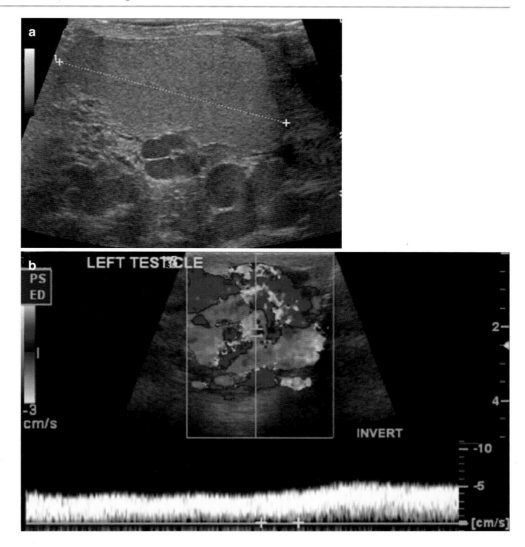

Other imaging techniques are usually not necessary. MR imaging may show increased, decreased, or normal signal in epididymis and testis with associated hypervascularity and hydrocele [8]. Abscess may be present and seen as complex scrotal fluid collection.

Fournier Gangrene

It is a rapidly progressing polymicrobial necrotizing fasciitis, seen most commonly in 50–60-year-old men. It involves the perineal, perianal, or genital regions and requires immediate surgical debridement as well as aggressive antibiotic treatment.

It is an infection, caused by multiple bacteria (average of more than three organisms), most commonly *Escherichia coli*, *Bacteroides*, and streptococcal species [9, 10]. Usually the infection spreads from abscess (perianal, perirectal, and ischiorectal), anal fissures or colonic perforations, urinary tract infections, and epididymitis. The predisposing factors are diabetes mellitus, alcohol abuse, urinary bladder instrumentation, trauma, surgical procedure, tumors, steroid therapy, chemotherapy, radiation therapy, prolonged hospitalization, and HIV infection [9].

On ultrasound, the findings include thickening of the scrotal skin, normal testicles, and hyperechoic soft tissue gas with reverberation artifacts. CT allows the evaluation of soft tissue inflammation, collections, and gas as well as complications, such as subcutaneous emphysema, abscess formation, and retroperitoneal extension (Fig. 8.5). It is also helpful in differentiating Fournier gangrene from inguinal hernia, soft tissue edema, and cellulitis.

The complications include abscess extension to thigh or abdomen, coagulopathy, diabetic ketoacidosis, sepsis, and multiple organ failure. The treatment includes hemodynamic stabilization, intravenous antibiotics, and surgical debridement of the necrotic tissues. Hyperbaric oxygen has also been used as adjuvant treatment, in patients who do not respond well to surgery.

Testicular Torsion

Spermatic cord torsion is a surgical emergency which affects 1 in 125 males in the USA and requires urgent surgery. The torsion results in vascular compromise, first of the veins and then arteries.

Intravaginal torsion is the most common type and is associated with abnormal suspension of the testis by tunica vaginalis, resulting in bell-clapper deformity. This abnormality has a 2 % prevalence (40–80 % bilateral) and allows the testicle to rotate freely within the hemiscrotum.

Extravaginal torsion is most frequent in newborn, where the testicle is poorly or not at all attached to the scrotal wall, permitting rotational mobility of the testicle. The resulting spermatic cord torsion is at the external inguinal ring level.

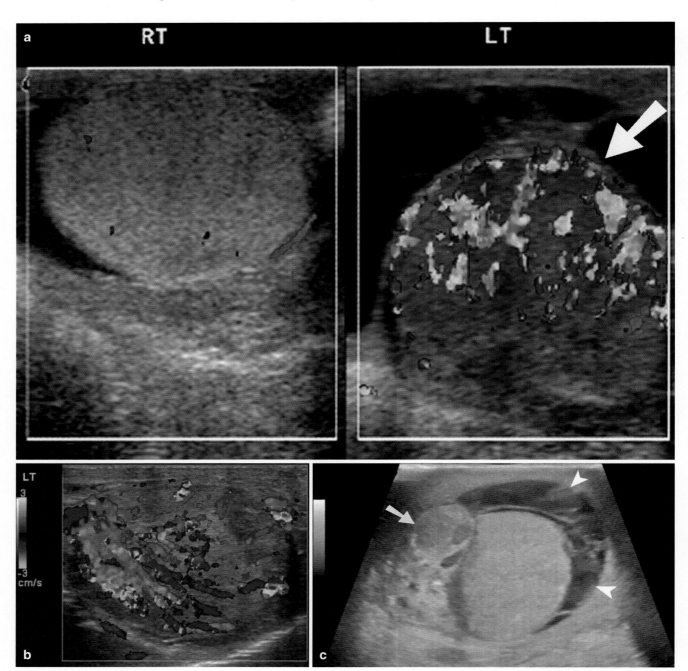

Fig. 8.4 Acute orchitis and epididymitis. (**a**, **b**) Ultrasound of the testicle demonstrates markedly increased color Doppler flow within the testicular parenchyma (*arrow*). The testicular echogenicity is mildly heterogeneous. (**c**, **d**) Ultrasound of the scrotum demonstrates enlarged epididymis (*arrow*) with increased color Doppler flow and complex hydrocele (*arrowheads*)

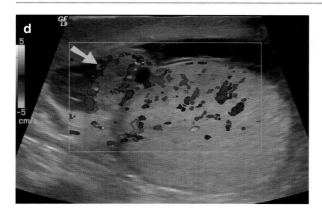

Fig. 8.4 (continued)

Ultrasound is the first-line imaging technique which shows low or absent vascular flow into the symptomatic cord and organs. Other findings include enlargement of the testis as well as epididymis in the first hours of onset. Although the testicular echogenicity is initially normal, with time the testis becomes heterogeneous and hypoechoic, indicating possible nonviability (Fig. 8.6). Hydrocele is frequently present on the affected side. Infarction and hemorrhage develop 24 h after torsion onset and give the testicle a heterogeneous appearance. The diagnosis may be difficult in cases with intermittent torsion where the blood flow may be normal or there may be postischemic hyperemia.

If not treated, the torsion leads to irreversible ischemia and lost of the testicle. If torsion is surgically detrosed within 6 h of symptom onset, salvage rate is as high as 80–100 %. However, salvage rate drops to 20 % after 12 h [2].

Scrotal Trauma

Trauma is the third most common cause of acute scrotal pain after torsion and inflammation. The primary causes are blunt, penetrating, degloving, electrical burn and postsurgical injuries. Scrotal trauma accounts for less than 1 % of all trauma-related injuries because of the anatomic location and mobility of the scrotum. The peak occurrence of scrotal trauma is in the age range of 10–30 years [11].

Blunt trauma is the most common cause of testicular injury and usually results from athletic injury (50 %), motor vehicle collision (9–17 %), or assault [8]. Penetrating trauma is usually due to gunshot wounds and less commonly due to stab wounds, animal attacks, and self-mutilation. In degloving injury the scrotal skin shears off, and skin grafting may be required. The right testis is injured more often than the left one because of its greater propensity to be trapped against the pubis or inner thigh.

Ultrasonography is commonly performed for the assessment of scrotal trauma, as it shows testicular integrity, scrotal collections, and blood flow. Ultrasound can detect scrotal hematoma, hydrocele, hematocele, testicular fracture, and testicular rupture. Color Doppler ultrasound can also be helpful in differentiating posttraumatic conditions from tumors, since tumors larger than 1.5 cm are hypervascular and hematomas are avascular.

Testicular Fracture and Rupture

Fracture of the testis is an uncommon condition which is most often secondary to blunt traumatic injury. Urgent diagnosis is imperative because of the high orchiectomy rate, if the surgery is delayed for more than 3 days.

On ultrasound, testicular fracture is seen as linear hypoechoic band that extends across the testicular parenchyma with intact testicular contour. Testicular rupture is seen as discontinuity of the echogenic tunica albuginea, poorly defined testicular margins, and heterogeneous echotexture due to hemorrhage or infarction (Fig. 8.7) [11, 12]. There may be associated scrotal wall thickening and hematocele. Color Doppler images may show decreased flow or no flow and is helpful in distinguishing normal parenchyma from hematoma.

MRI may be useful to show interruption of tunica albuginea and differentiate intratesticular hematoma (no tunica albuginea disruption) from testicular rupture, which needs surgical treatment. The tunica albuginea appears as a thin, low-signal membrane on both the proton-density and T2-weighted images. Testicular rupture is seen as discontinuity of this membrane, and intratesticular hematoma is seen as areas of high signal intensity on T1-weighted images and low signal intensity on T2-weighted images [10].

Testicular fractures are treated conservatively if normal flow is identified but require emergent surgery when there is no flow demonstrated. The timely diagnosis of rupture is critical because emergent surgery can salvage the testis in 80–90 % cases of rupture. The salvage rate is lower when surgery is delayed for more than 3 days. Testicular rupture from penetrating injury is managed in the same way as rupture from blunt injury.

Penile Fracture

Penile fracture results from external force on erect penis, causing rupture of corpus cavernosum and tear of tunica albuginea. It is usually posttraumatic, often from sexual intercourse, masturbation, falling on the erect penis, rolling over in bed with an erect penis, or direct injury. In majority of cases the tear occurs in only one of the corpora cavernosa, often affecting the distal two-thirds of the penis. In some

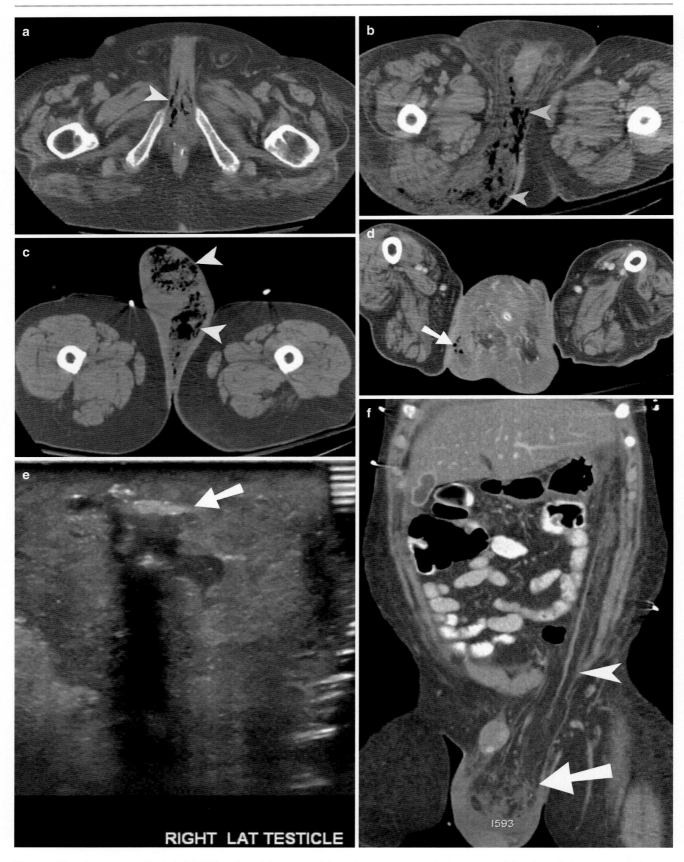

Fig. 8.5 Fournier gangrene. (**a–c**) Axial CT imaging of the lower pelvis demonstrates soft tissue air infiltrating in the perineum, penile shaft, and scrotal sac, secondary to anaerobic infection. (**d, e**) Ultrasound and CT demonstrate scrotal abscess containing foci of air (*arrow*). (**f**) Coronal CT reformation demonstrates omental fat passing through patulous left inguinal canal (*arrowhead*), into left scrotal hernia (*arrow*)

cases, the corpus spongiosum and the urethra (38 % cases) may also be involved [13, 14].

Patients with atypical clinical presentation or severe local pain which prohibits a physical examination may require imaging. Although cavernosography can identify a corpus cavernosal tear or urethrocavernous fistula, it is an invasive method with potential complications. Ultrasound allows depiction of normal penile anatomy, tear in the tunica albuginea, and soft tissue hematoma (Figs. 8.8 and 8.9). Because of its multiplanar capability and excellent tissue contrast,

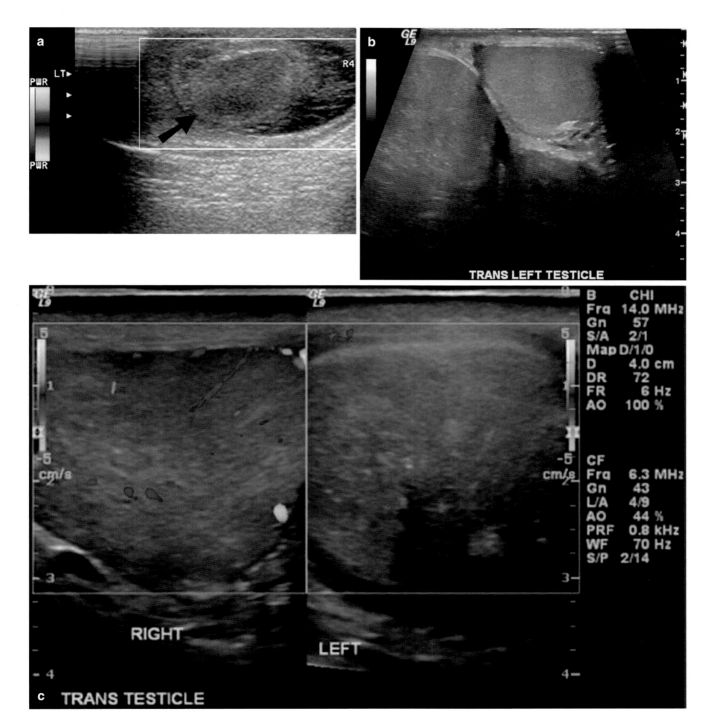

Fig. 8.6 Testicular torsion. (**a**, **b**) Grayscale ultrasound imaging demonstrates heterogeneously hypoechoic left testicle in relation to the normal echogenicity of the right testicle (**b**). (**c**, **d**) Power Doppler and color Doppler imaging of the testicle demonstrate complete absence of flow in the testicle parenchyma. There is complex hydrocele identified caudal to the testicle (**d**)

Fig. 8.6 (continued)

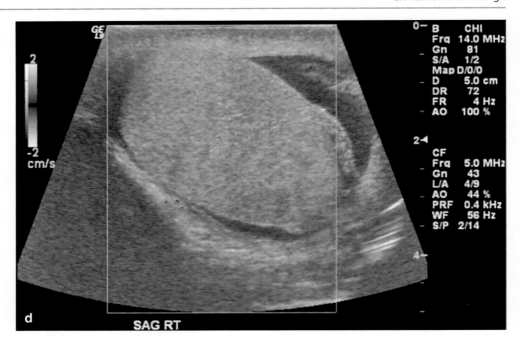

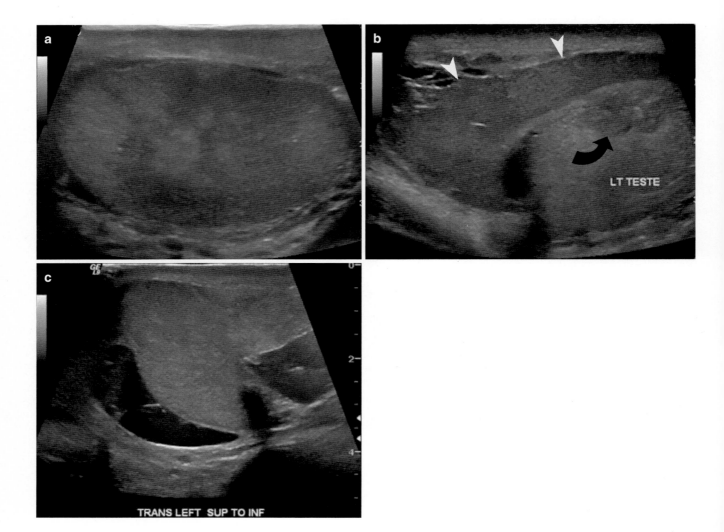

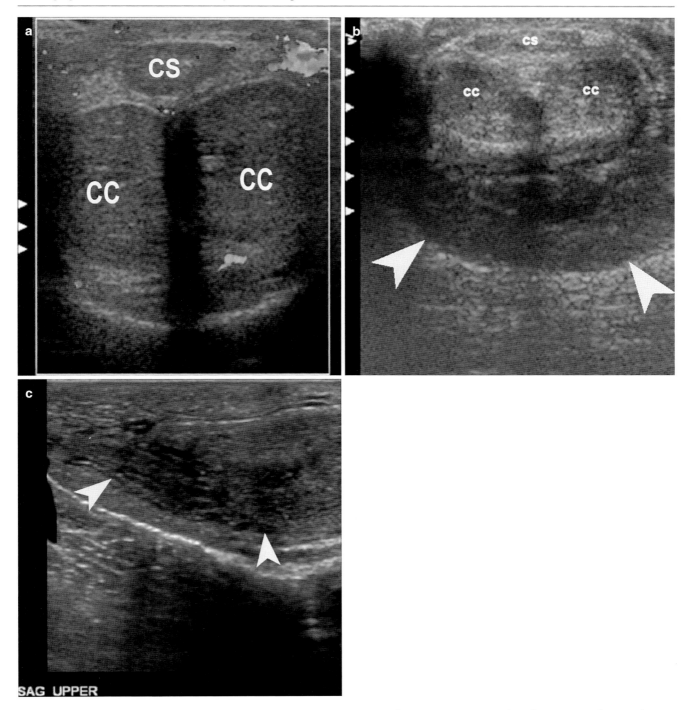

Fig. 8.8 Normal and abnormal ultrasound anatomy of the penile shaft. (**a**) Normal anatomy. Transverse ultrasound of the penile shaft demonstrates paired corpora cavernosa (*CC*) and single corpus spongiosum (*CS*). (**b**) Transverse ultrasound of the penile shaft in a patient with history of trauma demonstrates a large hematoma on the ventral aspect of the penile shaft, displacing the corpus callosum superiorly. (**c**) Sagittal image, a patient with corpora cavernosa hematoma demonstrating widening of the corpora cavernosa (*arrowheads*)

Fig. 8.7 Testicular contusion after trauma. (**a**, **b**) Ultrasound of the testicle demonstrates heterogeneous areas of low echogenicity in the testicular parenchyma, secondary to testicular contusion (*curved arrow*). There is no discontinuity identified outline of the testicle. There is associated echogenic fluid identified around the testicle, consistent with a hematocele (*arrowheads*). (**c**) Ultrasound demonstrates discontinuity of the testicular outline in a patient with testicular fracture

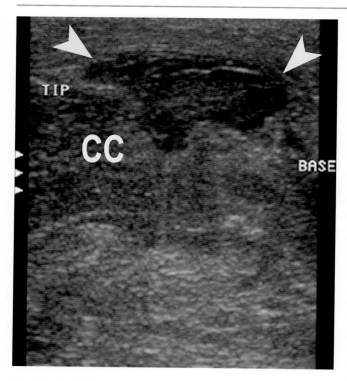

Fig. 8.9 Penile fracture. Ultrasound image in a patient with penile fracture demonstrates a hematoma located on the dorsal aspect of the corpora cavernosa with discontinuity of corpus spongiosum

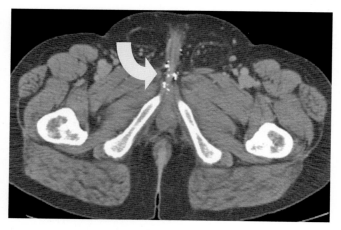

Fig. 8.10 Gunshot injury to the penile shaft. CT of the pelvis demonstrates multiple metallic fragments (*curved arrow*) seen in the penile shaft, secondary to gunshot injury. Note the limitation of CT in depiction of internal anatomy of the penile shaft

MR imaging can be useful in demonstrating the tunica albuginea [14]. CT is generally not performed for penile injury because of its limitation in depicting internal penile anatomy (Fig. 8.10).

Surgical repair is generally recommended for patients with a suspected tear of the tunica albuginea or urethral injury. Early surgical intervention can prevent late complications such as plaque formation and erectile dysfunction [15].

Urethral Injury

Urethral injury is a common complication of pelvic trauma (motor vehicle injury and fall from height), occurring in as many as 24 % of adults with pelvic fractures [16]. The urethra is vulnerable because of its close proximity to the pubic bones and the puboprostatic ligaments. The distal membranous urethra is especially at risk, and its injury may disrupt the active continence mechanism.

The most common site of urethral injury is the posterior urethra (3–25 % of patients with pelvic fractures), followed by anterior urethral injury [16]. Approximately one-fifth of these patients have urinary bladder injury [14].

If urethral injury is suspected, then imaging should be performed to rule out urethral injury before a transurethral catheter is inserted. Retrograde urethrography is the most widely accepted technique to determine urethral integrity and classify urethral injury. Accurate classification of urethral injury is important because it allows effective treatment planning (Table 8.1).

CT imaging demonstrates stretched urethra, altered prostatic position, obliteration of periprostatic fat plane, and muscle hematomas (type I); extravasation of contrast agent above urogenital diaphragm is typical of type II injury and extravasation of contrast below urogenital diaphragm in type III injury [15, 17]. Urinary bladder extravasation is seen in type IV injury (Fig. 8.11).

Late complications associated with posterior urethral injury include impotence, incontinence, strictures, and fistula, whereas those associated with anterior urethral injury include strictures and impotence. While abrupt, short-segment strictures are usually traumatic, long-segment strictures may be traumatic or postinflammatory. The diagnosis of urethral stricture is usually made by retrograde urethrography that defines location, length, number strictures, as well as the periurethral abnormalities such as stones, false tract, and diverticula [14, 15].

Immediate surgery is necessary in type IV and type V injuries because of the potential for urinary incontinence. While type I injury may be conservatively managed, complete urethral disruption (types II–III) may require immediate surgery because of risk of stricture formation in the future. In presence of short strictures, the first-line treatment is dilatation by catheter or urethrotomy, while longer and recurrent strictures require surgical resection [15].

Teaching Points

1. Fournier gangrene is an infection, caused by multiple bacteria, most commonly *Escherichia coli*, Bacteroides, and streptococcal species.

Table 8.1 Classification of urethral injury on retrograde urethrography

Injury type	Anatomical description	Radiological findings
I	Stretched/elongated posterior urethra	Urethra is stretched but not injured
II	Disruption of the posterior urethra above urogenital diaphragm	Extravasation above the urogenital diaphragm
III	Disruption of the membranous urethra	Extravasation above and below the urogenital diaphragm
IV	Injury of the bladder neck and the proximal urethra	Extravasation into the extraperitoneal spaces and disruption of the bladder neck
IV A	Injury of the bladder base with intact urethra (simulating type IV)	Extravasation into the urethral space associated to the lesion of the bladder base
V	Injury of the anterior urethra	Extravasation below the urogenital diaphragm

According to Goldman [2, 9]

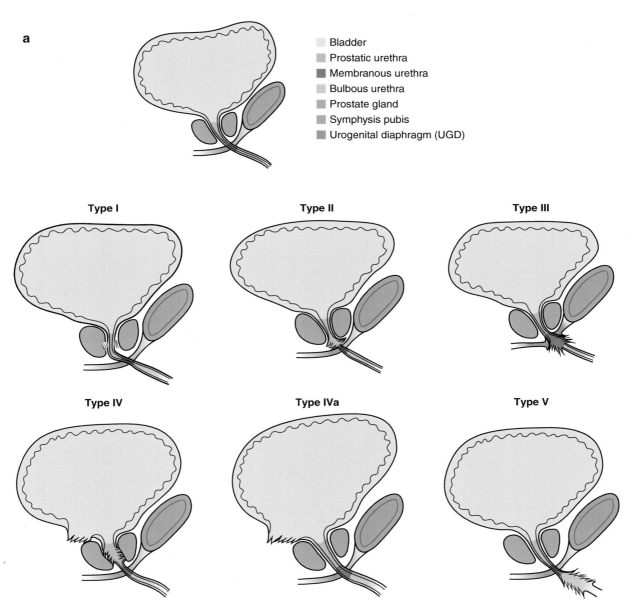

Fig. 8.11 Urethral injury. (**a**) Normal urethral anatomy and classification of urethral injury (Goldman's classification). (**b**) Cysto-urethrogram study demonstrates focal urethral stricture (*arrowhead*) and extravasation (*curved arrow*) of contrast from the proximal penile urethra in the first patient and leakage of contrast (*curved arrow*) from the penile urethra in the second patient with urethral injury

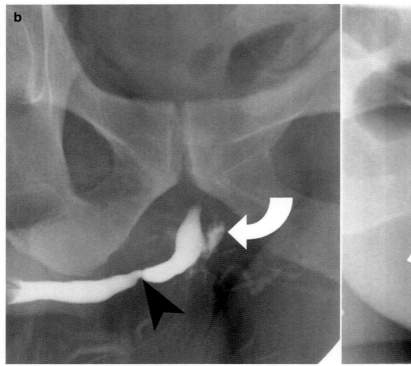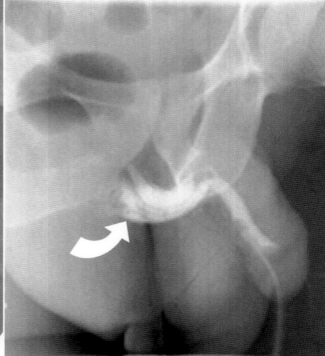

Fig. 8.11 (continued)

2. Intravaginal testicular torsion is the most common type of torsion and is associated with abnormal suspension of the testis by tunica vaginalis, resulting in bell-clapper deformity.
3. On retrograde urethrography, extravasation of contrast agent above urogenital diaphragm is seen with type II injury and extravasation of contrast below urogenital diaphragm is seen with type III urethral injury.

References

1. Garriga V, Serrano A, Marin A, Medrano S, Roson N, Pruna X. US of the tunica vaginalis testis: anatomic relationships and pathologic conditions. Radiographics. 2009;29:2017–32.
2. Cokkinos DD, Antypa E, Tserotas P, Kratimenou E, Kyratzi E, Deligiannis I, et al. Emergency ultrasound of the scrotum: a review of the commonest pathologic conditions. Curr Probl Diagn Radiol. 2011;40(1):1–14.
3. Brant WE, Helms CA. Helms, Fundamentals of diagnostic radiology. 2nd ed. Philadelphia: Lippincott Williams & Wilkins; 1999. p. 869–77.
4. Horstman WG, Middleton WD, Leland Melson G, Siegel BA. Color Doppler US of the scrotum. RadioGraphics. 1991;11:941–57.
5. Mazzucato F. Anatomia Radiologica – tecniche e metodologie in radiodiagnostica. IIIth ed. Milano: Piccin Editore; 2009. p. 2419–20, cap.39.
6. Tessler FN, Tublin ME, Rzfldn MD. US case of the day. Radiographics. 1998;18:251–3.
7. Muttarak M, Lojanapiwat B. The painful scrotum: an ultrasonographical approach to diagnosis. Singapore Med J. 2005;46(7):352.
8. Brant WE, Helms CA. Fundamentals of diagnostic radiology. 2nd ed. Philadelphia: Lippincott Williams & Wilkins; 1999. p. 823–6.
9. Levenson RB, Singh AK, Novelline RA. Fournier gangrene: role of imaging. Radiographics. 2008;28:519–28.
10. Cramer BM, Schlegel EA, Thueroff JW. MR imaging in the differential diagnosis of scrotal and testicular disease. Radiographics. 1991;11(1):9–21.
11. Deurdulian C, Mittelstaedt CA, Chong WK, Fielding JR. US of acute scrotal trauma: optimal technique, imaging findings, and management. Radiographics. 2007;27:357–69.
12. Bertolotto M, Pavlica P, Serafini G, Quaia E, Zappetti R. Painful penile induration: imaging findings and management. Radiographics. 2009;29:477–93.
13. Choi M-H, Kim B, Ryu J-A, Lee SW, Lee KS. MR imaging of acute penile fracture. Radiographics. 2000;20:1397–405.
14. Kawashima A, Sandler CM, Wasserman NF, LeRoy AJ, King Jr BF, Goldman SM. Imaging of urethral disease: a pictorial review. RadioGraphics. 2004;24:S195–216.
15. Kirkham APS, Illing RO, Minhas S, Allen C. MR imaging of nonmalignant penile lesions. RadioGraphics. 2008;28:837–53.
16. Ingram MD, Watson SG, Skippage PL, Patel U. Urethral injuries after pelvic trauma: evaluation with urethrography. Radiographics. 2008;28:1631–43.
17. Ali M, Safriel Y, Sclafani SJA, Schulze R. CT signs of urethral injury. RadioGraphics. 2003;23:951–66.

Paul F. von Herrmann, David J. Nickels, and Ajay Singh

Introduction

Trauma is the leading cause of morbidity and mortality among people younger than 45 years of age. Traumatic injury to the abdominal organs, with ensuing exsanguination, is the primary cause of death [1]. Of all abdominal traumatic injuries presenting to hospitals, blunt trauma comprises approximately 90 % and typically results from a motor vehicle collision or a fall. Penetrating trauma accounts for the remaining 10 % and is often a result of a bullet or knife injury. The evaluation of blunt or penetrating abdominal trauma can be one of the most challenging and resource-exhaustive aspects of acute trauma care.

In 1988, the American Association for the Surgery of Trauma (AAST) devised a set of organ injury scales (OISs) based on findings at surgical exploration. The OISs have now been defined by computed tomography (CT) criteria [2]. Accurate noninvasive assessment of injuries with CT is beneficial and can guide management. Since the development and application of these CT-based criteria, nonoperative management for blunt abdominal trauma has become increasingly common, particularly in hemodynamically stable patients. The accumulated evidence has demonstrated that minimally invasive management of blunt abdominal trauma, instead of laparotomy, results in improved survival rates. Analogously, managing penetrating abdominal trauma with laparotomy results in a negative or nontherapeutic procedure in 15–25 % of cases, prompting a movement toward more conservative management algorithms [3].

Currently, multidetector computed tomography (MDCT) with intravenous contrast is the "gold standard" diagnostic imaging examination in hemodynamically stable patients who have intra-abdominal fluid by focused assessment with sonography for trauma (FAST) [4]. Many studies have reported that MDCT has high sensitivity, specificity, positive predictive value, negative predictive value, and accuracy in injuries to the liver, spleen, kidney and urinary bladder, hollow viscus, and major vascular structures [2–5].

FAST

FAST is a useful diagnostic tool when performed in the acute setting because it can demonstrate intra-abdominal fluid, a finding that suggests significant organ injury, with a sensitivity of 90–93 % [4]. FAST is often performed after the secondary assessment or during resuscitation efforts. Identification of intra-abdominal free fluid on FAST in a hemodynamically unstable patient is regarded as synonymous with hemoperitoneum, thereby directing the surgeon to consider the abdomen as the major source of blood loss and prompting emergent laparotomy instead of CT. Conversely, a positive FAST in a hemodynamically stable patient should be followed by a CT scan to determine the source of the fluid.

Shortcomings of FAST include its inability to qualitatively grade the extent of organ injury and its low (34–55 %) sensitivity for direct demonstration of blunt abdominal injury [4]. Other limiting factors include inability to demonstrate small amounts of free fluid, operator dependence, limited accuracy in the retroperitoneum, and large body habitus.

P.F. von Herrmann, MD
Department of Radiology,
University of Kentucky,
Lexington, KY, USA

D.J. Nickels, MD, MBA
Department of Radiology,
Division of Emergency Radiology,
University of Kentucky,
Lexington, KY, USA

A. Singh, MD (✉)
Department of Radiology,
Massachusetts General Hospital, Harvard Medical School,
10 Museum Way, # 524, Boston, MA 02141, USA
e-mail: asingh1@partners.org

A. Singh (ed.), *Emergency Radiology*,
DOI 10.1007/978-1-4419-9592-6_9, © Springer Science+Business Media New York 2013

Liver

The liver is the most frequently injured solid abdominal organ in blunt and penetrating trauma. Hepatic injury in patients who have sustained blunt trauma has been reported to occur in 1–8 % and in penetrating trauma in up to 39 % [1, 6]. However, with utilization of abdominal CT in the severely injured patient, hepatic injuries can be detected in up to 25 % of those with blunt trauma [7]. Mortality rates from blunt or penetrating liver injury have been reported to range from 2.8 to 11.7 % [6, 8].

Nonsurgical management is the preferred strategy for hemodynamically stable patients with blunt liver injury. Accurate characterization of the extent of the injury by CT assists the managing provider with specific information that can be followed and categorized by the AAST OIS criteria (Table 9.1).

Hepatic injuries detected by CT can be classified as lacerations, hematomas, active hemorrhage, and juxtahepatic venous injuries. Hepatic laceration is the most common type of parenchymal liver injury; it appears as an irregular, linear, or branching low-attenuation region on contrast-enhanced CT (CECT) (Fig. 9.1). Lacerations are further divided into superficial (<3 cm) or deep (>3 cm).

Hematomas that present in blunt liver trauma are designated as subscapular or intraparenchymal. On CECT, a subcapsular hematoma appears as an elliptical collection of low-attenuation blood between the capsule of the liver and the enhancing liver parenchyma (Fig. 9.2). Intraparenchymal hematomas are characterized by focal low-attenuation regions with poorly defined, irregular margins in the liver parenchyma on CECT (Fig. 9.1). Active hemorrhage is diagnosed by identification of a focal high-attenuation area representing a collection of extravasated contrast. Active vascular extravasation can often be differentiated from clotted blood by measuring the CT attenuation coefficient. The attenuation of clotted blood ranges from 28 to 82 Hounsfield units (HU) (mean, 54 HU), whereas active arterial extravasation ranges from 91 to 274 HU (mean, 155 HU) [10]. Active contrast extravasation (ACE) changes its appearance over time; such a pattern can be demonstrated with multiphase vascular imaging, that is, during the arterial, portal venous, or delayed phases. On later vascular phase imaging, a region of ACE will increase in size and often pool or mix with non-contrasted blood in the adjacent hematoma.

Hepatic lacerations or hematomas that extend into a major venous structure indicate a severe injury and have been reported to require surgical management approximately 6.5 times more frequently than injuries not involving the hepatic veins or inferior vena cava (IVC) [11]. A CT finding that may indicate liver injury is periportal low attenuation paralleling the portal vein and its branches. Periportal low attenuation adjacent to a hepatic laceration may represent extension of hemorrhage into the periportal connective tissue, although this finding is nonspecific. It can also represent distention of the periportal lymphatic vessels as can be seen after aggressive fluid resuscitation, tension pneumothorax, or pericardial tamponade [12].

Table 9.1 AAST organ injury scale for liver

Grade	Description
I	Hematoma: subcapsular, <10 % surface area
	Laceration: capsular tear, <1 cm in parenchymal depth
II	Hematoma: subcapsular, 10–50 % surface area; intraparenchymal, <10 cm in diameter
	Laceration: 1–3 cm in parenchymal depth, <10 cm in length
III	Hematoma: subcapsular, >50 % surface area or expanding or ruptured subcapsular parenchymal hematoma; intraparenchymal hematoma >10 cm or expanding or ruptured
	Laceration: >3 cm in parenchymal depth
IV	Laceration: parenchymal disruption involving 25–75 % hepatic lobe or 1–3 Couinaud segments
V	Laceration: parenchymal disruption involving >75 % of a hepatic lobe or >3 Couinaud segments within a single lobe
	Vascular: juxtahepatic venous injuries (i.e., central major hepatic veins or retrohepatic vena cava)
VI	Vascular: hepatic avulsion

Source: Tinkoff et al. [9]

Spleen

Currently, 60–80 % of patients who sustain blunt splenic injury are managed nonoperatively with a success rate near 95 % [2]. Nonoperative management of isolated splenic injury is contingent on hemodynamic stability. Inevitably, failure of nonoperative management correlates with the presence of ACE on CT scan as well as with the radiological grade of the injury per the AAST criteria [9] (Table 9.2).

CECT can accurately diagnose the four common types of splenic injury: hematoma, laceration, active hemorrhage, and vascular injuries [13]. Splenic hematomas may be classified as subcapsular or intraparenchymal. On CECT, a subcapsular hematoma appears as an elliptical, low-attenuating collection between the splenic capsule and the enhancing splenic parenchyma (Fig. 9.3). Acute lacerations have a jagged or sharp margin and appear on CECT as a linear or branching low-attenuation area.

Active hemorrhage in the spleen is represented as an irregular or linear focus of contrast extravasation on CECT. Active hemorrhage may be seen in several locations: within splenic parenchyma or subcapsular space or intraperitoneally. Differentiating between ACE (range 85–350 HU, mean 132 HU) and hematoma or clotted blood (range 40–70 HU, mean 51 HU) is accomplished by measuring the attenuation coefficient [13].

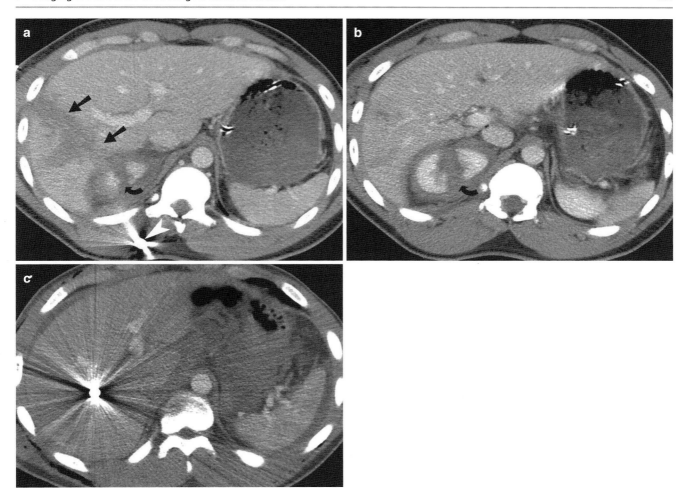

Fig. 9.1 Hepatic laceration from gunshot wound. (**a** and **b**) Contrast-enhanced CT demonstrates a deep hepatic (*straight arrow*) as well a right renal laceration (*curved arrow*). There is a bullet fragment (*white arrowhead*) located in the right posterior abdominal wall. (**c**) Contrast-enhanced CT demonstrates a metallic density bullet fragment located centrally with in the right lobe of liver. The liver laceration is obscured by the extensive beam-hardening artifact produced by the bullet fragment

Splenic vascular injuries include post-traumatic pseudoaneurysms and arteriovenous (AV) fistulas. A splenic pseudoaneurysm will appear as a well-circumscribed focus of increased attenuation in comparison to the enhancing splenic parenchyma (Fig. 9.4). An AV fistula is best demonstrated by early splenic vein enhancement. Both of these vascular injuries are best seen on arterial phase imaging and can be difficult to detect on portal venous phase or delayed (renal excretory phase) imaging. If a splenic pseudoaneurysm is suspected on early arterial phase imaging, it is helpful to distinguish this finding from ACE by noting the characteristics on delayed imaging. Specifically, on delayed imaging, a pseudoaneurysm will remain the same size and demonstrate similar density to the aorta, but ACE will increase in size and remain with high density. Splenic vascular lesions can be managed successfully by splenic arteriographic embolization, which improves the success rate of nonoperative management of blunt splenic injuries from 87 to 94 % [14, 15].

Pancreas

Pancreatic injuries have been reported as high as 12 % in victims of blunt trauma and 6 % in those with penetrating trauma. Typically, pancreatic injuries are associated with other intra-abdominal injuries 50–98 % of the time [13]. The clinical diagnosis of pancreatic injury may be difficult, particularly when isolated. Owing to the retroperitoneal location of the pancreas, peritonitis from a pancreatic injury may take hours to days to manifest. In addition, serum and urinary amylase levels are unreliable markers for the diagnosis of pancreatic injury [16].

CECT is the modality of choice for diagnosing pancreatic injury; its reported sensitivity and specificity is as high as 85 % [17]. CECT findings of pancreatic injury may be subtle, and the pancreas may appear normal immediately post-injury. Of primary importance is evaluation of the pancreatic duct because its integrity or lack of integrity directs management.

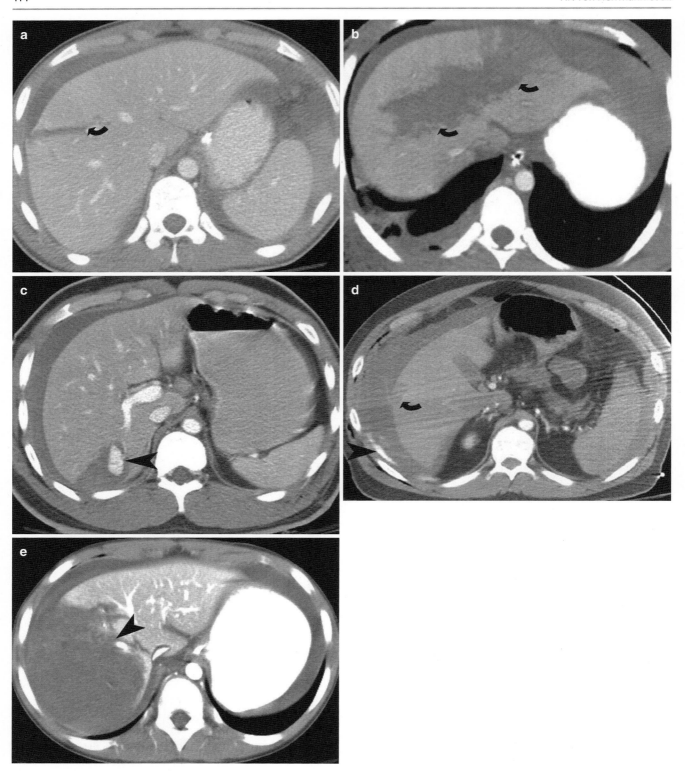

Fig. 9.2 Hepatic lacerations. (**a** and **b**) Contrast-enhanced CT in two different patients show a deep (>3 cm) hepatic laceration (grade III and grade IV liver injury) (*curved arrows*) due to stab injury. (**c**) Contrast-enhanced CT shows a wedge shaped liver laceration due to stab injury with subcapsular hematoma and enhancing pseudoaneurysm (*arrowhead*). (**d**) Contrast-enhanced CT shows a large perihepatic hematoma and active extravasation (*arrowhead*) arising from a gunshot injury related superficial liver laceration (*curved arrow*). (**e**) Contrast-enhanced CT shows grade IV liver injury with devascularization of >25 % of the right lobe of the liver (*arrowhead*)

Table 9.2 AAST organ injury scale for spleen

Grade	Description
I	Hematoma: subcapsular, <10 % surface area
	Laceration: capsular tear, <1 cm in parenchymal depth
II	Hematoma: subcapsular, 10–50 % surface area; intraparenchymal, <5 cm in diameter
	Laceration: capsular tear, 1–3 cm in parenchymal depth, not involving a trabecular vessel
III	Hematoma: subcapsular, >50 % surface area or expanding; ruptured subcapsular or parenchymal hematoma; intraparenchymal hematoma >5 cm or expanding
	Laceration: >3 cm in parenchymal depth or involving trabecular vessels
IV	Laceration: involving segmental or hilar vessels producing major devascularization (>25 % of spleen)
V	Hematoma: completely shattered spleen
	Laceration: hilar vascular injury that devascularizes spleen

Source: Tinkoff et al. [9]

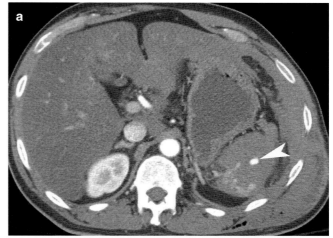

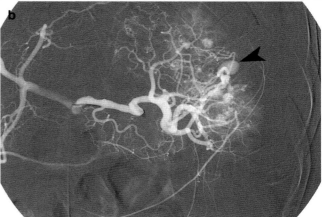

Fig. 9.4 Splenic pseudoaneurysm. (**a**) Contrast-enhanced CT demonstrates a pseudoaneurysm (*arrowhead*) within the splenic parenchymal laceration. (**b**) Conventional splenic artery angiogram demonstrates the splenic arterial branch pseudoaneurysm (*arrowhead*)

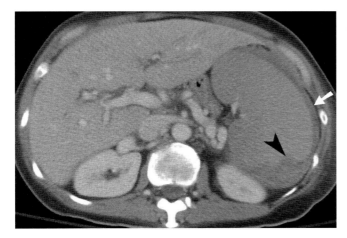

Fig. 9.3 Splenic laceration. Contrast-enhanced CT shows subcapsular hematoma (*arrow*) and intraparenchymal laceration (*arrowhead*) with hematoma

A pancreatic injury can be categorized as contusion, laceration, or transection. A pancreatic contusion may appear as diffuse enlargement of the pancreas or as focal low attenuation or heterogeneity. Pancreatic lacerations are demonstrated by linear, irregular low-attenuation areas within the normally enhancing parenchyma (Fig. 9.5). A pancreatic transection may be difficult to diagnose with CT unless there is low-attenuation fluid collection separating the two edges of the transected pancreas.

The position of the pancreatic laceration in relation to the superior mesenteric artery as well as the depth of the laceration helps predict pancreatic ductal disruption, which occurs in up to 15 % of pancreatic trauma [13, 17]. The superior mesenteric vessels provide a landmark for dividing the pancreas into proximal and distal portions with injury to the

proximal pancreas usually associated with more severe injury. A laceration of the pancreas involving >50 % of the anteroposterior diameter of the pancreatic body or tail is often associated with ductal disruption.

There are several nonspecific CT findings associated with pancreatic trauma, the most common of which is thickening or infiltration of the anterior pararenal fascia. Additional nonspecific CT findings include blood/fluid tracking along the mesenteric vessels, fluid in the lesser sac, fluid between the pancreas and splenic vein, or infiltration of the peripancreatic fat with fluid or hemorrhage [13].

Kidney

The kidney is the most commonly injured urogenital organ in trauma. Approximately 10 % of all significant blunt abdominal traumatic injuries include a renal injury, and of those, 80–90 % are managed nonoperatively. The goal of

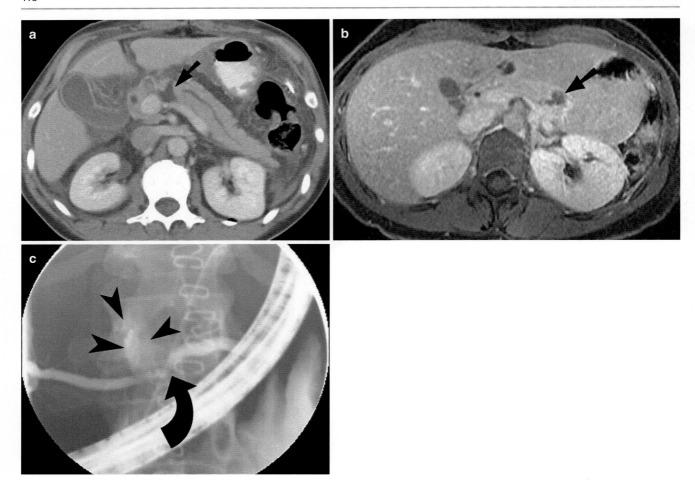

Fig. 9.5 Pancreatic injury. (**a** and **b**) Contrast-enhanced CT demonstrates pancreatic laceration (*arrow*) with disruption of the main pancreatic duct. (**c**) Endoscopic retrograde cholangiopancreatography image showing pancreatic duct discontinuity (*curved arrow*) and extravasation of contrast from the ductal disruption (*arrowheads*)

conservative management is to preserve organ integrity and reduce the complication rate. Historical evidence shows that hemodynamically stable patients with kidney injuries who undergo surgical exploration have a much higher incidence of nephrectomy [4]. Blunt trauma accounts for approximately 90 % of renal trauma, while penetrating trauma accounts for approximately 10 %. Nonsurgical management is more commonly advocated in blunt renal injuries, but conservative protocols have also been applied to penetrating renal injuries [18, 19]. However, penetrating trauma is more frequently associated with major renal injury and frequently requires invasive treatment, as it is more often associated with hemodynamic instability and damage to surrounding abdominal organs [20]. Indications for renal imaging include gross hematuria and penetrating or blunt trauma with hematuria. The imaging modality of choice to evaluate the kidneys after trauma is CECT.

Renal injuries may be classified as lacerations, contusions, or renovascular injuries, which determine the radiological grade of the injury per AAST criteria (Table 9.3).

Renal contusions are visualized as poorly marginated, round or ovoid areas of low-attenuation and show a delayed or persistent nephrogram when compared to normal adjacent renal parenchyma. Hematomas can be categorized as subcapsular or perinephric. On an unenhanced CT, a subcapsular hematoma (Fig. 9.6) is seen as an eccentric hyperattenuating fluid collection confined between the renal parenchyma and renal capsule. However, on a CECT a subcapsular hematoma will be hypoattenuating compared to the normal enhancing renal parenchyma. A subcapsular hematoma may also exert a mass effect on the renal contour and can cause decreased perfusion in extreme cases. A perinephric hematoma is a poorly marginated, hyperattenuating fluid collection (45–90 HU) that is confined between the renal parenchyma and the Gerota fascia [21]. Other findings associated with a perinephric hematoma are thickening of the lateroconal fascia, compression of the colon, and displacement of the kidney.

Renal lacerations are visualized as hypoattenuating, irregular wedge-shaped, or linear parenchymal defects or clefts (Figs. 9.7 and 9.8). The most severe form of renal laceration,

Table 9.3 AAST organ injury scale for kidney

Grade	Description
I	Hematoma: subcapsular, nonexpanding without parenchymal laceration
	Contusion: microscopic or gross hematuria, urologic studies normal
II	Hematoma: nonexpanding perirenal hematoma confirmed to renal retroperitoneum
	Laceration: <1 cm parenchymal depth of renal cortex without urinary extravasation
III	Laceration: >1 cm in parenchymal depth of renal cortex without collecting system rupture or urinary extravagation
IV	Laceration: parenchymal laceration extending through renal cortex, medulla, and collecting system
	Vascular: main renal artery or vein injury with contained hemorrhage
V	Hematoma: completely shattered kidney
	Vascular: avulsion of renal hilum that devascularizes kidney

Source: Tinkoff et al. [9]

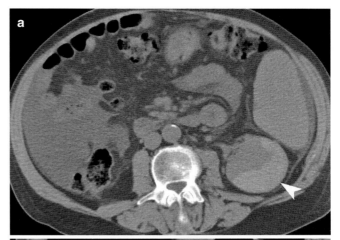

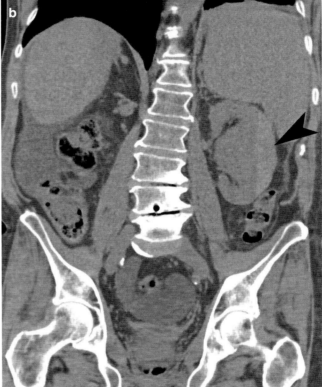

Fig. 9.6 Page kidney. (**a** and **b**) Axial and coronal contrast-enhanced CT images demonstrate subcapsular hematoma (*arrowhead*) compressing the left renal cortex

termed a "shattered kidney," represents a kidney that is fractured into multiple fragments. It is often associated with devitalized renal tissue, injuries to the collecting system, severe hemorrhage, active arterial bleeding, and compromise in the excretion of contrast material [21].

The depth of a renal laceration is important as it relates to the renal collecting system. If a laceration extends into the collecting system, this is consistent with a higher-grade injury (IV or V instead of III). Renal pelvis or collecting system involvement can be demonstrated by urine extravasation, which is seen as a perinephric low-density fluid collection on arterial or portal venous phase imaging. Suspected urine extravasation can be differentiated from hematoma by the presence of contrast extravasation, which is only seen on the delayed renal excretory phase images.

Urinary Bladder

Bladder injuries are caused by blunt or penetrating trauma. Blunt trauma accounts for 60–85 % of bladder injuries, whereas penetrating trauma accounts for 15–40 % [22]. The conventional mechanism of injury to the bladder in blunt abdominal trauma is rapid increase of the intravesical pressure resulting in a tear along the intraperitoneal portion of the bladder wall. Bladder injury is more common among those sustaining a seatbelt or steering wheel injury.

Bladder rupture should be suspected when a patient presents with gross hematuria, pelvic fluid, and/or pelvic fractures. Certain types of pelvic fractures are associated with bladder rupture; these include sacral, iliac, and pubic rami fractures as well as pubic symphysis diastasis and sacroiliac joint diastasis [23]. In patients with pelvic fractures, bladder injury occurs in approximately 10 %; however, traumatic extraperitoneal ruptures of the bladder are predominantly associated with pelvic fractures [24]. CT cystography or conventional fluoroscopic cystography should be performed following CT of the abdomen and pelvis in hemodynamically stable trauma patients with (1) gross hematuria, (2) pelvic fracture (other than an isolated acetabular fracture) plus microhematuria (>25 RBC/HPC), or (3) microhematuria and pelvic fluid.

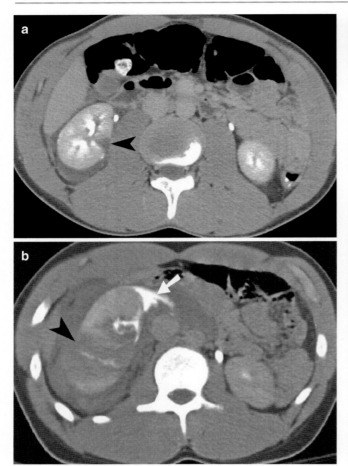

Fig. 9.7 Renal laceration. (**a**) Axial contrast-enhanced CT demonstrating a grade II laceration (*arrowhead*) with small perinephric hematoma. (**b**) Axial contrast-enhanced CT demonstrates grade V shattered kidney (*arrowhead*) and extravasation of urine (*white arrow*) into the perinephric space

CT cystography has a similar sensitivity and specificity to conventional fluoroscopic cystography and provides a more complete and more sensitive evaluation of the urinary bladder than a conventional abdominal and pelvic CT [25].

On abdominal CT, findings suggestive of urinary bladder injury or rupture include the presence of free fluid in the pelvis with no obvious source, urinary contrast extravasation, bladder wall discontinuity, and the presence of any foreign body within the bladder wall (Figs. 9.9, 9.10, and 9.11). On CT cystography, extraperitoneal injuries can be distinguished from intraperitoneal injuries by the location of the extravasation in relation to the peritoneal reflection. An extraperitoneal injury is below the peritoneal reflection and will demonstrate contrast extravasation in the classic "flame-shaped" or "molar tooth" configuration as the contrast penetrates into the paravesical tissues. In the case of intraperitoneal bladder injuries, the perforation is above the peritoneal reflection and extravasated contrast will outline bowel loops. Injuries to the neck of the bladder will show

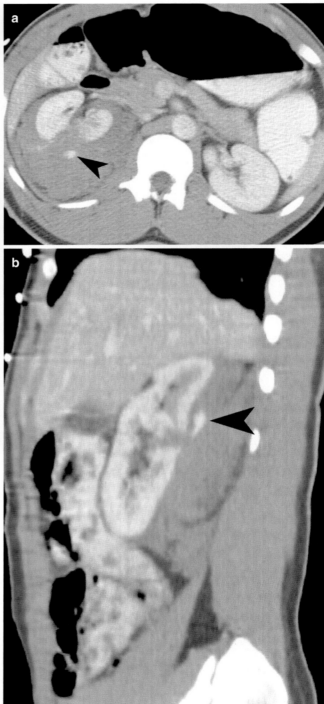

Fig. 9.8 Renal injury, CECT. (**a** and **b**) Axial and sagittal contrast-enhanced CT demonstrate right renal laceration with extravasation of contrast (*arrowhead*) into a perinephric hematoma

extravasation near the base of the bladder. The pattern of contrast extravasation on cystography is of foremost importance and will guide management of the patient.

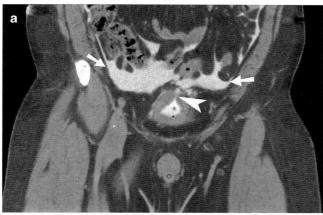

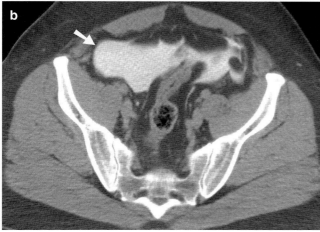

Fig. 9.9 Intraperitoneal bladder rupture. (**a** and **b**) Coronal CT cystogram image demonstrating large amount of intraperitoneal contrast (*arrows*) leaking from the dome of the urinary bladder (*arrowhead*) and outlining the small bowel loops

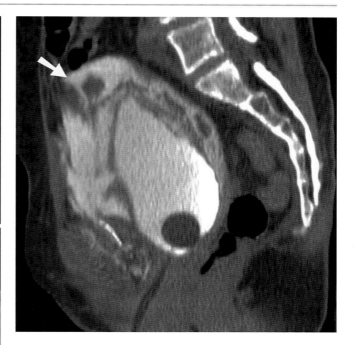

Fig. 9.10 Intraperitoneal rupture of the urinary bladder. Sagittal CT cystogram image demonstrating intraperitoneal contrast (*arrow*) outlining the pelvis

Urethra

Injuries to the urethra are most often caused by a displaced anterior arch pelvic fracture or iatrogenic manipulation [26]. Approximately 10–25 % of patients with a pelvic fracture also have urethral trauma. Urethral injury is most often diagnosed with a retrograde urethrogram (RUG), which should be performed prior to insertion of a urethral catheter to avoid further injury. The ultimate goal of an RUG following trauma is to evaluate the integrity of the urethra and to determine if the urethra is "watertight." Contrast extravasation during an RUG is diagnostic for urethral injury (Fig. 9.12). An RUG can also demonstrate strictures, which can be long-term sequelae of urethral injury.

Urethral injuries are divided into two categories based on the anatomical site of the injury. Posterior urethral injuries are located in the membranous and prostatic urethra. Anterior urethral injuries are located distal to the membranous urethra. Typically, both posterior and anterior urethral injuries

are the result of blunt trauma. Penetrating trauma, which includes gunshot and stab wounds, most often affects the penile urethra (Fig. 9.13).

Radiologists employ two different classification systems for grading urethral injuries. The Goldman classification (Table 9.4) is most commonly used by urologists and includes urethral injuries as well as bladder injuries that simulate posterior urethral injury. The second classification system is the AAST Organ Injury Scale for urethral injuries (Table 9.5). Imaging of the urethra with an RUG is the reference standard for urethral injury; however, with the widespread use of CT, it is vital to be familiar with CT findings indicative of urethral injury. These findings include indistinct urogenital diaphragmatic fat plane, indistinct prostatic contour, hematoma of the ischiocavernosus and obturator internus muscles, and obscuration of the bulbocavernosus muscle [27–29].

Bowel and Mesentery

Unidentified bowel and mesenteric injuries carry significant morbidity and mortality secondary to complications arising from peritonitis. Injuries to the bowel and mesentery occur in approximately 5 % of patients sustaining blunt abdominal trauma and 30 % in patients sustaining penetrating trauma to the abdomen [2, 6, 13]. Similar to pancreatic injury, the initial physical examination on a patient with mesenteric injury may be misleadingly normal. Classic peritoneal signs may be present in only one-third of patients [30].

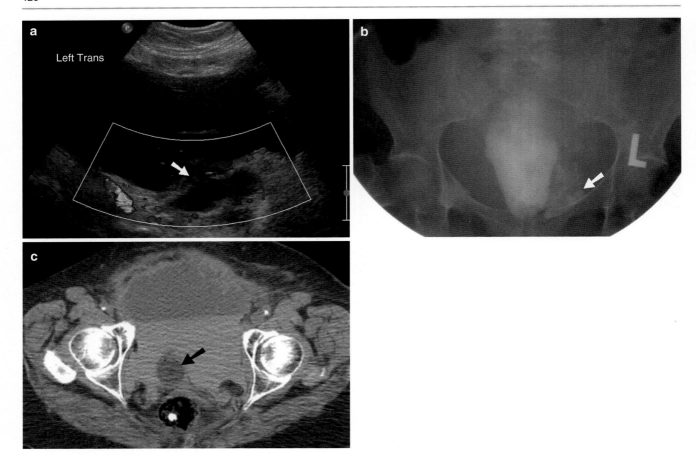

Fig. 9.11 Urinary bladder rupture. (**a**) Ultrasound image of the pelvis demonstrating direct transperitoneal communication (*arrow*) between urinary bladder and a large pelvic urinoma. (**b**) Cystogram study depicts extravasation of contrast from the urinary bladder into the extraperitoneal space (*arrow*). (**c**) CT cystogram demonstrating Foley catheter bulb (*arrow*) located outside the urinary bladder in a large pelvic fluid collection

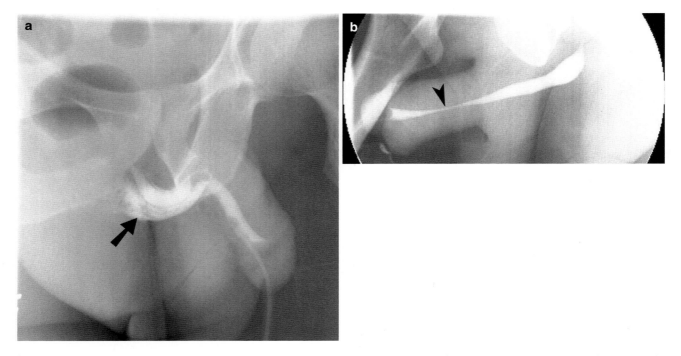

Fig. 9.12 Urethral injuries by RUG. (**a**) RUG demonstrating extravasation of contrast (*arrow*) from the bulbous urethra. (**b**) RUG demonstrating urethral narrowing (*arrowhead*) due to extrinsic compression from a penile shaft hematoma

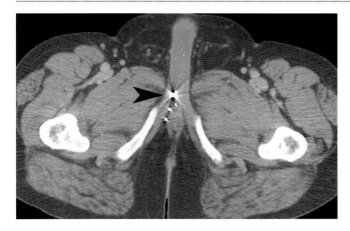

Fig. 9.13 Penile and urethral injury from shotgun pellets. Contrast-enhanced CT demonstrates multiple metallic foreign bodies (*arrowheads*) in the corpora cavernosa and spongiosum of the penis

Table 9.4 Goldman classification for urethral injuries

Grade	Description
I	Posterior urethra intact but stretched and elongated. Prostate and bladder apex displaced superiorly
II	Urethra disrupted above urogenital diaphragm in prostatic segment. Membranous urethra intact
III	Membranous urethra disrupted. Extension of injury to the proximal bulbous urethra and/or disruption of urogenital diaphragm
IV	Bladder neck injury with extension into the proximal urethra
IVA	Injury at the base of the bladder with periurethral extravasation simulating a type IV urethral injury
V	Partial or complete pure anterior urethral injury

Source: Ali et al. [27]

Table 9.5 AAST organ injury scale for urethra

Grade	Injury type	Description
I	Contusion	Blood at urethral meatus, urethrography normal
II	Stretch injury	Elongation of urethra without extravasation on urethrography
III	Partial disruption	Extravasation of urethrography contrast at injury site. Contrast visualized in bladder
IV	Complete disruption	Extravasation of urethrography contrast at injury site without contrast in bladder <2 cm of urethral separation
V	Complete disruption	Complete transection with >2 cm of urethral separation or extension into the prostate or vagina

Source: Ingram et al. [28]

Injury to the bowel and mesentery is most often diagnosed with CECT. However, there is no single CT sign that is considered both sensitive and specific for bowel or mesenteric injury. CT findings suggestive of a mesenteric injury include ACE into the mesentery, focal mesenteric hematoma or infiltration (Fig. 9.14), bowel wall thickening, or abnormal

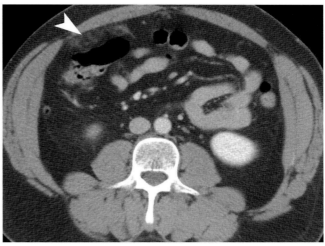

Fig. 9.14 Omental contusion. Contrast-enhanced CT demonstrates fat stranding in omental fat (*arrowhead*) due to traumatic omental contusion

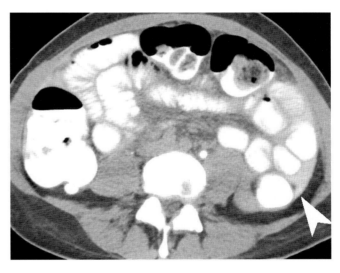

Fig. 9.15 Small bowel perforation. Contrast-enhanced CT shows extravasation of oral contrast (*arrowhead*) secondary to small bowel perforation caused by trocar during laparoscopic surgery

enhancement with mesenteric hematoma. In the presence of bowel perforation (Fig. 9.15), CT findings may include extraluminal air or oral contrast (if administered), or moderate to large volumes of free intraperitoneal fluid without an obvious source such as solid organ injury [5].

Shock bowel or diffuse small bowel ischemia (Figs. 9.16 and 9.17) can occur when a patient becomes severely hypotensive following hemorrhage. Shock develops from decreased circulating blood volume, which is often complicated by derangement of circulatory control and release of vasoconstrictors such as angiotensin II, adrenaline, and noradrenaline. The blood supply to the intestinal mucosa is drastically reduced during marked sympathetic stimulation and is diverted to other crucial organs such as the brain and heart.

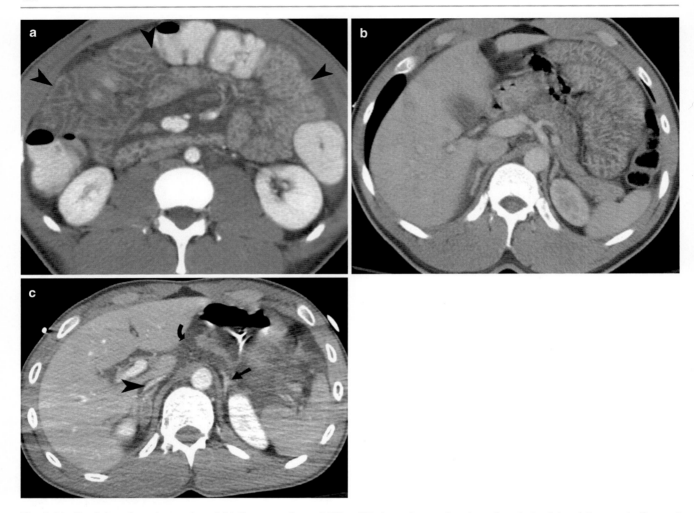

Fig. 9.16 Shock bowel syndrome. (**a** and **b**) Contrast-enhanced CT shows hyperenhancing small bowel walls (*arrowheads*) in a patient with hypovolemia after motor vehicle accident. (**c**) Contrast-enhanced CT shows hyperenhancing adrenal gland (*straight arrow*), flattened IVC (*arrowhead*), and peripancreatic fluid (*curved arrow*)

The resulting splanchnic vasoconstriction leads to intestinal hypoperfusion and, in advanced cases, intestinal ischemia. Mesenteric arterial vasoconstriction and venous constriction of the bowel wall develop after release of angiotensin II, adrenaline, and noradrenaline. The resultant decrease in both arterial perfusion and venous outflow contributes to the enhancement of the bowel mucosa in shock bowel [31]. Bowel hypoperfusion most profoundly affects the intestinal mucosa, which can lead to "third space" fluid loss into the gastrointestinal tract. CT characteristics of shock bowel are diffuse thickening of the small bowel wall (7–15 mm), fluid-filled dilated small bowel, increased contrast enhancement of the small bowel wall, and flattened vena cava. The large bowel will often appear normal in the setting of small bowel ischemia.

In addition to the aforementioned effects of the hypoperfusion complex on the bowel and mesentery, shock adrenal glands play a role in the increased sympathetic stimulation and demonstrate symmetric hyperenhancement on CT. Hypoperfusion results in the release of angiotensin II which stimulates the adrenal cortex of the adrenal glands to produce aldosterone and the adrenal medulla to produce adrenaline and noradrenaline.

Teaching Points

- Findings suggestive of mesenteric injury include ACE into the mesentery, focal mesenteric hematoma or infiltration, bowel wall thickening, or abnormal enhancement with mesenteric hematoma.
- RUG is the study of choice for the diagnosis of urethral injury.
- CT cystography or conventional cystography should be performed following abdomen/pelvis CT if bladder injury is suspected.

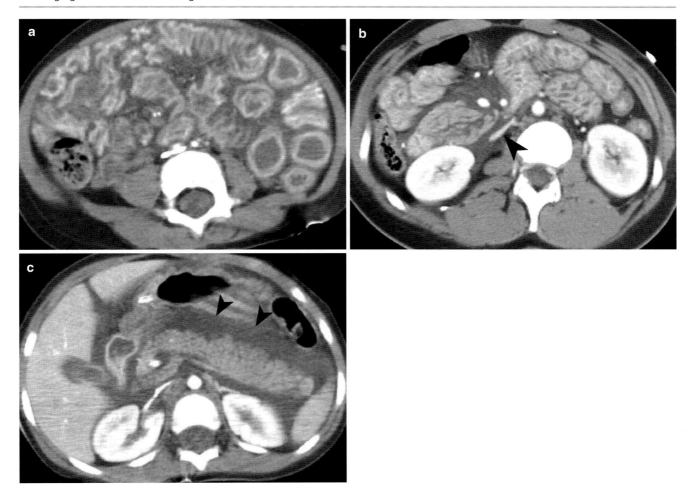

Fig. 9.17 Shock bowel syndrome. (**a** and **b**) Contrast-enhanced CT shows hyperenhancing small bowel walls and ascites. The IVC (*arrowhead*) is flattened secondary to hypovolemia. (**c**) Contrast-enhanced CT shows peripancreatic fluid (*arrowheads*) and flattened IVC

- Bowel perforation may show extraluminal air or oral contrast, or moderate to large volume of intraperitoneal free fluid without an obvious source.
- Shock bowel appears as diffuse thickening of the small bowel wall (7–15 mm), fluid-filled dilated small bowel, increased contrast enhancement of the small bowel wall, and flattened vena cava.

References

1. Sauaia A, Moore FA, Moore EE, Moser KS, Brennan R, Read RA, et al. Epidemiology of trauma deaths: a reassessment. J Trauma. 1995;38:185–93.
2. Milia DJ, Brasel K. Current use of CT in the evaluation and management of injured patients. Surg Clin North Am. 2011;91:233–48.
3. Melo EL, de Menezes MR, Cerri GG. Abdominal gunshot wounds: multi-detector-row CT findings compared with laparotomy-a prospective study. Emerg Radiol. 2012;19:35–41.
4. van der Vlies CH, Olthof DC, Gaakeer M, Ponsen KJ, van Delden OM, Goslings JC. Changing patterns in diagnostic strategies and the treatment of blunt injury to solid abdominal organs. Int J Emerg Med. 2011;4:47.
5. Butela ST, Federle MP, Chang PJ, Thaete FL, Peterson MS, Dorvault CJ, et al. Performance of CT in detection of bowel injury. AJR Am J Roentgenol. 2001;176:129–35.
6. Feliciano DV, Rozycki GS. The management of penetrating abdominal trauma. Adv Surg. 1995;28:1–39.
7. Matthes G, Stengel D, Seifert J, Rademacher G, Mutze S, Ekkernkamp A. Blunt liver injuries in polytrauma: results from a cohort study with the regular use of whole-body helical computed tomography. World J Surg. 2003;27:1124–30.
8. Yoon W, Jeong YY, Kim JK, Seo JJ, Lim HS, Shin SS, et al. CT in blunt liver trauma. Radiographics. 2005;25:87–104.
9. Tinkoff G, Esposito TJ, Reed J, Kilgo P, Fildes J, Pasquale M, et al. American association for the surgery of trauma organ injury scale: spleen, liver, and kidney, validation based on the national trauma data bank. J Am Coll Surg. 2008;207:646–55.
10. Willmann JK, Roos JE, Platz A, Pfammatter T, Hilfiker PR, Marincek B, et al. Multidetector CT: detection of active hemorrhage in patients with blunt abdominal trauma. AJR Am J Roentgenol. 2002;179:437–44.
11. Poletti PA, Mirvis SE, Shanmuganathan K, Killeen KL, Coldwell D. CT criteria for management of blunt liver trauma: correlation with angiographic and surgical findings. Radiology. 2000;216: 418–27.

12. Shanmuganathan K, Mirvis SE. CT scan evaluation of blunt hepatic trauma. Radiol Clin North Am. 1998;36:399–411.
13. Shanmuganathan K. Multi-detector row CT imaging of blunt abdominal trauma. Semin Ultrasound CT MR. 2004;25:180–204.
14. Davis KA, Fabian TC, Croce MA, Gavant ML, Flick PA, Minard G, et al. Improved success in nonoperative management of blunt splenic injuries: embolization of splenic artery pseudoaneurysms. J Trauma. 1998;44:1008–13; discussion 1013–5.
15. Shanmuganathan K, Mirvis SE, Boyd-Kranis R, Takada T, Scalea TM. Nonsurgical management of blunt splenic injury: use of CT criteria to select patients for splenic arteriography and potential endovascular therapy. Radiology. 2000;217:75–82.
16. Craig MH, Talton DS, Hauser CJ, Poole GV. Pancreatic injuries from blunt trauma. Am Surg. 1995;61:125–8.
17. Fisher M, Brasel K. Evolving management of pancreatic injury. Curr Opin Crit Care. 2011;17:613–7.
18. Broghammer JA, Fisher MB, Santucci RA. Conservative management of renal trauma: a review. Urology. 2007;70:623–9.
19. Meng MV, Brandes SB, McAninch JW. Renal trauma: indications and techniques for surgical exploration. World J Urol. 1999;17:71–7.
20. Sica G, Bocchini G, Guida F, Tanga M, Guaglione M, Scaglione M. Multidetector computed tomography in the diagnosis and management of renal trauma. Radiol Med. 2010;115:936–49.
21. Alonso RC, Nacenta SB, Martinez PD, Guerrero AS, Fuentes CG. Kidney in danger: CT findings of blunt and penetrating renal trauma. Radiographics. 2009;29:2033–53.
22. Cass AS, Luxenberg M. Features of 164 bladder ruptures. J Urol. 1987;138:743–5.
23. Morgan DE, Nallamala LK, Kenney PJ, Mayo MS, Rue 3rd LW. CT cystography: radiographic and clinical predictors of bladder rupture. AJR Am J Roentgenol. 2000;174:89–95.
24. Tonkin JB, Tisdale BE, Jordan GH. Assessment and initial management of urologic trauma. Med Clin North Am. 2011;95:245–51.
25. Wirth GJ, Peter R, Poletti PA, Iselin CE. Advances in the management of blunt traumatic bladder rupture: experience with 36 cases. BJU Int. 2010;106:1344–9.
26. Koraitim MM, Marzouk ME, Atta MA, Orabi SS. Risk factors and mechanism of urethral injury in pelvic fractures. Br J Urol. 1996;77:876–80.
27. Ali M, Safriel Y, Sclafani SJ, Schulze R. CT signs of urethral injury. Radiographics. 2003;23:951–63; discussion 963–6.
28. Ingram MD, Watson SG, Skippage PL, Patel U. Urethral injuries after pelvic trauma: evaluation with urethrography. Radiographics. 2008;28:1631–43.
29. Ramchandani P, Buckler PM. Imaging of genitourinary trauma. AJR Am J Roentgenol. 2009;192:1514–23.
30. Donohue JH, Crass RA, Trunkey DD. The management of duodenal and other small intestinal trauma. World J Surg. 1985;9:904–13.
31. Lubner M, Demertzis J, Lee JY, Appleton CM, Bhalla S, Menias CO. CT evaluation of shock viscera: a pictorial review. Emerg Radiol. 2008;15:1–11.

Acute Nontraumatic Imaging in the Liver and Spleen

Dale E. Hansen III, Sridhar Shankar, and Ajay Singh

Introduction

Each year, more than 120 million patients visit the emergency room in the USA. The single most common cause of presentation in the emergency room patient is abdominal pain. Our job as radiologists is to help pinpoint a diagnosis and triage patients in the right direction. The following review covers acute nontraumatic disease processes of the liver and spleen.

Acute Hepatitis

Broadly speaking, acute hepatitis is any acute insult to the liver resulting in the influx of inflammatory cells [1]. The differential diagnosis for hepatitis is long, ranging from an acute viral hepatitis to autoimmune hepatitis [2]. The imaging findings of the various causes of hepatitis are relatively nonspecific, and teasing out a specific diagnosis must often be left to the clinician. The imaging findings in acute viral hepatitis are discussed below, though these findings could be seen in any acute hepatitis.

The "classic" ER case of acute hepatitis is one with right upper quadrant pain, jaundice, and fever [2]. In severe cases of fulminant hepatic failure, patients may present with severe coagulopathy and mental status changes [2]. Laboratory evaluation can help determine the diagnosis of hepatitis and possibly a specific cause. The aminotransferases are nearly always elevated, usually significantly so. Viral hepatitis panels help determine if an acute viral infection is the cause.

D.E. Hansen III, MD (✉) • S. Shankar, MD, MBA
Department of Radiology,
University of Tennessee,
Memphis, TN, USA

A. Singh, MD
Department of Radiology,
Massachusetts General Hospital, Harvard Medical School,
10 Museum Way, # 524, Boston, MA 02141, USA
e-mail: asingh1@partners.org

Finally, history is crucial in determining any patient's risk for hepatitis. Historical factors suggesting acute hepatitis include IV drug use, food poisoning, other autoimmune disease, alcoholism, obesity, diabetes, acetaminophen overdose, or radiation.

Imaging

As mentioned earlier, imaging of acute hepatitis is fairly nonspecific. Ultrasound will often demonstrate hepatomegaly with diffuse decreased echogenicity of the hepatic parenchyma [3]. This decreased echogenicity leads to a relative hyperechoic appearance of the portal branches, resulting in the classic "starry sky" appearance (Fig. 10.1a). There may be associated reactionary gallbladder wall thickening as well. Unfortunately, a normal appearance to the liver does not exclude acute hepatitis [3].

Contrast-enhanced CT study will often demonstrate a heterogeneous appearing liver [3]. The hypoattenuating regions represent areas of necrosis or periportal edema. The more hyperattenuating regions usually represent focal areas of sparing or, in the more chronic case, areas of nodular regeneration. Other findings include hepatomegaly, periportal edema, gallbladder wall thickening, and ascites (Fig. 10.2b, c). On MRI, T2-weighted images will show hyperintense regions of periportal edema; these same areas will be low intensity on T1 images [3].

Fulminant hepatitis, the most devastating and life-threatening form, is characterized by a small liver with massive areas of hypoattenuation associated with expansive necrosis [4, 5]. Secondary findings of ascites, splenomegaly, and portal vein dilatation may be noted. Although generally not intended to diagnose hepatitis, HIDA scans in patients with right upper quadrant pain and suspected cholecystitis can be useful in determining the cause of gallbladder wall thickening (Fig. 10.2). Impaired clearance of the blood pool with no excretion of radiotracer into the biliary system suggests marked hepatocellular dysfunction consistent with acute hepatitis.

A. Singh (ed.), *Emergency Radiology*,
DOI 10.1007/978-1-4419-9592-6_10, © Springer Science+Business Media New York 2013

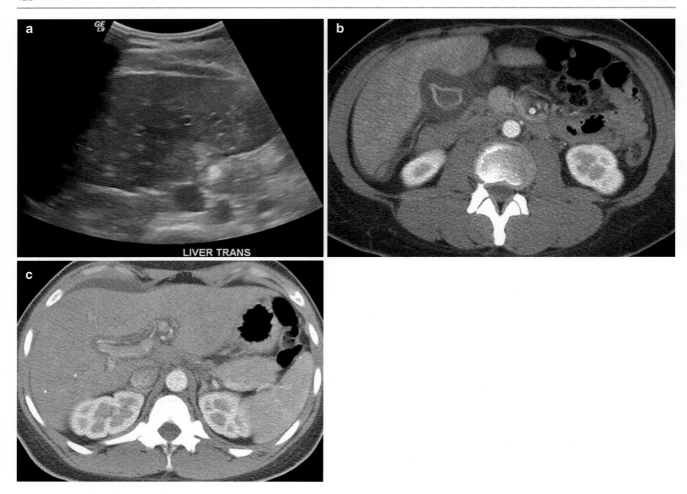

Fig. 10.1 Acute hepatitis C. (**a**) Ultrasound of the liver shows "starry sky" appearance due to decreased parenchymal echogenicity and relative increase in periportal echogenicity. (**b** and **c**) Contrast-enhanced CT demonstrates periportal edema, gallbladder wall edema, and pericholecystic fluid

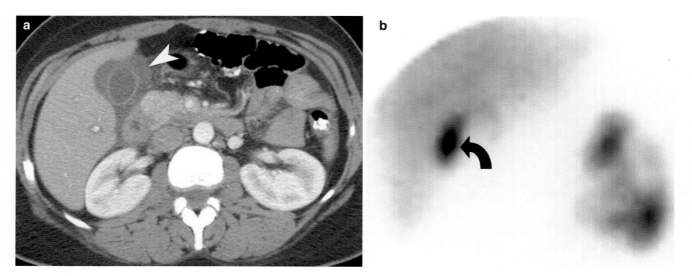

Fig. 10.2 Acute hepatitis B. (**a**) Contrast-enhanced CT demonstrates gallbladder wall edema (*arrowhead*) and pericholecystic fluid. The gallbladder wall, though prominent, is not as thickened as in the previ-ous case. (**b**) HIDA scan showing uptake in the gallbladder (*curved arrow*) and excretion into small bowel loops. The presence of radiotracer into the gallbladder lumen rules out cystic duct

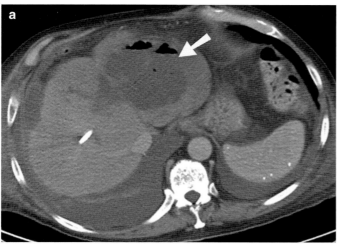
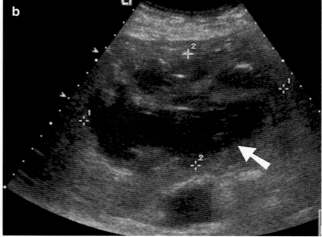

Fig. 10.3 Pyogenic hepatic abscess after liver transplant. (**a**) Contrast-enhanced CT through the liver demonstrates a large, irregular hypodense collection (*arrow*) in the left lobe of liver, containing air. This is virtually diagnostic of an abscess. An internal biliary stent is also seen. (**b**) Gray-scale ultrasound in the same patient showing a complex collection (*arrow*) within the liver. This patient went on to have percutaneous drainage of the abscess under CT guidance

Hepatic Abscess

Liver abscesses can be polymicrobial, with *Escherichia coli* being by far the most common pathogen, or they can be due to fungal infection or *Entamoeba histolytica*. Fungal infection of the liver is most commonly seen in the patient with AIDS, hematologic malignancy, or organ transplant [3]. Candida is the most frequent causative organism. Cryptococcus, histoplasmosis, aspergillus, and mucormycosis are less commonly seen. Liver abscesses are most often caused by spread of biliary infection or by hematogenous spread, superinfection of necrotic liver, or iatrogenic causes. Overall, pyogenic abscesses are a fairly dangerous entity, with an associated 2 % mortality rate [3].

Pyogenic abscesses are generally treated by radiologists, with CT-guided drainage being the mainstay of treatment.

Imaging

Pyogenic Abscess

Pyogenic abscesses can further be subdivided into two categories: microabscesses versus macroabscesses, with 2 cm being the cutoff between the two [3]. Ultrasound and CT are the mainstays of imaging.

In the setting of microabscesses, ultrasound will show a small (<2 cm), possibly scattered hypoechoic focus or foci, or heterogeneous echotexture. With macroabscesses, the ultrasound appearance can be quite varied, ranging from hypoechoic to hyperechoic with varying degrees of internal septation and debris. Internal gas, indicated by high-intensity echoes and dirty posterior shadowing, helps seal the diagnosis [3].

CT, with microabscesses, will demonstrate small, hypoattenuating lesions with faint peripheral enhancement and surrounding edema [3]. Larger abscesses will also be hypoattenuating, often with irregular margins, rim enhancement, and internal gas (Figs. 10.3 and 10.4).

Fungal Abscess

At ultrasound four appearances of fungal infection have been described:

1. A "wheel within a wheel" appearance featuring a central hypoechoic zone of fungal necrosis surrounded by echogenic inflammatory cells. There may also be a thin hypoechoic rim of fibrosis.
2. A "bull's-eye" appearance with a central echogenic Nidus with a surrounding hypoechoic region. This appearance is seen in patients with active infection.
3. Simply a hypoechoic nodule without other distinguishing features. Unfortunately, this is the most common appearance and also the least specific.
4. An echogenic focus with posterior shadowing. This appearance is typically seen during early resolution.

At contrast-enhanced CT, the typical finding is multiple, small, hypoattenuating lesions throughout the liver. The lesions typically enhance centrally (though less than the surrounding liver) and may occasionally enhance peripherally. MRI will demonstrate multiple small lesions throughout the liver which are extremely T2 hyperintense and mildly hypointense on T1-weighted images (Fig. 10.5). Gadolinium-enhanced T1-weighted images will show hypointense lesions when compared to the surrounding liver.

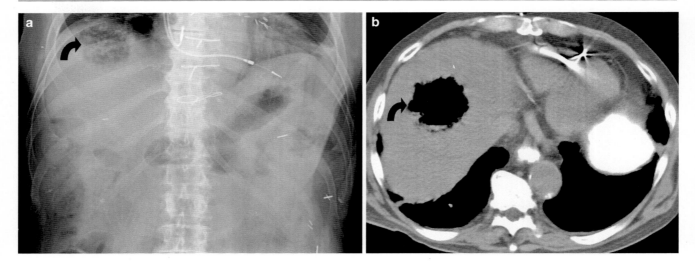

Fig. 10.4 Hepatic abscess. (**a**) Plain film of the upper abdomen demonstrates a round collection of gas in the right upper quadrant (*curved arrow*). This would be an atypical appearance and location of bowel gas. (**b**) Contrast-enhanced CT through the upper abdomen confirms a large collection of air within the liver with some layering debris (*curved arrow*), diagnostic of abscess

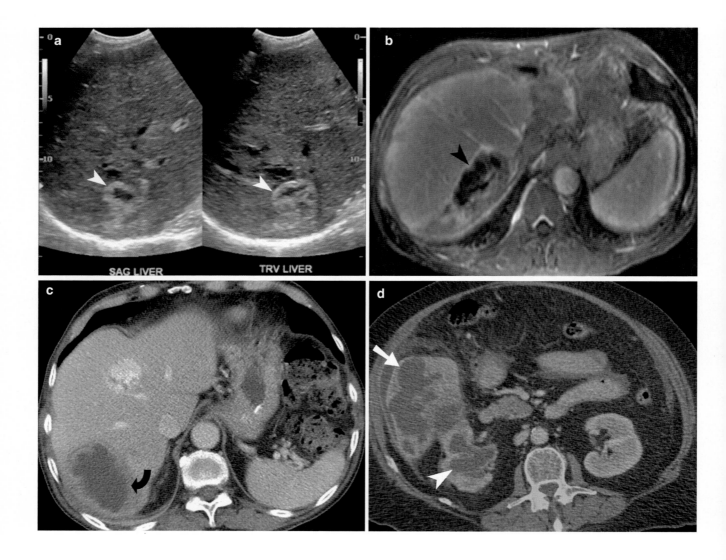

Amebic Abscess

Although amebic abscesses may appear very similar to pyogenic abscesses, one helpful clue is the tendency for amebic abscesses to spread beyond the liver. Findings of a right pleural effusion or intraperitoneal rupture suggest the diagnosis of amebic abscess [6].

Amebic abscesses are typically oval abscesses seen near the capsule, generally hypoechoic on ultrasound, with low level internal echoes and no wall echoes. There may be increased through transmission. Contrast-enhanced CT will show a complex fluid collection with rim enhancement and peripheral edema. Internal septa or fluid-debris levels may be identified [3, 6]. MRI, if utilized, will generally show a high-intensity T2 lesion with low intensity on T1. Fifty percent will have surrounding edema, best appreciated on the T2 sequence [3].

Hydatid Cyst

Though rarely seen in the USA, hydatid cysts are endemic to the Mediterranean Basin. The disease is spread through ingesting the eggs of Echinococcus granulosus, a tapeworm. Dogs act as a reservoir for the spread of disease. Hydatid cysts often go undetected, but patients may present secondary to cyst rupture, mass effect of the cyst, or superimposed infection [2].

Histologically, hydatid cysts consist of three layers. The outer pericyst is composed of compressed liver; the middle ectocyst, a thin membrane; and the inner endocyst, a germinal layer [3].

Imaging

Imaging characteristics of hydatid cysts vary from a cystic lesion to a solid pseudotumor. The classic appearance is the "water lily sign," which is actually wavy bands of delaminated endocyst. Daughter cysts and peripheral calcifications are commonly seen.

On CT, hydatid cysts will generally present as hypoattenuating lesions with a distinguishable wall. Fifty percent will have peripheral wall calcifications, and a daughter cyst can be identified in 75 % (Fig. 10.6) [3]. MRI is excellent for delineating the pericyst, which will be hypointense on both T1- and T2-weighted images secondary to fibrosis and

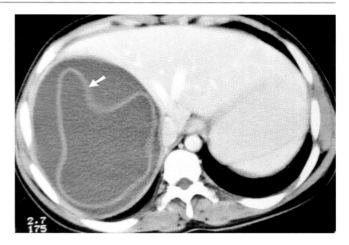

Fig. 10.6 Hydatid cyst. Contrast-enhanced CT of the abdomen demonstrates a large, cystic lesion within the right lobe of the liver. Internally, there is a delaminated endocyst (*arrow*); this is equivalent to the water lily sign described on ultrasound

calcification. The hydatid matrix will generally be extremely T2 hyperintense and T1 hypointense. The daughter cyst, if identified, will be T1 and T2 hypointense.

Fitz-Hugh-Curtis Syndrome

Fitz-Hugh-Curtis syndrome is a fairly uncommon sequel of advanced pelvic inflammatory disease in which there is intraperitoneal spread of infection from the pelvis into the right upper quadrant. These patients present with fever, vaginal discharge, cervical motion tenderness, and right upper quadrant pain [2]. The differential diagnosis includes other causes of "perihepatitis" such as perforated cholecystitis, radiation changes, and perforated abscess [7].

Imaging findings include early arterial enhancement of the anterior surface of the liver on contrasted CT with findings of PID in pelvis (pyosalpinx, inflammation) [7, 8]. Ultrasound will typically appear normal [2].

Hepatic Infarct

Hepatic infarcts are generally rare because of the dual blood supply of the liver [9]. They are generally seen after insult to the hepatic artery or portal vein thrombus in the setting of chronic hepatic arterial insufficiency [10]. However, the one

Fig. 10.5 Hepatic abscesses. (**a**) Transverse and sagittal gray-scale ultrasound images of the liver demonstrate a hypoechoic lesion with a hyperechoic rim (*white arrowhead*). (**b**) Gadolinium-enhanced T1-weighted MRI in the same patient shows a necrotic lesion (*black arrowhead*) in the right lobe of the liver with faint peripheral enhancement. This is a case of treated enterococcal abscess. (**c**) Contrast-enhanced CT of the abdomen shows a fluid density lesion with an irregular wall, consistent with abscess (*curved arrow*). Incidentally note is made of a hemangioma, located more anteriorly in the right lobe of liver. (**d**) Contrast-enhanced CT abdomen through the inferior aspect of the liver demonstrates an irregular abscess (*arrow*), communicating with pyonephrosis (*arrowhead*)

occasion when hepatic infarcts are more common is after liver transplant. In this setting, the hepatic artery plays a larger role in supplying blood to the liver. Any insult to the hepatic artery, without the "backup" of the portal vein, will therefore result in infarction.

The causes of hepatic infarction include trauma, shock, hypercoagulable state, post-TIPS, and posttransplant status. Because the hepatic artery is the sole blood supply to the bile ducts, hepatic arterial occlusion can lead to biliary necrosis with the eventual formation of bile lakes [10, 11].

Imaging

On CT, hepatic infarcts are generally seen as wedge-shaped peripheral areas of hypoattenuation, often paralleling the bile ducts (Fig. 10.7a) [9–11]. These areas may show heterogeneous enhancement, with lack of enhancement in any necrotic regions. Gas may be seen within the infarct, secondary to either necrosis or superinfection. Bile lakes, or bilomas after biliary necrosis, may be seen as irregular, hypoattenuating regions, often in posttransplant patients with hepatic arterial compromise (Fig. 10.7b). Arterial phase imaging can be used to evaluate the hepatic artery for any insult. Conversely, portal venous phase imaging will help assess for any portal vein thrombus. One etiologic clue is to search for associated splenic infarcts, which would suggest either systemic hypoperfusion (shock) or embolic disease.

Budd-Chiari Syndrome

Budd-Chiari syndrome is caused by occlusion of the hepatic veins or inferior vena cava. This impairs venous outflow, causing hepatic congestion, decreased portal venous flow, and eventual necrosis and atrophy [12]. There are multiple causes of Budd-Chiari, the most common being a hypercoagulable state. Nearly all patients have some degree of abdominal pain, and ascites is nearly always present.

The most common form is the subacute form, in which there has been some time to develop collateral vessels. Rarely, patients can present with fulminant hepatic failure with massive necrosis, ascites, and encephalopathy. The changes consistent with portal hypertension (splenomegaly and varices) may be seen in more subacute to chronic forms. The caudate lobe of the liver is generally spared secondary to separate venous drainage into the IVC.

Imaging

Ultrasound, CT, and MRI are all useful in imaging Budd-Chiari syndrome. Color Doppler ultrasound is extremely helpful in detecting diminished or absent venous outflow from the liver as well as in detecting echogenic thrombus with the hepatic veins or IVC. The secondary findings of splenomegaly and ascites may be seen as well.

In the acute phase of Budd-Chiari syndrome, unenhanced CT will generally show an enlarged liver with decreased attenuation [10, 12]. The IVC may appear hyperattenuating on noncontrast imaging secondary to the presence of a thrombus [9]. After contrast enhancement, the classic pattern is early arterial enhancement of the caudate lobe and central liver with diffuse peripheral hypoattenuation secondary to necrosis and/or steatosis (Fig. 10.8). On the portal venous phase images, there may be a "flip-flop," with contrast washout from the central liver and peripheral enhancement due to flow from capsular veins [10]. Hypoattenuating clot may be seen within the hepatic veins or IVC. More chronically, the liver will appear dysmorphic with peripheral atrophy, caudate hypertrophy, and heterogeneous enhancement secondary to fibrosis and nodular regeneration [10, 12]. Secondary findings of portal hypertension including splenomegaly, ascites, and varices may be seen as well.

On MRI, acute phase imaging will show decreased T1 signal and heterogeneously increased T2 signal at the liver periphery [12]. Chronically, effected portions of the liver will become fibrotic, resulting in hypointensity on both T1- and T2-weighted images.

Spontaneous Nontraumatic Hepatic Hematoma

Spontaneous hepatic hematoma without trauma is a fairly rare entity, usually seen in the setting of hepatic neoplasm. By far the two most common etiologies are hemorrhage into a hepatic adenoma and hepatocellular carcinoma, though several other less common etiologies include focal nodular hyperplasia, amebic abscess, metastases, and hemangioma [13].

The findings on CT include hyperattenuating hematoma seen within the liver in the acute phase, though in more chronic phases this may become hypoattenuating.

Adenomas are classically related to females taking oral contraceptives (4 cases/10,000 users) [13]. They may also rarely be seen in the setting of diabetes, glycogen storage disease, iron deposition disease, and anabolic steroid use. Eighty percent of adenomas are solitary, and they are nearly always asymptomatic until they rupture [14]. Because adenomas generally have poor connective tissue support, incomplete capsules, and high peripheral vascularity, they are a perfect setup for extensive hemorrhage.

Unenhanced CT will show a hypoattenuating tumor containing areas of hyperattenuating blood (Fig. 10.9). Subcapsular hematoma and intraperitoneal hematoma may also be visualized. Ten percent of adenomas will contain fat [14].

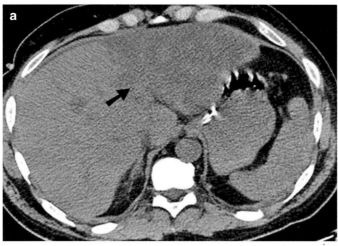
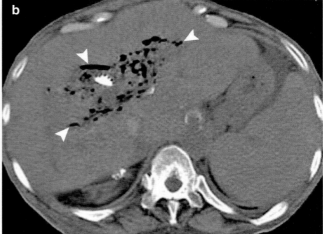

Fig. 10.7 Liver infarct after Whipple procedure and liver transplant. (**a**) Noncontrast CT demonstrates a large, hypoattenuating region occupying the left lobe of the liver, consistent with a large hepatic infarct. *Arrow* denotes a well-delineated transition between normal liver and infarcted liver. (**b**) Noncontrast CT of the transplant liver shows debris with in a dilated biliary tree (*arrowheads*). The patient had hepatic arterial thrombosis, resulting in biliary necrosis

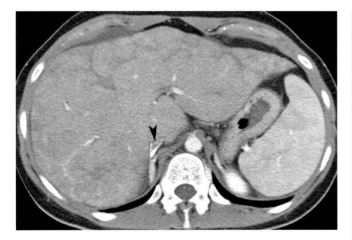

Fig. 10.8 Budd-Chiari syndrome. Contrast-enhanced CT shows areas of hypoattenuating fibrosis and multiple regenerating nodules as well as trace ascites anteriorly. A thrombus (*arrowhead*) can be seen within the inferior vena cava with some contrast passing around the thrombus

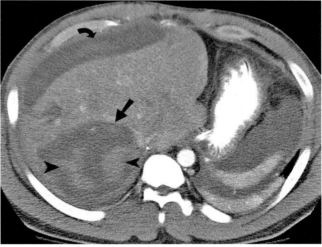

Fig. 10.9 Hemorrhagic adenoma. Contrast-enhanced CT of the abdomen demonstrates areas of mixed attenuation adenoma (*arrow*) within the right lobe of the liver (*arrowheads*), containing hemorrhagic areas (*arrowheads*). There is also subcapsular hematoma (*curved arrow*) anterior to the liver and fluid around the spleen from hemoperitoneum

The appearance on MRI is variable depending on the age of the hematoma.

Treatment of a hemorrhagic adenoma is generally surgical resection of the tumor with a margin of normal liver. Nonhemorrhagic adenomas are generally prophylactically removed if they are larger than 4 cm [14].

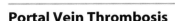

Portal Vein Thrombosis

Portal vein thrombosis is most commonly seen in cirrhotic patients, often as a complication of hepatocellular carcinoma. Other entities such as hypercoagulable states, myeloprolifera-tive disease, embolic phenomenon, and infection can also result in portal vein thrombosis [15]. As discussed previously, patients with portal vein thrombosis may also present with a liver infarct if there is superimposed hepatic arterial insufficiency.

Imaging

Ultrasound is perhaps the most commonly used technique for identifying portal vein thrombosis and discriminating the source. Bland thrombus can be distinguished from tumor

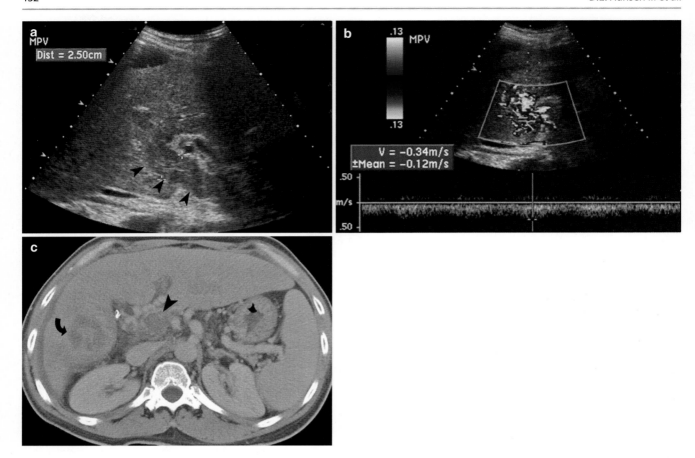

Fig. 10.10 Hepatocellular carcinoma and portal vein thrombus in a patient with hepatitis C. (**a** and **b**) Gray-scale and color Doppler ultrasound of portal vein thrombosis. There is echogenic thrombus within an enlarged portal vein (*arrowheads*). There is arterial flow within the thrombus, consistent with tumor thrombus. (**c**) Contrast-enhanced CT of the same patient shows low-density thrombus within the portal vein (*arrowhead*) as well as a hepatocellular carcinoma in the right lobe of the liver (*curved arrow*)

thrombus because bland thrombus will have no internal flow, whereas tumor thrombus will have internal flow (Fig. 10.10). Secondary findings of cirrhosis, hepatic mass, splenomegaly, and ascites may be seen and help determine the etiology.

On unenhanced CT, hyperattenuating thrombus can be seen within the portal vein. After contrast administration, obstruction of contrast flow can be seen in the portal vein on the portal venous images with the thrombus visualized as a filling defect [15]. If there is any hepatic lesion seen in the setting of cirrhosis and portal vein thrombosis, one should be very careful about calling it anything other than hepatocellular carcinoma.

Splenic Infarct

Though uncommon, splenic infarction is a recognized cause of abdominal pain. Embolic cause from atrial fibrillation is the most common cause of splenic infarct. Other infarcted organs, including the liver, may be seen as well in patients with embolic infarcts of the spleen. Other causes include malignancy and hypercoagulable states [16].

Imaging

The imaging modality of choice for imaging splenic infarction is contrast-enhanced CT (Figs. 10.11 and 10.12). The CT appearance is typically a wedge-shaped, hypoattenuating region within the spleen. Perisplenic fluid, a left-sided pleural effusion, and associated infarcts in other organs are other signs, each present in 30 % of cases. Care must be taken to differentiate a splenic infarction from early, heterogeneous perfusion of the spleen; more delayed images will help differentiate the two. Ultrasound may show wedge-shaped, hypoechoic regions within the spleen but is not very sensitive [16, 17]. MRI will show a region of low T1 and T2 intensity which does not enhance [18].

Fig. 10.11 Splenic infarct before and after. Left-side image shows a normal spleen. Image on the right in the same patient demonstrates diffuse decreased density within the spleen (*arrow*) secondary to infarct of the entire spleen

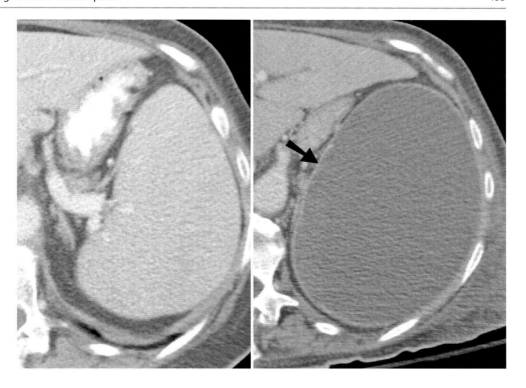

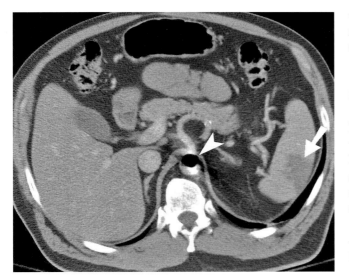

Fig. 10.12 Splenic infarct secondary to intra-aortic balloon pump. Contrast-enhanced CT demonstrates a wedge-shaped hypodense region within the spleen consistent with infarct (*arrow*). Intra-aortic balloon pump (*arrowhead*) is seen in the aorta adjacent to the origin of the celiac trunk

Splenic Torsion

Splenic torsion is a very uncommon diagnosis, usually seen in the setting of a wandering spleen. With wandering spleen, the spleen can "wander" outside of its usual position in the left upper quadrant due to laxity of splenic ligaments. Patients with a wandering spleen can get spontaneous torsion and may present with an acute abdomen secondary to torsion splenic ischemia [19].

Imaging

Like torsion to other organs, splenic torsion is diagnosed when there is evidence of decreased blood flow. Color Doppler ultrasound will show decreased vascular flow to a spleen which may be in an ectopic position. CT may show an ectopic spleen with poor enhancement and decreased attenuation on noncontrasted studies (Fig. 10.13).

Hematoma

Spontaneous, nontraumatic splenic hematoma or rupture is a rare pathology, seen most often in patients with splenomegaly, from either malignancy (leukemia or lymphoma) or infection (infectious mononucleosis, CMV infection, and malaria) [20].

Like hematomas in other locations, spontaneous splenic hematomas are most easily diagnosed with CT as heterogeneous pseudo-masses within the spleen and often extending outside of the splenic parenchyma. The spleen itself may be enlarged with a sizeable hematoma, giving onion skin appearance (Fig. 10.14). Hemoperitoneum may also be present if there is extension of hematoma outside of the spleen.

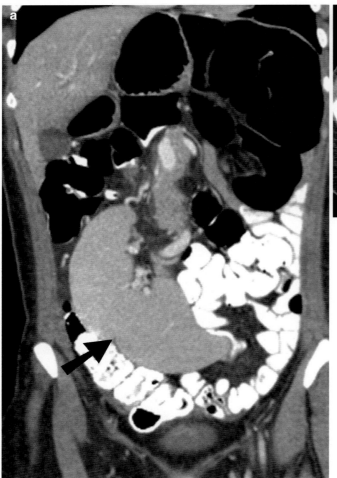

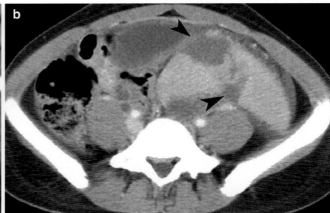

Fig. 10.13 Wandering spleen and splenic torsion. (**a**) Coronal CT reformation with oral and IV contrast demonstrates an ectopic location of the spleen (*arrow*) within the pelvis due to ligamentous laxity. There is normal enhancement of the spleen. (**b**) Contrast-enhanced CT through the pelvis demonstrates an ectopic location of the spleen. Additionally, there are multiple hypodense regions within the spleen (*arrowheads*) consistent with infarcts from vascular compromise

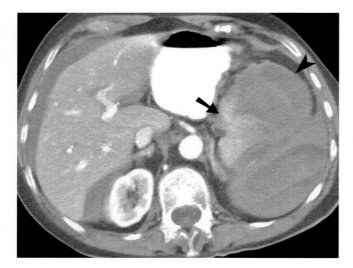

Fig. 10.14 Spontaneous splenic hematoma. Contrast-enhanced CT of the abdomen demonstrates a large subcapsular splenic hematoma (*arrowhead*) compressing the spleen (*arrow*) in a patient with no history of trauma. There is associated high-density fluid around the liver, hemoperitoneum

Teaching Points

- The most common ultrasound appearance of a fungal infection in the liver is a hypoechoic nodule.
- The imaging findings of acute hepatitis include increased echogenicity of the portal tracts and gallbladder wall thickening.
- Common findings associated with splenic infarction include wedge-shaped hypodensity, perisplenic fluid, left-sided pleural effusion, and infarcts in other organs.
- Hepatocellular carcinoma should be suspected in a patient with cirrhosis with portal vein thrombus, intrahepatic hematoma, and subcapsular hematoma.
- Imaging findings in acute Budd-Chiari include contrast washout from the central areas of the liver on enhanced CT during the portal venous phase and sparing of the caudate lobe.

References

1. Kumar V, Abbas AK, Fausto N. Robins and Cotran: pathologic basis of disease. 7th ed. Philadelphia: Saunders; 2004.
2. Kasper DL et al. Harrison's principles of internal medicine. 16th ed. New York: McGraw-Hill; 2005.
3. Mortele KJ, Segatto E, Ros PR. The infected liver: radiologic-pathologic correlation. Radiographics. 2004;4:937–55.
4. Itai Y, Sekiyama K, Ahmadi T, Obuchi M, Yoshiba M. Fulminant hepatic failure: observation with serial CT. Radiology. 1997;202: 379–82.
5. Murakami T, Baron RL, Peterson MS. Liver necrosis and regeneration after fulminant hepatitis: pathologic correlation with CT and MR findings. Radiology. 1996;198:239–42.
6. Radin DR, Ralls PW, Colletti PM, Halls JM. CT of amebic liver abscess. AJR Am J Roentgenol. 1988;150:1297–301.
7. Kim S, Kim TU, Lee JW, Lee TH, Lee SH, Jeon TY, et al. The perihepatic space: comprehensive anatomy and ct features of pathologic conditions. Radiographics. 2007;27:129–43.
8. Joo SH, Kim MJ, Lim JS, Kim JH, Kim KW. CT diagnosis of Fitz-Hugh and Curtis syndrome: value of the arterial phase scan. Korean J Radiol. 2007;8:40–7.
9. Kawamoto S, Soyer PA, Fishman EK, Bluemke DA. Nonneoplastic liver disease: evaluation with CT and MR imaging. Radiographics. 1998;18:827–48.
10. Torabi M, Hosseinzadeh K, Federle MP. CT of nonneoplastic hepatic vascular and perfusion disorders. Radiographics. 2008;28: 1967–82.
11. Smith GS, Birnbaum BA, Jacobs JE. Hepatic infarction secondary to arterial insufficiency in native livers: CT findings in 10 patients. Radiology. 1998;208:223–9.
12. Cura M, Haskal Z, Lopera J. Diagnostic and interventional radiology for Budd Chiari syndrome. Radiographics. 2009;29:669–81.
13. Casillas VJ, Amendola MA, Gascue A, Pinar N, Levi JU, Perez JM. Imaging of nontraumatic hemorrhagic hepatic lesions. Radiographics. 2000;20:367–8.
14. Grazioli L, Federle MP, Brancatelli G, Ichikawa T, Olivetti L, Blachar A. Hepatic adenomas: imaging and pathologic findings. Radiographics. 2001;21:877–94.
15. Gallego C, Velasco M, Marcuello P, Tejedor D, Campo LD, Friera A. Congenital and acquired anomalies of the portal venous system. Radiographics. 2002;22:141–59.
16. Antopolsky M, Hiller N, Salameh S, Goldshtein B, Stalnikowicz R. Splenic infarction: 10 years of experience. Am J Emerg Med. 2009;27:262–5.
17. Goerg C, Schwerk W. Splenic infarction: sonographic patterns, diagnosis, follow-up, and complications. Radiology. 1990;174: 803–7.
18. Elsayes KM, Narra VR, Mukundan G, Lewis JS, Menias CO, Heiken JP. MR imaging of the spleen: spectrum of abnormalities. Radiographics. 2005;25:967–82.
19. Herman TE, Siegel MJ. CT of acute splenic torsion in children with wandering spleen. AJR Am J Roentgenol. 1991;156:151–3.
20. Furlan A, Fakhran S, Federle MP. Sponateous abdominal hemorrhage: causes, CT findings, and clinical implications. AJR Am J Roentgenol. 2009;193:1077–87.

Caterina Missiroli and Ajay Singh

Acute pancreatitis is the most common inflammatory process affecting the pancreas [1]. In the USA, more than 200,000 patients are admitted for acute pancreatitis per year, costing more than $2 billion annually. The frequency of hospital admission for acute pancreatitis has been progressively increasing, resulting in higher medical care cost. Certain groups of population (blacks and older patients) have disproportionately high hospitalization rates for pancreatitis.

Acute Pancreatitis

The cause of acute pancreatitis is believed to be pancreatic autodigestion by pancreatic enzymes. In adults, 70–80 % of cases of pancreatitis are due to biliary stones or alcohol [2, 3]. In children the most frequent causes are blunt trauma, drugs (steroids and furosemide), infection (mumps, coxsackievirus, ascariasis, *E. coli*), or hereditary disorders, such as hemolytic-uremic syndrome, gene mutation (cationic trypsinogen), and biliary tract anomalies [1, 4].

Classification

The Atlanta classification for acute pancreatitis was introduced in 1992 and classified acute pancreatitis into mild and severe groups [5]. Mild pancreatitis results in edematous

C. Missiroli, MD
Diagnostic Imaging Department,
Azienda Ospedaliera della Provincia di
Lecco – Presidio Ospedaliero A. Manzoni,
Lecco, Italy

A. Singh, MD (✉)
Department of Radiology,
Massachusetts General Hospital,
Harvard Medical School,
10 Museum Way, # 524, Boston, MA 02141, USA
e-mail: asingh1@partners.org

pancreatic parenchyma, which results in uneventful recovery with conservative management. Severe pancreatitis is associated with organ failure and complications such as pseudocyst formation, pancreatic necrosis, and pancreatic abscess formation. In 2008, Acute Pancreatitis Classification Working Group revised the Atlanta classification system to improve clinical assessment as well as clarify appropriate terms for pancreatic/peripancreatic fluid collections. This classification defines pancreatitis in two categories, including interstitial edematous pancreatitis and necrotizing pancreatitis with pancreatic parenchymal necrosis and/or peripancreatic necrosis.

The classification defines four types of collections associated with pancreatitis. These are acute peripancreatic fluid collection (<4-week-old), pseudocyst (>4-week-old), acute postnecrotic collection (<4-week-old), and walled-off necrosis (>4-week-old).

Balthazar et al. described CT severity index, giving scores from 0 to 4 for various findings of acute pancreatitis (Table 11.1) [6]. A composite score of 6 is associated with >50 % frequency of pancreatic necrosis.

Table 11.1 CT severity index

CT finding	CT grade	Score
Normal pancreas	A	0
Focal or diffuse enlargement of the pancreas	B	1
Inflammatory changes in peripancreatic fat	C	2
Single fluid collection	D	3
≥2 collections and/or gas in/ adjacent to pancreas	E	4
Necrosis (%)		Score
<30		2
30–50		4
>50		6

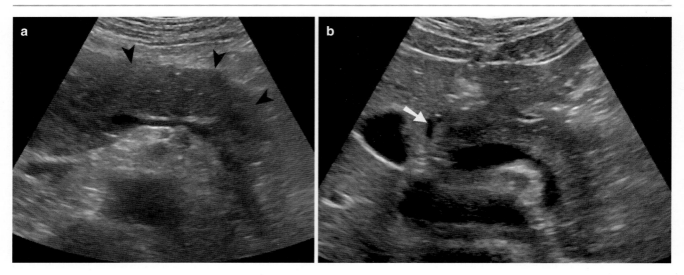

Fig. 11.1 Acute edematous pancreatitis. (**a**) Ultrasound shows pancreatic enlargement (*arrowheads*) with hypoechogenicity of the pancreatic parenchyma caused by pancreatic parenchymal edema. (**b**) Ultrasound shows hypoechoic pancreatic parenchyma and small peripancreatic fluid (*white arrow*)

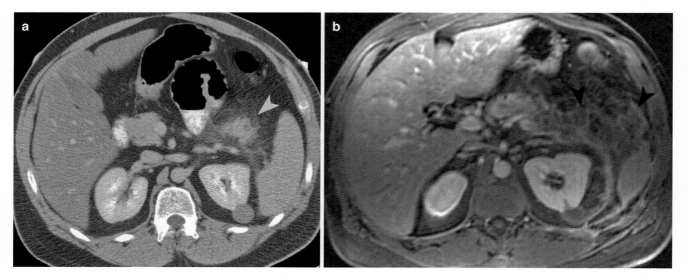

Fig. 11.2 Acute edematous pancreatitis. (**a**) Contrast-enhanced CT image shows fat stranding around the pancreatic tail (*arrowhead*) due to oedematous pancreatitis. (**b**) Contrast-enhanced MR shows heterogeneous inflammation (*arrowhead*) around the pancreatic tail with thickening of the lateroconal fascia

Imaging

When imaging is required, contrast-enhanced CT and ultrasound are both considered first-line imaging modality for the initial assessment of acute pancreatitis in patients with elevated amylase and/or lipase but no fever or evidence of fluid loss (Fig. 11.1). Ultrasound is primarily used to assess for gallstones, and contrast-enhanced CT is the most appropriate imaging modality for the assessment of pancreatic parenchyma in children and adults. For the assessment of pancreatitis in patients who are not improving after 48 h of presentation, contrast-enhanced CT and MRI with MRCP are both considered the equally appropriate first-line imaging modalities (Fig. 11.2).

Ultrasound is often limited by technical factors such as obesity and bowel gas, thereby limiting its usefulness for purposes other than biliary assessment. The CT imaging findings of acute pancreatitis include pancreatic enlargement, ill definition of the peripancreatic fat planes, extrapancreatic fluid collection, dilated pancreatic duct, and pancreatobiliary calculus (Figs. 11.3 and 11.4). Interstitial edematous pancreatitis is seen on CT as localized or diffuse pancreatic enlargement with homogeneous or heterogeneous enhancement. Necrotizing pancreatitis is characterized by lack of pancreatic parenchymal enhancement. The extent of pancreatic necrosis is categorized as less than 30 %, 30–50 %, and more than 50 % of the pancreas. Areas of no or poor

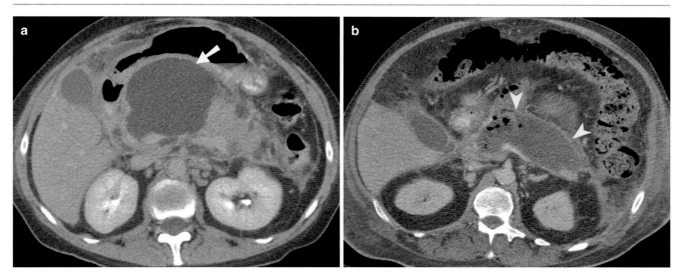

Fig. 11.3 Pancreatic collections. (**a**) Contrast-enhanced CT shows pancreatic enlargment due to a dominant pancreatic head collection (*arrow*). (**b**) Contrast-enhanced CT shows pancreatic parenchymal necrosis with intrapancreatic fluid (*arrowheads*) and air

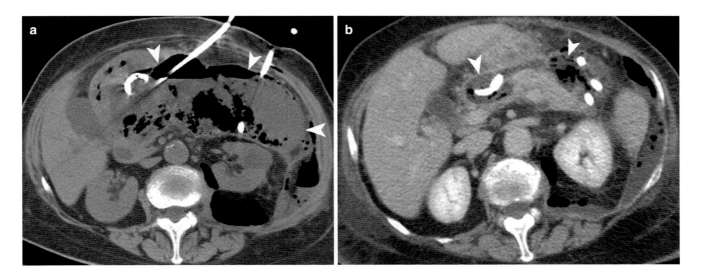

Fig. 11.4 Pancreatic collection. (**a**) Noncontrast CT obtained immediately after image-guided pigtail catheter placement demonstrates a large lesser sac fluid- and air-containing collection (*white arrowheads*). There are collections also seen in left posterior pararenal space and left paracolic gutter. (**b**) Follow-up contrast-enhanced CT image shows marked improvement in the lesser sac fluid collection (*white arrowheads*)

enhancement in less than 30 % of the pancreas categorized as necrosis may on a follow-up CT actually represent changes of edematous pancreatitis rather than necrosis.

MRI is useful in stable patients because of the capacity of identifying as well as grading the inflammatory process and detecting ducts and their obstruction or disruption when present [2, 3, 7]. The detection of the type fluid composition is also possible on MRI in patients with complicated pancreatitis (e.g., hemorrhagic, necrotic) (Figs. 11.5 and 11.6).

The complications of acute pancreatitis include hemorrhage, necrosis, abscesses, pseudocyst, and pseudoaneurysm [3] (Figs. 11.7, 11.8, 11.9, and 11.10). Symptomatic collections and pseudocysts are often best treated with image-guided catheter drainage. ERCP is used for diagnosis as well

as treatment of stone-related pancreatitis and is often used when a stone is seen obstructing the pancreatobiliary duct on MRCP (Figs. 11.11 and 11.12).

Acute Pancreatitis in Pancreatic Cancer

Pancreatic inflammation is possible in the presence of a neoplasm, usually adenocarcinoma, lymphoma, or metastasis. Acute pancreatitis is caused by neoplasm in 1–2 % of the cases [1]. The pancreatitis is usually due to ductal obstruction by a pancreatic head mass.

In patients over the age of 40 with first episode of pancreatitis and no identifiable cause, contrast-enhanced CT

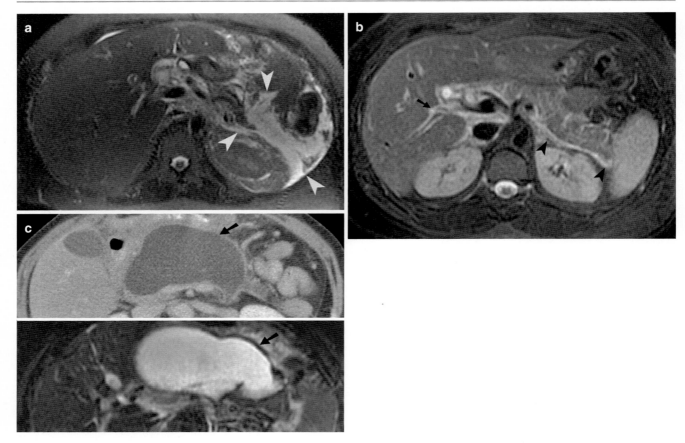

Fig. 11.5 Acute pancreatitis on MRI. (**a**) TSE-T2-weighted sequence shows extensive hyperintense peripancreatic inflammatory process (*arrowheads*) in the left anterior pararenal space. (**b**) Post-gadolinium T1-weighted sequence in a patient with amylase level of 2,300 units per liter shows peripancreatic inflammation (*arrowheads*) and periportal edema (*arrow*). (**c**) Contrast-enhanced CT and corresponding FSE-T2-weighted MRI sequence shows pancreatic necrosis and large homogeneous fluid collection (*arrows*) within the pancreas

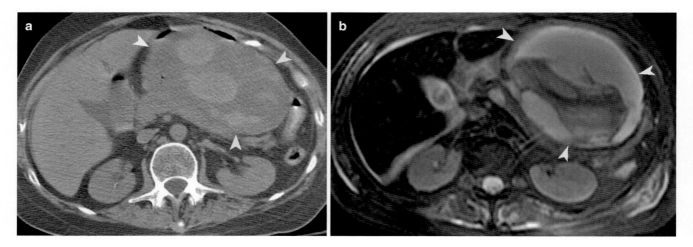

Fig. 11.6 Pseudocyst with bleeding. (**a**, **b**) Noncontrast-enhanced CT and T2-weighted MR image shows a large lesser sac pseudocyst (*arrowheads*) containing blood clots from recent bleeding

should be used to exclude an underlying neoplastic process. The diagnosis of the pancreatic neoplasm is usually delayed because of the inflammatory changes masking the tumor. Imaging findings useful in making the diagnosis of underlying neoplasm include significant enlargement of ducts, pancreatic head enlargement disproportionate to the rest of the gland, lymphadenopathy, metastasis, and vascular involvement. The definite diagnosis can be made with endoscopic or image-guided biopsy.

Traumatic Injuries

Pancreatic injury is relatively uncommon, accounting for 2 % of all abdominal traumas. In patients with pancreatic injury, the mortality is high, ranging from 9 to 34 % [4, 8]. Majority of the patients have associated other visceral organ

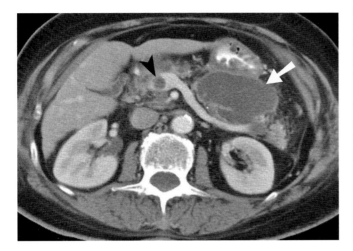

Fig. 11.7 Portal vein thrombosis. Contrast-enhanced CT image shows a thrombus in the main portal vein (*arrowhead*) which developed secondary to acute pancreatitis. There is an intrapancreatic collection (*arrow*) seen within the pancreatic body

injury, which is the major cause of mortality within 48 h after injury.

The pancreatic injury may involve the duct (type I) or duct as well as pancreatic parenchyma (type II) (Table 11.2) (Fig. 11.13). In children the common causes of pancreatic injury include bicycle accident and abuse. In adults motor vehicle accident is the most common cause, followed by less common causes such as sports injury, fall, and blow to the abdomen [8].

Contrast-enhanced CT is the most frequently used imaging tool in trauma patients and is the best technique for the diagnosis of pancreatic injuries in stable patients [9]. The sensitivity of CT in detecting pancreatic trauma is approximately 80 %. CT tends to underestimate the severity of pancreatic injury. The CT findings of pancreatic trauma include pancreatic lacerations (seen as linear hypodensity), edema, or hemorrhage.

Pancreatic contusions are seen as focal or diffuse hypodensity in the pancreas (Fig. 11.14). A pancreatic laceration of more than one-half the diameter of the pancreatic thickness indicates the presence of main pancreatic ductal injury. The presence of fluid between the splenic vein and the pancreas is a helpful CT finding for the diagnosis of pancreatic injury after blunt abdominal trauma [10].

Documenting the integrity of the pancreatic duct is important for triaging the patient and predicting the prognosis. MRCP is the best noninvasive modality in the evaluation of the pancreatic duct. T2-weighted MRI sequence is sensitive in the detection of pancreatic parenchymal injury as well as peripancreatic inflammation (Fig. 11.15). ERCP allows evaluation of the pancreatic

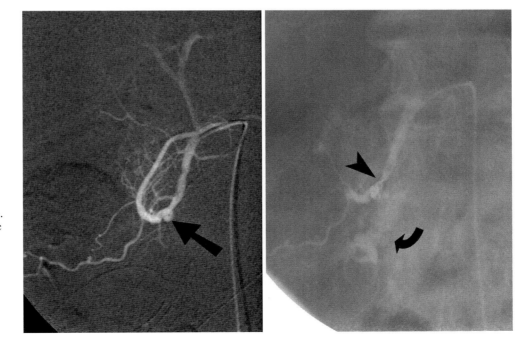

Fig. 11.8 Postpancreatitis gastroduodenal artery aneurysm. Digital subtraction angiographic images show the presence of an aneurysm (*arrow*) along the course of the gastroduodenal artery. The second image obtained after aneurysm coiling (*arrowhead*) demonstrates contrast extravasation (*curved arrow*)

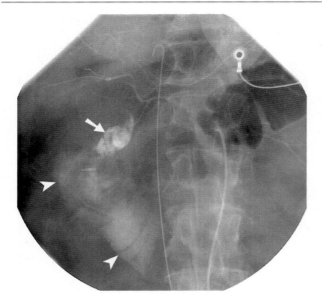

Fig. 11.9 Gastroduodenal artery aneurysm. Conventional angiogram demonstrates contrast extravasation (*arrowheads*) into the duodenal lumen from a large gastroduodenal artery aneurysm (*arrow*)

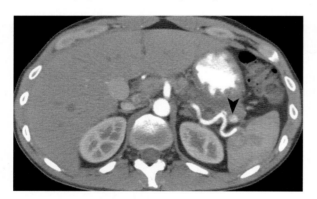

Fig. 11.10 Splenic artery aneurysm. Contrast-enhanced CT shows a subcentimeter pseudoaneurysm (*arrowhead*) within the pancreatic tail, adjacent to the splenic artery

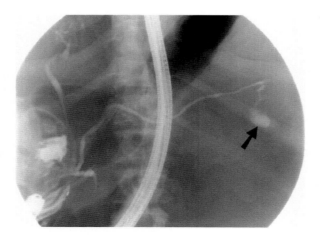

Fig. 11.11 Pancreatic duct leak. ERCP spot film shows the presence of contrast leaking (*arrow*) the main pancreatic duct, in the tail of the pancreas. The resultant collection was drained using image-guided pigtail catheter drainage

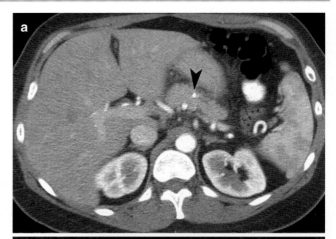

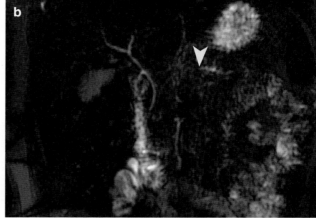

Fig. 11.12 Pancreatic duct stone. (**a**) Contrast-enhanced CT shows a small calculus (*arrowhead*) in the main pancreatic duct, causing ductal obstruction and pancreatitis. (**b**) MRCP shows main pancreatic ductal obstruction (*arrowhead*) caused by the calculus, located 8 cm from the ampulla

Table 11.2 Grading of pancreatic injury

	Grading of injuries
I	No ductal injury, hematoma and minor laceration
II	Hematoma and major laceration/contusion, no ductal injury
III	Distal laceration/transaction with duct injury
IV	Proximal laceration/transaction with biliary duct injury and ampullar lesion
V	Massive head injury

duct integrity and placement of patent. The imaging findings of pancreatic trauma include pancreatic enlargement, hypoattenuating laceration/contusion, pancreatic duct discontinuity, peripancreatic stranding, fluid collection, and hematoma.

Complications occur in 30–60 % of patients with pancreatic injury and include fistulas, pancreatitis, pseudocysts, abscess, hemorrhage, sepsis, and multiorgan failure. Surgical

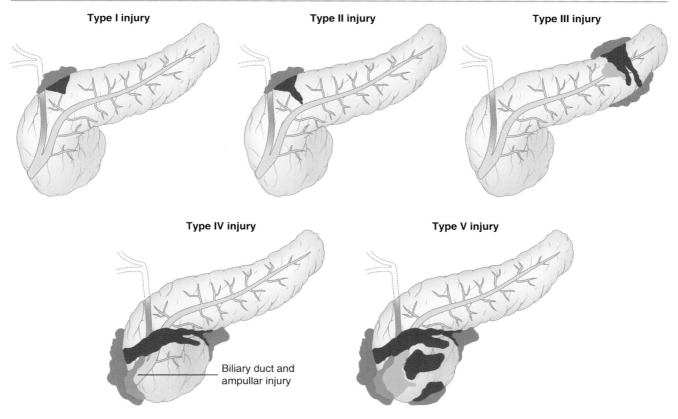

Fig. 11.13 Grading of pancreatic injury

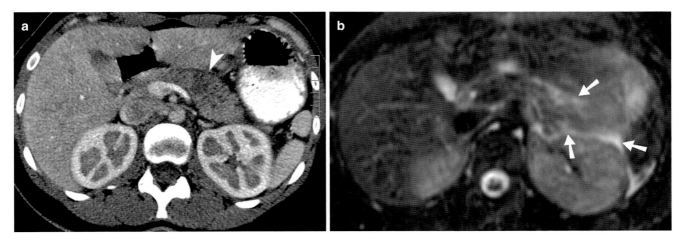

Fig. 11.14 Pancreatic contusion. (**a**) Contrast-enhanced CT demonstrates a low-density contusion (*arrowhead*) in the pancreatic body in a patient with history of blunt trauma. (**b**) T2-weighted sequence demonstrates prepancreatic hyperintensity (*arrows*) produced by edema in the retroperitoneum

treatment is required for penetrating traumas and severe blunt injuries (grades III–V), active hemorrhage, and ductal transection [11]. Image-guided drainage can be used for pseudocyst, infected collection, and postoperative seroma.

Summary

• In adults, 70–80 % of cases of pancreatitis are due to biliary stones or alcohol.

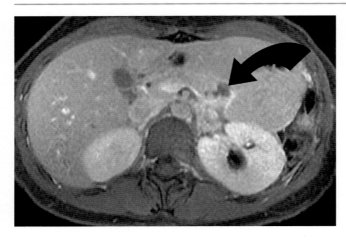

Fig. 11.15 Pancreatic laceration. Contrast-enhanced MRI study demonstrates pancreatic laceration (*arrow*) which had disrupted the main pancreatic duct

- The revised Atlanta classification system divides acute pancreatitis into acute edematous pancreatitis and necrotizing pancreatitis.
- In patients over the age of 40 with first episode of pancreatitis and no identifiable cause, contrast-enhanced CT should be used to exclude an underlying neoplastic process.
- According to CT severity index, a composite score of 6 is associated with >50 % frequency of pancreatic necrosis.

References

1. Shanbhogue AKP, Fasih N, Surabhi VR, Doherty GP, Shanbhogue DKP, Sethi SK. A clinical and radiologic review of uncommon types and causes of pancreatitis. Radiographics. 2009;29:1003–26.
2. Kim YS, Kim Y, Kim SK, Rhim H. Computed tomographic differentiation between alcoholic and gallstone pancreatitis: significance of distribution of infiltration or fluid collection. World J Gastroenterol. 2006;12(28):4524–8.
3. Xiao B, Zhang XM, Tang W, Zeng NL, Zhai ZH. Magnetic resonance imaging for local complications of acute pancreatitis: a pictorial review. World J Gastroenterol. 2010;16(22):2735–42.
4. Vaughn DD, Jabra AA, Fishman EK. Pancreatic disease in children and young adults: evaluation with CT. Radiographics. 1998;18:1171–87.
5. Thoeni RF. The revised Atlanta classification of acute pancreatitis: its importance for the radiologist and its effect on treatment. Radiology. 2012;262(3):751–64.
6. Balthazar EJ, Robinson DL, Megibow AJ, Ranson JHC. Acute pancreatitis: value of CT in establishing prognosis. Radiology. 1990;174:331–6.
7. Vanzulli GA. Role of MR imaging in the diagnostic work-up of acute pancreatitis. JOP. 2006;7(1):110–2.
8. Linsenmaier U, Wirth S, Reiser M, Körner M. Diagnosis and classification of pancreatic and duodenal injuries in emergency radiology. Radiographics. 2008;28:1591–601.
9. Gupta A, Stuhlfaut JW, Fleming KW, Lucey BC, Soto JA. Blunt trauma of the pancreas and biliary tract: a multimodality imaging approach to diagnosis. Radiographics. 2004;24:1381–95.
10. Lane MJ, Mindelzun RE, Sandhu JS, McCormick VD, Jeffrey RB. CT diagnosis of blunt pancreatic trauma: importance of detecting fluid between the pancreas and the splenic vein. AJR Am J Roentgenol. 1994;163(4):833–5.
11. Henarejos A, Cohen DM, Moossa AR. Management of pancreatic trauma. Ann R Coll Surg Engl. 1983;65:297–300.

Ajay Singh

The aims of a first-trimester ultrasound study include localization of the gestational sac, detection of embryonic demise, detection of multiple pregnancies, and confirmation of gestational age. The American College of Obstetrics and Gynecology and American College of Radiology do not recommend routine ultrasound screening in the first trimester of pregnancy. Typically the endovaginal probes used for assessment of first trimester of pregnancy give more information than transabdominal probes and are typically 5–7.5 MHz [1]. Transabdominal probes used in first trimester are often 3.5–5 MHz.

Gestational Age

Fertilization typically occurs within 24 h on the fallopian tube. The zygote migrates and implants on days 22–25 of the menstrual cycle, 4 days prior to the first missed period. The gestational sac progressively increases in size at the age of 1–1.5 mm per day for the first 2 months.

The gestational age is not same as the fertilization age. The fertilization age is counted from the time of fertilization, while the gestational age is 2 weeks more than the fertilization age.

Menstrual age = 30 days + gestational sac diameter (1 mm is equal to 1 day)

Once the embryonic pole is detected, the crown-rump length measurement is considered the most accurate measurement of gestational age. The mean sac diameter is used to measure the gestational age between 5 and 6 weeks of pregnancy or when the embryo is not identified. The biparietal diameter and the femur length are used for the measurement of gestational age in the second trimester of pregnancy.

Normal Pregnancy

Intradecidual sign refers to focal anechoic eccentrically positioned focus within the endometrium, surrounded by thick echogenic wall (Fig. 12.1a). It is due to the presence of a blastocyst embedded in thickened endometrium. Although it can be seen as early as 3.5 weeks of menstrual age, Laing et al. found low sensitivity of 34–66 % for this sign [2]. It is a useful sign, especially when the endometrial cavity can be reliably separated from the gestational sac [3, 4].

The gestational sac is eccentric to the endometrial canal and measures 1 mm in diameter when a 4-week blastocyst cavity is present. It is possible to see the gestational sac along with the yolk sac (in chorionic cavity) on ultrasound at 4.5–5-week gestational age, when it measures up to 1 cm in diameter. The embryo and the amniotic cavity are very small at this gestational age. The gestational sac typically grows at the rate 1.1 mm/day and measures 1.6 cm by 6 weeks.

Double decidual sac sign refers to the presence of two concentric rings: the inner representing chorion and outer one representing the decidua (Fig. 12.1b). The presence of double decidual sign does not exclude the presence of ectopic pregnancy. It is seen in majority of the pregnancies and is best seen when the gestational sac is approximately 10 mm in diameter.

Yolk sac is the first element identified within the gestational sac, typically at 5 weeks of gestation. It is usually less than 5 mm in diameter and spherical in shape (Fig. 12.1c). A yolk sac which is too small or too large is considered to be abnormal (Table 12.1). The number of yolk sac is equal to the number of amniotic sac.

A. Singh, MD
Department of Radiology,
Massachusetts General Hospital,
Harvard Medical School,
10 Museum Way, # 524, Boston, MA 02141, USA
e-mail: asingh1@partners.org

A. Singh (ed.), *Emergency Radiology*,
DOI 10.1007/978-1-4419-9592-6_12, © Springer Science+Business Media New York 2013

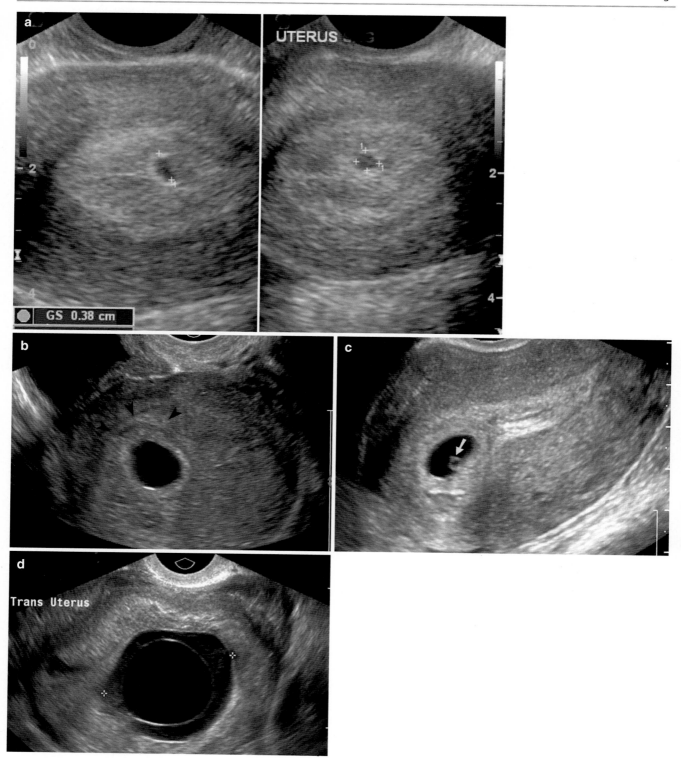

Fig. 12.1 Normal pregnancy. (**a**) Intradecidual sac sign: ultrasound demonstrating a 4-week gestational sac in thickened endometrium, without any identifiable yolk sac or embryo. (**b**) Double decidual sac sign: ultrasound demonstrating concentric hyperechoic rings produced by chorion and decidua (*arrowheads*), around the gestational sac. (**c**) Six weeks: ultrasound demonstrates a yolk sac (*arrow*) and tiny embryo within a 6-week-old pregnancy. (**d**) Nine weeks: ultrasound demonstrates the anechoic amniotic cavity separated from chorionic cavity by the amnion. The chorionic cavity has low-level echoes due to the presence of high protein concentration

Table 12.1 Criteria for abnormal yolk sac

1. More than 5.6 mm (between 5 and 10 weeks) in diameter
2. Less than 2 mm in diameter (between 8 and 12 weeks)
3. Absence of yolk sac in a gestational sac more than 8 mm in diameter
4. Absence of yolk sac in presence of embryo during early pregnancy

Table 12.2 Morphologic findings of pregnancy and the corresponding gestational ages when they appear

Gestational sac	4.5 weeks (in all by 5 weeks)
Yolk sac	5 weeks
Embryo	5.7–6.1 weeks
Embryonic cardiac pulsations	6.2 weeks

The amnion is barely appreciable when the crown-rump length is 2 mm, at gestational age of 6 weeks. It is normal to see an amnion as a separate membrane between 2 and 4 months of gestation (Fig. 12.1d). The chorionic fluid is more echogenic than the amniotic fluid because of the presence of a high protein concentration. The amniotic cavity progressively increases in size and fills the subchorionic cavity by 14–16 weeks. Double bleb refers to the visualization of two concentric blebs due to the presence of a yolk sac and amniotic sac.

Although the embryonic cardiac activity begins at day 26 of menstrual age, they are first seen on sonography when the crown-rump length is 5 mm, at approximately 6.2 weeks. If the crown-rump length is less than 5 mm and no embryonic cardiac pulsations are demonstrated, then the ultrasound should be repeated. The embryonic cardiac activity of less than 80 beats per minute is associated with high risk of embryonic demise.

The reliable criteria to verify the presence of early intrauterine pregnancy include demonstration of yolk sac within the gestational sac and presence of an embryo with cardiac activity (Table 12.2).

Typically transabdominal ultrasound is positive for pregnancy when beta-hCG level is more than 3,600. Intrauterine pregnancies should be seen on transvaginal ultrasound in all when the beta-hCG level is more than 2,000.

Abnormal Gestational Sac

Anembryonic gestation refers to the presence of gestational sac without an embryo. It is due to embryonic death with continued development of the trophoblast and is often due to underlying chromosomal abnormality.

The most important criteria for detection of anembryonic pregnancy are the absence of embryo when the mean sac diameter on transvaginal ultrasound study is more than 18 mm and the absence of yolk sac when the mean sac diameter is more than 13 mm on transvaginal sonography (Fig. 12.2a) (Table 12.3). Since these criteria are not full proof, a follow-up ultrasound should be performed in 7–10 days' time to rule out the possibility of normal pregnancy.

When the fetal pole is more than 6 mm in diameter and no fetal cardiac pulsations are demonstrated, the findings are suggestive of silent miscarriage. If the fetal pole is less than 6 mm in diameter and no fetal cardiac pulsations are demonstrated, then the patient should be rescanned in a week's time to distinguish live from failed pregnancy. If no fetal cardiac activity is seen on 1 week follow-up ultrasound study, then the findings indicate a silent miscarriage. Small sac size, defined by difference of less than 5 mm between mean sac diameter and crown-rump length, is associated with high miscarriage rates. Missed abortion refers to retention of pregnancy for more than or equal to 2 months.

Pregnancy Termination Failure

Termination of pregnancy could be performed within 72 h with more than 80 % success rate with the use of oral misoprostol and mifepristone. In case of failed termination, the sonographic features include presence of intrauterine mass and increased vascularity. The lack of blood flow however does not exclude the presence of retained products of conception. The absence of color Doppler flow favors that the products of conception are nonviable and therefore will pass out spontaneously without the use of dilatation and curettage (Fig. 12.3a, b). Retained products of conception typically produce irregular interface between endometrium and myometrium. If no endometrial mass or fluid is seen and the endometrial stripe thickness is less than 10 mm, retained products of conception are very unlikely. MR imaging may show intracavitary uterine mass with variable enhancement and junctional zone obliteration (Fig. 12.3c, d).

Subchorionic Hemorrhage

Subchorionic hemorrhage refers to separation of the chorionic membrane from the decidua vera by a hematoma. The subchorionic hemorrhage is initially isoechoic or hyperechoic to the placenta and progressively becomes hypoechoic (Fig. 12.4). The earlier the gestational age and larger the size of the hemorrhage, more are the chances of pregnancy loss from subchorionic hemorrhage. We typically describe the size of subchorionic hemorrhage in relation to the proportion (<1/3, 1/3 to 2/3, >2/3, etc.) of circumference of the

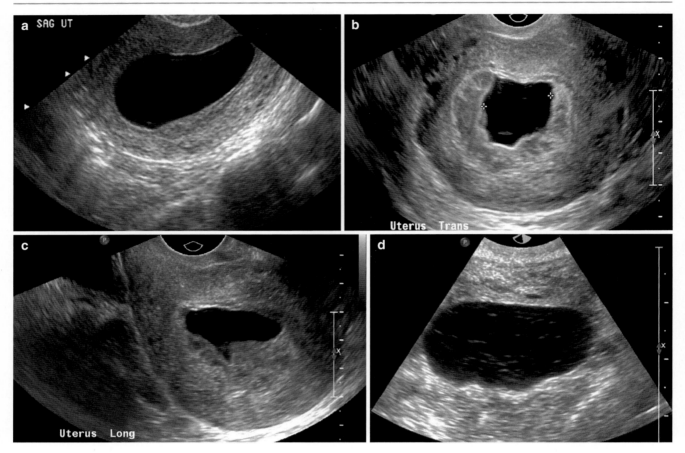

Fig. 12.2 Abnormal gestational sac: anembryonic pregnancy. (**a**) Ultrasound demonstrates anembryonic gestational sac in 8-week-old pregnancy. Lack of embryo in a gestational sac measuring more than 13 mm in diameter is considered abnormal on transvaginal ultrasound. (**b, c**) Ultrasound shows irregular outline of the anembryonic gestational sac on transvaginal ultrasound. (**d**) Ultrasound shows anembryonic 8-week gestational sac, containing low-level internal echoes

Table 12.3 Imaging findings of anembryonic pregnancy

1. Absent embryo when mean sac diameter is 18 mm
2. Absent yolk sac when the mean sac diameter is 13 mm
3. Low-lying gestational sac
4. Irregular shape of the gestational sac (Fig. 12.2b, c)
5. Thin decidual reaction of less than 2 mm thickness
6. Absence of double decidual sac sign
7. Presence of fluid-fluid level or debris within the gestational sac (Fig. 12.2d)

gestational sac covered by the hematoma. The frequency of abortion is higher for larger subchorionic hemorrhage.

Ectopic Pregnancy

The most common location of ectopic pregnancy is in the ampulla, followed by isthmus, fimbria, and cornua of the fallopian tube, in descending frequency. The second most scommon site of ectopic pregnancy which occurs in approximately 2 % is in the intramural portion of the fallopian tube. The presence of a mass within the ovary is unlikely to be ectopic pregnancy because of the rarity of ectopic pregnancy within the ovary. The risk factors for ectopic pregnancy include pelvic inflammatory disease, history of ectopic pregnancy, endometriosis, pelvic surgery, infertility treatment early age at first intercourse, and uterotubal abnormalities. The use of intrauterine device does not increase the risk of ectopic pregnancy.

Ectopic gestational sac can be seen on ultrasound study in anywhere from one-fourth to two-thirds of the cases. The combination of adnexal mass and pelvic free fluid in patients with suspicion of ectopic pregnancy has a high positive predictive value. In up to one-third of patients with proven ectopic pregnancy, the adnexal ultrasound study is normal, while in one-fifth of the cases, a live embryo can be seen within the adnexa. High suspicion of ectopic pregnancy should be raised when there is no intrauterine pregnancy identified on

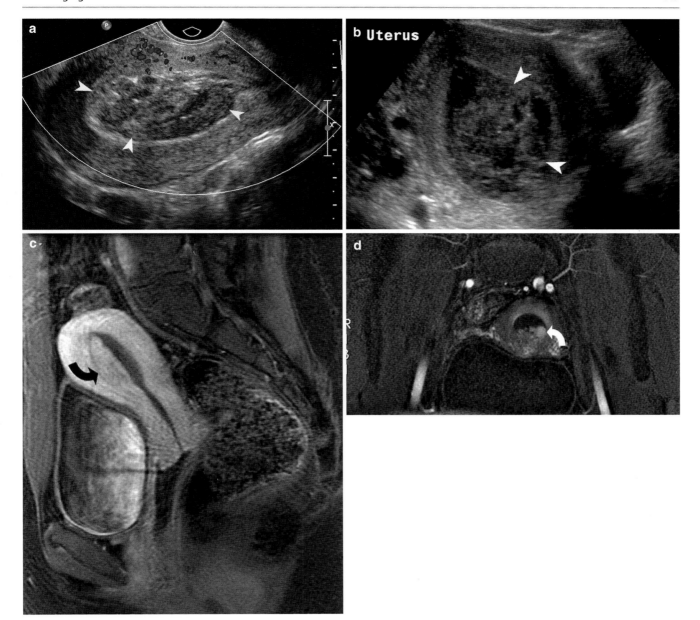

Fig. 12.3 Retained products of conception. Ultrasound demonstrates retained blood clots (**a**) (*arrowheads*) and products of conception (**b**) (*arrowheads*) present within the endometrial cavity. Gadolinium-enhanced MRI (**c**, **d**) demonstrates enhancement of the retained products of conception (*curved arrows*)

ultrasound, in a patient with menstrual age of more than 5 weeks and a positive beta-hCG level.

Ectopic tubal ring consists of a 2–4 mm echogenic rim surrounding a hypoechoic center and is present in 49–68 % cases [5, 6]. The echogenic rim is produced by trophoblast around the chorionic sac, which is more echogenic than the ovarian parenchyma (Figs. 12.5 and 12.6). The color Doppler flow in the fallopian tube on the affected side is typically high velocity with low impedance. The lower resistive index in the affected fallopian tube is believed to be due to invasion

of the trophoblast [7, 8]. The ring of fire sign refers to increased color Doppler flow which can be seen with ectopic pregnancy as well as corpus luteum. The presence of flow within the ectopic pregnancy indicates viable tissue and can be treated with either methotrexate or laparoscopic surgery. Since there are a significant number of patients who have intrauterine pregnancy even when the beta-hCG is more than 2,000 and ultrasound fails to demonstrate a gestational sac, these patients should not be automatically considered to have ectopic pregnancy.

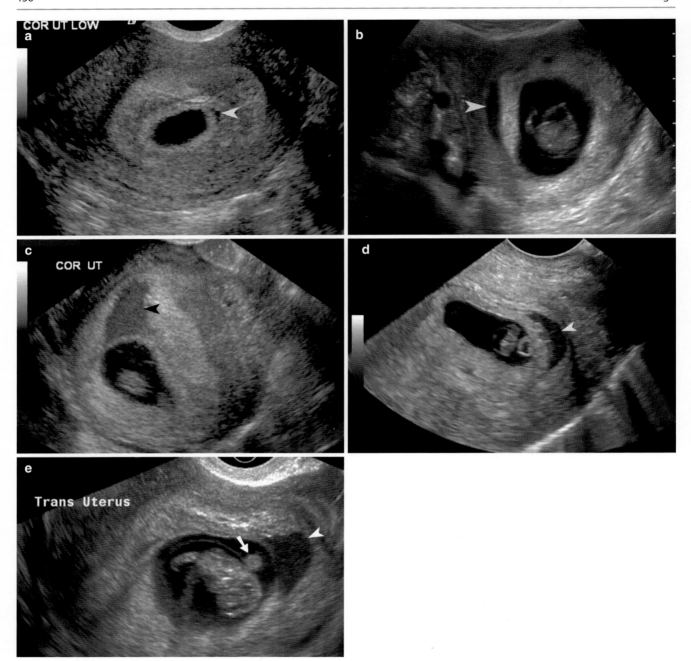

Fig. 12.4 Subchorionic hemorrhage. (**a–e**) Ultrasound demonstrates sickle-shaped subchorionic hemorrhage (*arrowhead*) in five different patients. An abnormally large and echogenic yolk sac (*arrow*) is identified with in the chorionic cavity (**e**)

Interstitial Ectopic Pregnancy

In these patients, the pregnancy is in the intramural portion of the fallopian tube and is surrounded by myometrial tissue which has richer blood supply which allows the pregnancy to progress into the second trimester. The clinical significance of interstitial ectopic pregnancy is that it has a tendency to rupture later, leading to higher mortality than other cases of ectopic pregnancy.

The ultrasound finding of interstitial ectopic pregnancy is thinning of the myometrium on one side of the gestational sac which is present eccentrically in the fundus, in relation to the endometrial cavity. Typically the myometrial thickness on the outer aspect of the gestational sac is less than 5 mm (Fig. 12.7).

Interstitial line sign is characterized by extension of echogenic line from the interstitial ectopic pregnancy to the endometrial echo complex. It has an 80 % sensitivity in making

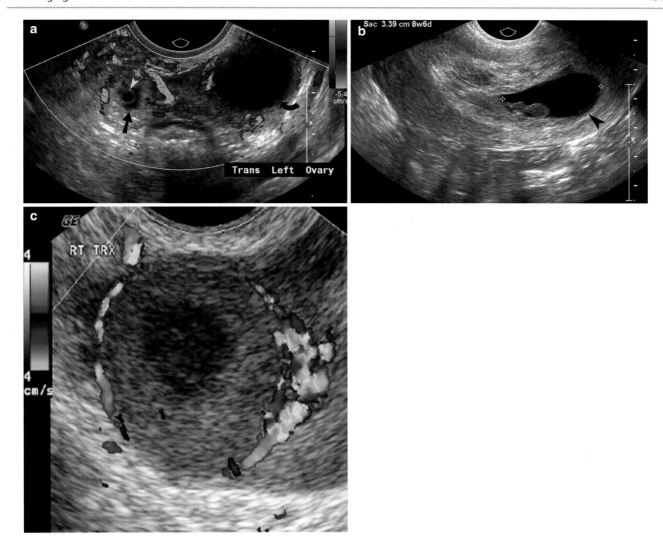

Fig. 12.5 Ectopic pregnancy. (**a**) Left adnexal ectopic pregnancy is indicated by the presence of gestational sac (*arrow*) and yolk sac (*arrowhead*), adjacent to the left ovary (*curved arrow*). (**b**) Sagittal ultrasound image demonstrates ectopic pregnancy in the cervical canal (*arrowhead*). (**c**) Hemorrhagic luteal cyst seen in the left ovary in a patient who had a recent abortion. The rarity of ectopic pregnancy within the ovary makes that diagnosis very unlikely in this case

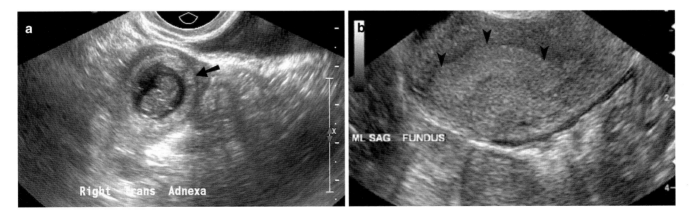

Fig. 12.6 Ectopic pregnancy. (**a**) Ectopic tubal ring is indicated by an ectopic gestational sac (*arrow*) surrounded by echogenic trophoblast in the right pelvic adnexa. (**b**) There is decidual reaction (*arrowheads*) identified within the uterus of the same patient with ectopic pregnancy

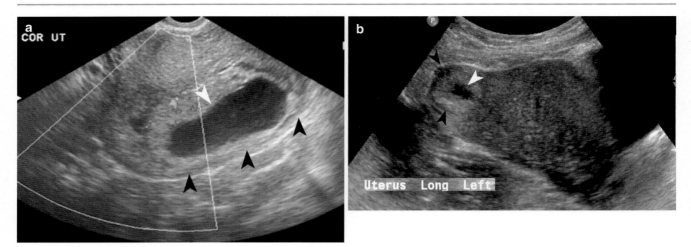

Fig. 12.7 Cornual ectopic pregnancy. (**a**, **b**) Ultrasound demonstrates eccentric gestational sac (*white arrowhead*) with thinning of the myometrium (*black arrowhead*) to less than 5 mm

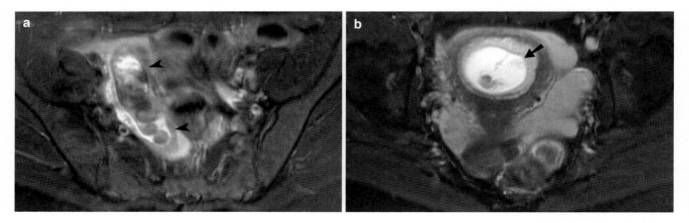

Fig. 12.8 Heterotropic pregnancy. (**a**, **b**) T2-weighted MRI demonstrates heterogeneous right adnexal ectopic pregnancy (*arrowheads*) and intrauterine pregnancy (*arrow*)

the diagnosis of an interstitial ectopic pregnancy, compared to 40 % sensitivity for eccentric gestational sac [9].

Heterotropic Pregnancy

Heterotropic pregnancy refers to the simultaneous presence of intrauterine as well as ectopic pregnancy (Fig. 12.8). The frequency of heterotrophic pregnancy has increased with the usage of ovulation induction medications. The extrauterine pregnancy is most commonly within the fallopian tube (94 %) [10]. The frequency if heterotrophic pregnancy which was estimated to be about 1 in 30,000 in general population has now increased to as much as 1 in 100, in patients undergoing fertility treatment. The current frequency of heterotrophic pregnancy is between 1 in 4,000 and 1 in 7,000 [11, 12].

Molar Pregnancy

Partial H mole is caused by two sperms penetrating the ovum, resulting in a total of 69 chromosomes, instead of 46. A complete H mole is usually caused by a single sperm fertilizing an ovum, which has lost its chromosomes. The sperm replicates its chromosomes to produce 46 chromosomes. Approximately 20 % of complete H moles and 2 % of partial H mole lead to gestational trophoblastic disease. Abnormal bleeding for more than 6 weeks after any pregnancy should be evaluated with beta HCG measurement to exclude a new pregnancy or gestational trophoblastic disease.

Ultrasound alone is not enough in diagnosing molar pregnancy and has a sensitivity of only 34 %. The sensitivity is higher for complete H mole (58 %) than partial H mole (17 %)

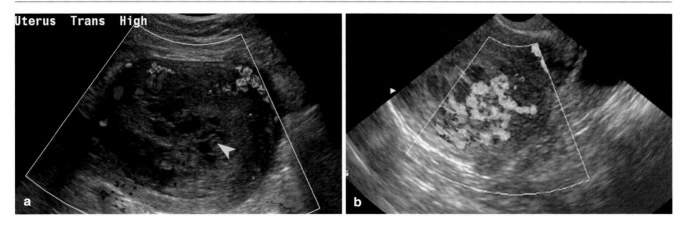

Fig. 12.9 Molar pregnancy. (**a, b**) Ultrasound demonstrates heterogeneous (*arrowhead*) solid as well as cystic (hydropic villi) areas distending the endometrial cavity with increased color Doppler flow

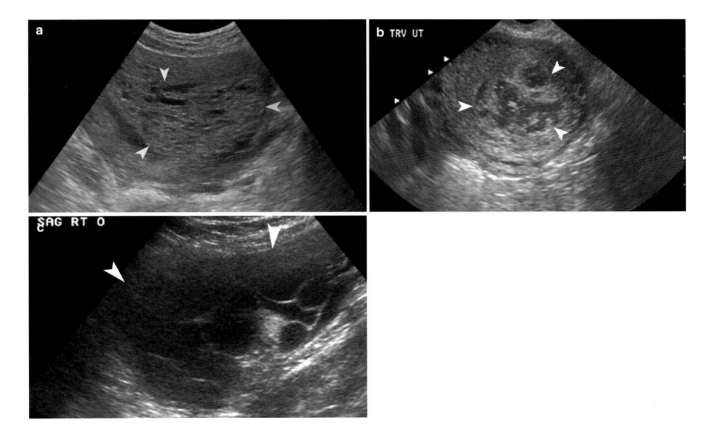

Fig. 12.10 Molar pregnancy. (**a, b**) Ultrasound of the uterus in two patients demonstrates heterogeneous echogenicity mass (*arrowheads*) located within the uterus. (**c**) Ultrasound of a patient with molar pregnancy demonstrates an enlarged ovary (*arrowheads*) measuring more than 8 cm in diameter and containing multiple large theca lutein cysts

[13]. Almost two-thirds of the molar pregnancy cases will be missed in ultrasound evaluation because the sonographic appearance is that of missed abortion or anembryonic pregnancy. The diagnostic ultrasound appearance of molar pregnancy is that of cystic spaces caused by hydropic villi. The heterogeneous mass produced by the molar pregnancy may have a snowstorm appearance (Figs. 12.9 and 12.10a, b). The ovaries are enlarged and theca lutein cysts are seen in up to 40 % cases due to overstimulation by beta HCG. Theca lutein cysts are typically multiloculated and bilateral (Fig. 12.10c).

Learning Points

1. The yolk sac and embryo should be visualized on transvaginal ultrasound when the mean sac diameter is 13 and 18 mm, respectively.
2. Lack of embryonic cardiac pulsations in an embryo measuring 6 mm in diameter warrants a follow-up ultrasound to evaluate for embryonic demise.
3. The crown-rump length is the preferred mode of measurement of gestational age in the first trimester of pregnancy, whenever possible.
4. Embryonic heart rate of less than 80 is associated with poor outcome in the first trimester.

References

1. Kaur A, Kaur A. Transvaginal ultrasonography in first trimester of pregnancy and its comparison with transabdominal ultrasonography. J Pharm Bioallied Sci. 2011;3(3):329–38.
2. Laing FC, Brown DL, Price JF, Teeger S, Wong ML. Intradecidual sign: is it effective in diagnosis of an early intrauterine pregnancy? Radiology. 1997;204:655–60.
3. Yeh HC. Efficacy of the intradecidual sign and fallacy of the double decidual sac sign in the diagnosis of early intrauterine pregnancy. Radiology. 1999;210(2):579–82.
4. Yeh HC, Goodman JD, Carr L, Rabinowitz JG. Intradecidual sign: a US criterion of early intrauterine pregnancy. Radiology. 1986;161:463–7.
5. Fleischer AC, Pennell RG, McKee MS, Worrell JA, Keefe B, Herbert CM, et al. Ectopic pregnancy: features at transvaginal sonography. Radiology. 1990;174(2):375–8.
6. Fleischer AC, Pennell RG, McKee MS, Worrell JA, Keefe B, Herbert CM, et al. Ectopic pregnancy: features at transvaginal sonography. Radiology. 1990;174:375–8.
7. Szabó I, Csabay L, Belics Z, Fekete T, Papp Z. Assessment of uterine circulation in ectopic pregnancy by transvaginal color Doppler. Eur J Obstet Gynecol Reprod Biol. 2003;106(2):203–8.
8. Kirchler HC, Kölle D, Schwegel P. Changes in tubal blood flow in evaluating ectopic pregnancy. Ultrasound Obstet Gynecol. 1992;2(4):283–8.
9. Ackerman TE, Levi CS, Dashefsky SM, Holt SC, Lindsay DJ. Interstitial line: sonographic finding in interstitial (cornual) ectopic pregnancy. Radiology. 1993;189:83–7.
10. Reece EA, Petrie RH, Sirmans MF, Finster M, Todd WD. Combined intrauterine and extrauterine gestations: a review. Am J Obstet Gynecol. 1998;146:323–30.
11. Hann LE, Bachman DM, McArdle CR. Coexistent intrauterine and ectopic pregnancy: a reevaluation. Radiology. 1984;152:151–4.
12. Rizk B, Tan SL, Morcos S. Heterotropic pregnancy after in vitro fertilization and embryo transfer. Am J Obstet Gynecol. 1991;164:161–4.
13. Sebire NJ, Rees H, Paradinas F, Seckl M, Newlands E. The diagnostic implications of routine ultrasound examination in histologically confirmed early molar pregnancies. Ultrasound Obstet Gynecol. 2001;18:662–5.

Imaging of Acute Gynecologic Disorders

Chris Malcom, Amisha Khicha, and Ajay Singh

Introduction

Pelvic pain is one of the most common causes for presentation to the emergency department. A variety of gynecological processes may be the etiology for pelvic pain; hemorrhagic ovarian cysts, pelvic inflammatory disease, ovarian torsion, endometriosis, cystitis, ovarian vein thrombosis, and ovarian hyperstimulation syndrome are a few of the most commonly encountered pathologies. Before medical imaging is performed for evaluation of pelvic pain, it is important to obtain relevant clinical history and review available laboratory information. The patient's age and pregnancy status are of particular importance in the differential diagnosis; therefore, serum beta-hCG laboratory evaluation is performed if there is even a remote possibility of pregnancy.

Transvaginal and transabdominal ultrasound are the workhorse modalities for the evaluation of pelvic pain when a gynecological etiology is suspected. Transvaginal and/or transabdominal ultrasound are both considered equally appropriate when evaluating pelvic pain; this is true whether the serum beta-hCG is positive or negative and whether a gynecologic or nongynecologic etiology is suspected.

Magnetic resonance imaging may be appropriate in the evaluation of pelvic pain in pregnant and nonpregnant women when ultrasound is nondiagnostic. The limitations of MR include limited availability, long imaging time, high cost, and motion artifacts from peristalsing bowel.

CT is not the frontline imaging modality in the evaluation of pelvic pain when a gynecologic etiology is suspected. It is the most appropriate imaging modality for acute pathologies of the gastrointestinal or urinary tract.

Functional Ovarian Cysts

The normal ovary in the preovulation period shows multiple simple follicles including a dominant follicle which usually measures less than 2.5 cm. At ovulation the dominant follicle ruptures, releasing an egg and a small amount of free fluid. Following ovulation, the dominant follicle becomes the corpus luteum cyst which usually measures less than 2.5 cm in maximal diameter and demonstrates a peripheral ring of increased vascularity on Doppler ultrasound. The regressing corpus luteum eventually forms the corpus albicans [1].

During the ovarian cycle, multiple events may occur which would prompt a visit to the emergency department. Many women experience varying degrees of pain during rupture of the dominant follicle at ovulation; the term mittelschmerz ("middle pain") is used to describe this pain accompanying rupture of the normal dominant follicle with release of the egg. A woman may experience pain from peritoneal irritation from the cyst rupture or pain due to hemorrhage into a cyst. Most ruptured ovarian cysts or hemorrhagic ovarian cysts are physiologic [2].

Imaging Findings

Simple ovarian cysts are anechoic without septations on ultrasound. In premenopausal women, if these simple cysts are less than or equal to 5 cm, they are mostly benign. In postmenopausal patients, simple cysts less than 1 cm do not require follow-up. If the features of an ovarian cyst are concerning for malignancy (i.e., thick septations, mural

C. Malcom, MD
Department of Radiology, William Beaumont Hospital,
Royal Oak, MI, USA

A. Khicha, MD
Department of Radiology, Wesley Medical Center,
University of Kansas School of Medicine,
Wichita, KS, USA

A. Singh, MD (✉)
Department of Radiology,
Massachusetts General Hospital,
Harvard Medical School,
10 Museum Way, # 524, Boston, MA 02141, USA
e-mail: asingh1@partners.org

A. Singh (ed.), *Emergency Radiology*,
DOI 10.1007/978-1-4419-9592-6_13, © Springer Science+Business Media New York 2013

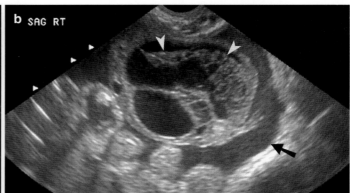

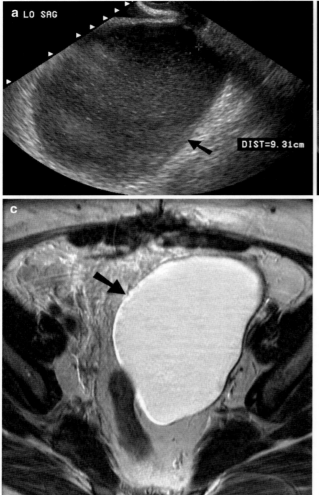

Fig. 13.1 Corpus luteal cyst. (**a**) Sagittal grayscale transabdominal ultrasound image of the pelvis demonstrates a large, cystic lesion (*arrow*) with relatively homogeneous internal echogenicity and posterior acoustic enhancement. (**b**) Ultrasound study demonstrates a hemorrhagic functional ovarian cyst containing a blood clot (*arrowhead*). There is surrounding hemorrhagic fluid (*straight arrow*) that is also seen in the adnexa. (**c**) Axial T2-weighted MR image of the pelvis shows a T2 hyperintense corpus luteal cyst in the left hemipelvis (*arrow*). Note the thin wall and lack of internal septations or nodularity

nodularity, or contrast enhancement), surgical consultation would be recommended regardless of the sonographic appearance.

A ruptured ovarian cyst does not have a specific appearance, and often the only finding is the presence of free fluid in the pelvis. Almost half of women will have some free fluid in the pouch of Douglas on ultrasound during normal ovulation; therefore, correlation with patient symptoms is necessary.

Hemorrhagic ovarian cysts on ultrasound classically have a hypoechoic appearance with a reticular pattern of internal echoes sometimes described as lacelike, spiderweb, or fishnet. Hemorrhagic cysts in premenopausal patients which measure greater than 5 cm should undergo follow-up imaging in 6–12 weeks on days 3–10 of the menstrual cycle (Fig. 13.1). Postmenopausal patients should never have a hemorrhagic cyst [1]. Hemoperitoneum resulting from

a ruptured hemorrhagic ovarian cyst may be demonstrated as a large amount of complex fluid in the pelvis on ultrasound. CT reveals hyperdense fluid within the peritoneal space and possible hyperdense sentinel clot adjacent to the hemorrhagic cyst. On MRI, hemorrhagic cyst is most often T2 hyperintense and hemorrhagic ascites is T1 hyperintense (Fig. 13.2) [3].

Pelvic Inflammatory Disease: Tubo-Ovarian Abscess and Pyosalpinx

Pelvic inflammatory disease (PID) is usually caused by bacterial infection with Chlamydia trachomatis or Neisseria gonorrhoeae [4]. Infection begins in the vagina and spreads to the endometrium causing endometritis. The infection then

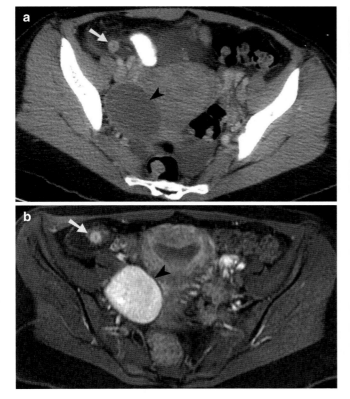

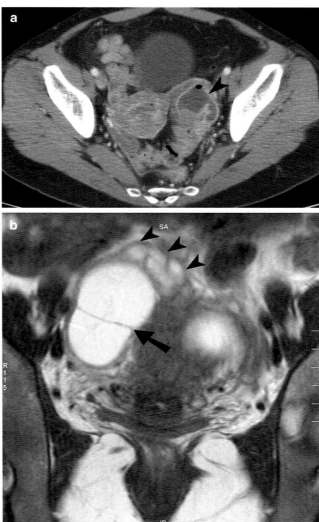

Fig. 13.2 Hemorrhagic ovarian cyst and appendicitis. (**a**) Contrast-enhanced axial CT image through the pelvis demonstrates an enlarged appendix with surrounded inflammatory fat stranding in the right lower quadrant (*arrow*). An oval, rim-enhancing ovarian cyst is identified to the right of the uterus (*arrowhead*), along with small amount of free fluid. (**b**) Axial contrast-enhanced, T1-weighted MR image with fat saturation obtained through the pelvis demonstrates a hyperenhancing, enlarged appendix with surrounding inflammatory changes in the adjacent mesenteric fat (*arrow*). The nonenhancing internal component of the hemorrhagic right ovarian cyst (*arrowhead*) is homogeneously T1 hyperintense, consistent with methemoglobin

Fig. 13.3 Tubo-ovarian abscess. (**a**) Axial contrast-enhanced CT image through the pelvis shows a left adnexal lesion containing a peripherally enhancing tubo-ovarian abscess (*arrowhead*) with a small focus of nondependent air. The ovary and fallopian tube are not distinguishable as separate structures. (**b**) Coronal noncontrast T2-weighted MR image of the pelvis demonstrates a large T2 hyperintense right adnexal abscess with a thick peripheral capsule and an internal septation (*arrow*). A mildly dilated, serpiginous fallopian tube (*arrowheads*) with a thick wall is seen extending in to the abscess

extends into the fallopian tube. The resulting inflammatory changes, edema, and exudate result in obstruction of the fallopian tube and formation of a pyosalpinx [5]. The infection then extends out along the fimbria and enters the ovary (often via a ruptured corpus luteum), leading to tubo-ovarian abscess [6]. The disease can spread in the peritoneal space to involve various organs including the liver and right paracolic gutter (Fitz-Hugh-Curtis syndrome).

The symptoms are often nonspecific and may include fever, pelvic pain, cervical/adnexal tenderness (chandelier sign), vaginal discharge, dyspareunia, nausea, and vomiting. Up to 35 % of the patients with PID have no symptoms [7].

Imaging

Pelvic ultrasound is the modality of choice when PID is suspected, due to high sensitivity and specificity with relatively

low cost. Because the symptoms of PID are nonspecific, CT is often the first study performed, especially when the differential diagnosis is wide and includes other suspected pathologies such as diverticulitis or appendicitis (Fig. 13.3a). Pelvic MRI also has high sensitivity and specificity for pelvic inflammatory disease; however, it is usually not considered a first-line imaging modality (Figs. 13.3b and 13.4) [4].

On ultrasound, the fallopian tubes often become distended with fluid in patients with PID. In acute disease, the fallopian tube walls measure 5 mm or thicker and demonstrate abundant

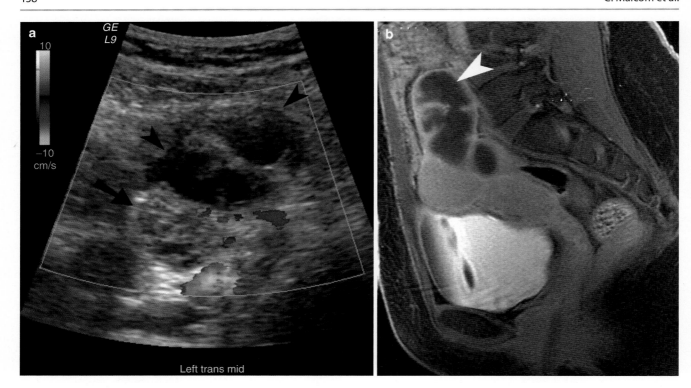

Fig. 13.4 Pyosalpinx (**a**) Transvaginal ultrasound image demonstrates a dilated fallopian tube (*arrowheads*) located adjacent to the ovary (*arrow*). (**b**) Sagittal contrast-enhanced T1-weighted MR image with fat saturation demonstrates a dilated fallopian tube (*arrowhead*) with incomplete internal septations and prominent contrast enhancement of the thickened tube wall

color flow with reduced flow resistance on the Doppler images (resistive index near 0.5). As the fluid-filled fallopian tubes distend, they become tortuous and fold on themselves; these folds have the appearance of incomplete septa. The thickened tube wall, fluid-filled lumen, and thickened mucosal folds can produce the "cogwheel sign" [5]. In pyosalpinx, fluid-debris levels are often visualized in the distended tubes. If the ovary cannot be visualized separate from this inflammatory mass, then the diagnosis of a tubo-ovarian abscess should be suggested rather than pyosalpinx. In chronic tubal disease, the luminal distention increases, the tube wall becomes thin, and mucosal folds are much more spread out resulting in a "beads-on-a-string" sign when visualized in cross section [5].

On CT, the findings of PID include dilated fallopian tubes, enlarged ovaries, inflammatory changes in the adjacent pelvic fat, thickening of the uterosacral ligaments, and peritoneal hyperenhancement [4, 7, 8]. The secondary findings which may include small bowel ileus/obstruction, perihepatitis (Fitz-Hugh-Curtis syndrome), and ureteral obstruction can be better evaluated on CT [4].

Pelvic infection with *Actinomyces israelii* is associated with the use of intrauterine contraceptive device. Tubo-ovarian abscesses with actinomycosis usually appear solid and may contain small rim-enhancing lesions. This infection spreads by direct extension, demonstrating linear, enhancing lesions which often have an appearance resembling carcinomatosis.

On MRI, a tubo-ovarian abscess usually presents as a mass which is T1 hypointense, often with hyperintense hemorrhage or proteinaceous debris. There is often a thin rim of T1 hyperintense signal along the inner portion of the abscess, secondary to hemorrhage within a layer of granulation tissue [8]. The abscess is usually hyperintense on T2-weighted sequence. On the postcontrast images, there is enhancement of the abscess wall and adjacent fat stranding [9]. Tubo-ovarian abscesses are hyperintense on diffusion-weighted images and demonstrate diffusion restriction [10].

Endometriosis

In endometriosis, endometrial tissue develops outside the uterine cavity, possibly due to metastatic implantation of endometrial cells from retrograde menstruation [11]. The most common locations for endometriosis include the ovaries (endometriomas), uterosacral ligament, rectosigmoid colon, vagina, and bladder. The ectopic endometrial tissue in endometriosis infiltrates adjacent structures causing an intense desmoplastic reaction, fibrosis, adhesions, and muscular hyperplasia. These changes can result in dysmenorrhea, dyspareunia, dyschezia, dysuria, back pain with menses, and hematuria [12–14].

Laparoscopy is the gold standard for the diagnosis, staging, and treatment of endometriosis; however, in cases where there is limited mobility of pelvic structures due to extensive fibrosis and adhesions, laparoscopic evaluation may be limited. The goal of imaging is lesion mapping for presurgical planning and postsurgical response evaluation. Transvaginal ultrasound is the first-line imaging technique for initial evaluation of suspected endometriosis.

Imaging

On ultrasound, deeply infiltrating endometrial implants are hypoechoic compared to myometrium. The endometriomas demonstrate diffuse low-level internal echoes and no internal blood flow.

MRI is probably the most specific imaging modality for diagnosing endometriomas. MRI is best for looking at hemorrhagic content, which is hyperintense on fat-suppressed T1-weighted images and hypointense on T2-weighted images (Fig. 13.5a). The surrounding desmoplastic reaction is hypointense on T1-weighted and T2-weighted sequence [12, 13]. Endometriomas are classically T1 hyperintense and T2 hypointense (described as "T2 shading") (Fig. 13.5b). Endometriosis may rarely be a cause of hemoperitoneum which can result from rupture of an endometrioma or infiltration and subsequent rupture of the uterine artery [14].

Ovarian Torsion

Ovarian torsion occurs when the adnexa twists on the vascular pedicle, often resulting in interruption of the venous flow and enlargement of the ovary. As the torsion progresses, the arterial blood flow is interrupted and ovarian ischemia occurs [15]. The ovary has a dual arterial blood supply which includes the ovarian artery and ovarian branches of the uterine artery. Any ovarian mass or large cyst may place the adnexa at risk of torsion [2, 16].

Torsion is most commonly seen in reproductive-age women with an ovarian mass or cyst found in up to 80 % of cases of torsion. Symptoms of torsion are nonspecific and most commonly include acute abnormal pain. Patients may also experience nausea and vomiting with fever occasionally developing several hours late [17]. Because the clinical presentation is nonspecific, correct diagnosis is often delayed [18].

Imaging

Ultrasound is the preferred initial imaging modality when ovarian torsion is suspected. If the ovaries appear normal in size and morphology on ultrasound, then torsion can be excluded [19]. The most common finding is ovarian enlargement of greater than 4 cm. The ovary may have a teardrop configuration with multiple small follicles displaced to the periphery of the ovary.

Although the absent vascular flow on color Doppler imaging is highly suggestive of torsion, normal Doppler flow does not exclude torsion because early torsion is often intermittent

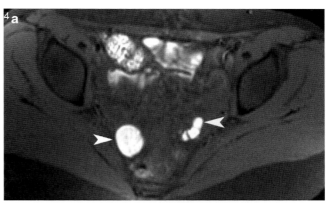
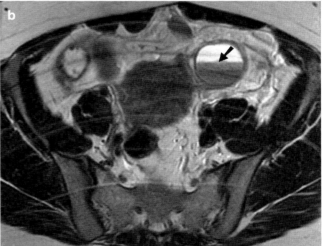

Fig. 13.5 Endometriosis. (**a**) Axial noncontrast T1-weighted MR image with fat saturation obtained through the pelvis showing multiple endometriotic cysts along bilateral pelvic side walls (*arrowheads*). The implants appear T1 hyperintense due to methemoglobin content. (**b**) Axial noncontrast T2-weighted MR image of the pelvis demonstrates a left ovarian endometrioma with a fluid/fluid level (*arrow*). The dependent contents of the endometrioma demonstrated characteristic "T2 shading" (hypointensity)

or partial [2, 16]. The "whirlpool sign" refers to visualization of twisted or circular vessels in the vascular pedicle; this is highly specific for adnexal torsion [15, 20].

Occasionally on CT and MRI, twisting of the vascular pedicle can be directly visualized; this finding is highly specific for adnexal torsion (Fig. 13.6) [21]. Most other findings are nonspecific and can include an adnexal mass, ipsilateral deviation of the uterus, lack of contrast enhancement, and ascites. On MRI, diffusion-weighted imaging reveals diffusion restriction when ischemia is present. Ovarian enlargement and edema from torsion result in T2 hyperintensity in the central ovarian stroma, which also shows multiple peripheral follicles.

Cystitis

Cystitis can be of multiple etiologies including bacterial infection, mechanical irritation (Foley catheter), medication effects (cyclophosphamide), radiation, or idiopathic

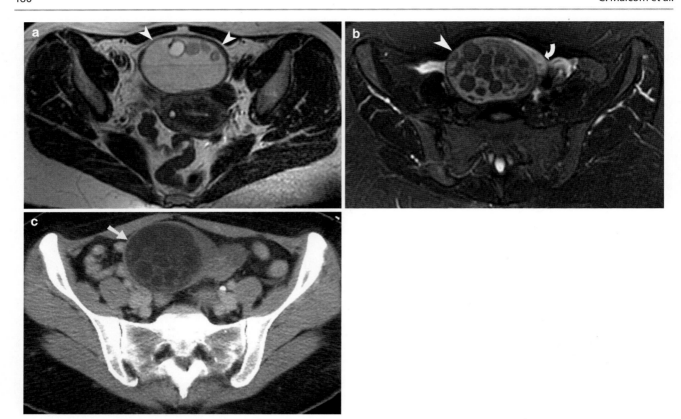

Fig. 13.6 Ovarian dermoid. (**a**) Axial noncontrast T2-weighted MR image of the pelvis demonstrates a well-circumscribed, round lesion (*arrowheads*) located anterior to the uterus. The majority of the contents of this mature teratoma appear T2 hyperintense, but there are multiple round lobules within the lesion. (**b**) Axial noncontrast STIR MR image of the pelvis again demonstrates a round, well-circumscribed ovarian dermoid located midline in the pelvis (*arrowhead*). There are multiple round, internal lobules which demonstrate signal dropout due to the fat content. A rim of edematous ovarian tissue lateral and anterior to the dermoid shows T2 hyperintensity (*curved arrow*). (**c**) Axial contrast-enhanced CT image of the pelvis again shows the immature teratoma with multiple internal fat density lobules demonstrating the characteristic fat attenuation which is diagnostic of an ovarian dermoid (*arrow*)

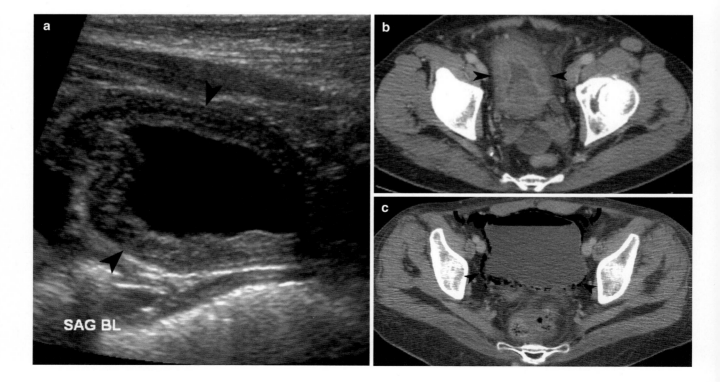

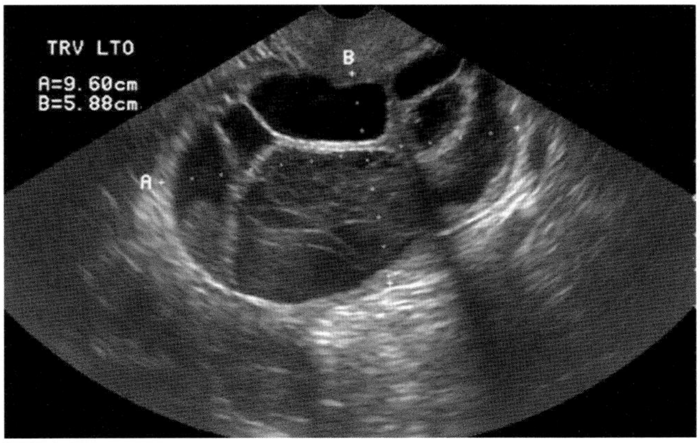

Fig. 13.8 Ovarian hyperstimulation syndrome. Ultrasound study demonstrates a markedly enlarged ovary measuring more than 9 cm in diameter and containing multiple cysts, some of which are hemorrhagic

(interstitial cystitis). When uncomplicated cystitis is suspected, no medical imaging is generally indicated [22]. However, imaging may be indicated if there is concern for malignancy, calculi, or urine flow obstruction.

The imaging findings of uncomplicated cystitis included diffuse bladder wall thickening and pericystic inflammation. The normal bladder wall thickness of the distended (>200 mL) urinary bladder is 1.1–4.5 mm [23]. Although bladder wall thickening can be evaluated with ultrasound, CT, or MRI, pericystic inflammation can only be appreciated on CT or MRI (Fig. 13.7a, b). Immunocompromised patients are at increased risk of emphysematous cystitis, which is best recognized by the presence of air within the urinary bladder wall (Fig. 13.7c) [24].

Ovarian Hyperstimulation Syndrome

Ovarian hyperstimulation syndrome (OHSS) is a rare complication which occurs in women undergoing infertility treatment with gonadotropic hormones. Symptoms include abdominal pain, nausea, vomiting, abdominal distention, and dizziness. The imaging findings include ascites and enlargement of ovaries which contain large peripheral cysts (Fig. 13.8). Pleural effusions may also be present [15, 25].

Ovarian Vein Thrombosis

Ovarian vein thrombosis most often occurs in postpartum or postoperative patients. The symptoms include fever and abdominal pain. Most cases involve the right ovarian vein

which appears enlarged with central filling defect and surrounding fat stranding. Contrast-enhanced CT is the most sensitive modality for diagnosis (Fig. 13.9) [25].

Symptomatic Fibroids

Uterine fibroids represent benign masses of uterine smooth muscle and connective tissue proliferation. Fibroids may be the cause for acute pelvic pain in the setting of infarction, torsion (pedunculated subserosal fibroid), or prolapse (pedunculated submucosal fibroid).

On ultrasound, the presence of cystic features within a fibroid indicates internal degeneration. The sensitivity and specificity for the detection of fibroid degeneration is higher with MRI (Figs. 13.10, 13.11, and 13.12). High T2 signal intensity of leiomyomas with poor or no enhancement on contrast-enhanced T1-weighted sequence suggests the presence of ischemia or hemorrhagic necrosis [26].

Red degeneration usually occurs in the setting of pregnancy or in patients on oral contraceptives and is due to obstruction of draining veins. Varying signal intensities are produced within the fibroid due to the presence of hemorrhagic products of different ages. The peripheral obstructed veins may be seen as a peripheral rim of low T2 and high T1 signal intensity. Postcontrast images will demonstrate no enhancement.

Hematometrocolpos and Hydrometrocolpos

While hematometrocolpos represents accumulation of blood within the vagina, hydrometrocolpos represents the presence of fluid within the vagina and uterus. The cause may be congenital imperforate hymen or acquired, such as neoplastic obstruction, postpartum infection, or iatrogenic cervical stenosis. Imaging by sonography, CT, or MRI will most commonly demonstrate cystic distension of the vagina and/or uterine cavity with a possible fluid-debris level posterior to the bladder (Fig. 13.13) [27, 28].

Teaching Points

1. Ultrasound is the primary modality utilized for imaging of acute pelvic disorders.
2. CT is the initial imaging study performed to evaluate for acute diverticulitis and appendicitis.

Fig. 13.7 Cystitis. (**a**) Transabdominal grayscale ultrasound image demonstrates inflammatory thickening of the urinary bladder wall (*arrowheads*). (**b**) Axial contrast-enhanced CT image of the pelvis shows marked thickening and hyperenhancement of the wall of the urinary bladder (*arrowheads*). There is also extensive inflammatory stranding in the adjacent fat. (**c**) Axial contrast-enhanced CT evidence of the pelvis demonstrates extensive emphysema within the urinary bladder wall (*arrowheads*). Extraluminal air is also seen anterior to the urinary bladder (*curved arrows*)

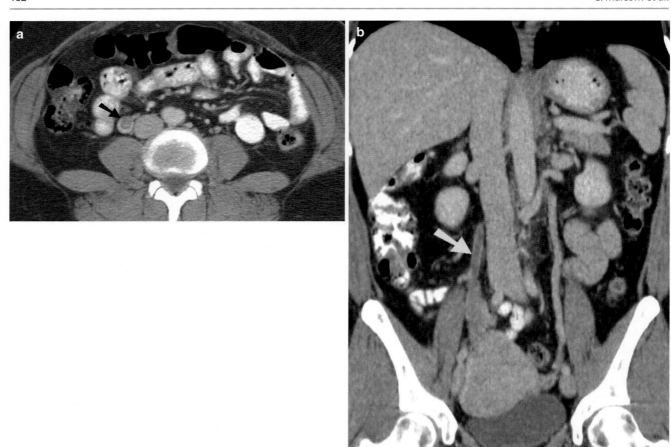

Fig. 13.9 Gonadal vein thrombosis. (**a**) Axial contrast-enhanced CT image of the abdomen demonstrates a low-density intraluminal thrombus within an abnormally expanded right gonadal vein (*arrow*). (**b**) Coronal contrast-enhanced CT image of the abdomen and pelvis shows a tubular intraluminal thrombus in a segment of the right gonadal vein (*arrow*). The vein is abnormally expanded and a small amount of contrast is seen surrounding the thrombus

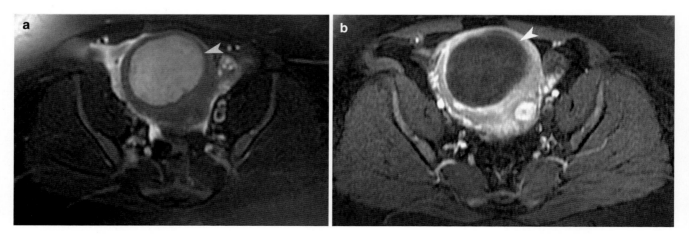

Fig. 13.10 Degenerating uterine fibroid. (**a**) Axial T2-weighted MR image with fat saturation obtained through the pelvis demonstrates a well-circumscribed, T2 hyperintense leiomyoma (*arrowhead*) with cystic degeneration. (**b**) Axial contrast-enhanced T1-weighted MR image with fat saturation shows no enhancement within the round, well-circumscribed leiomyoma (*arrowhead*)

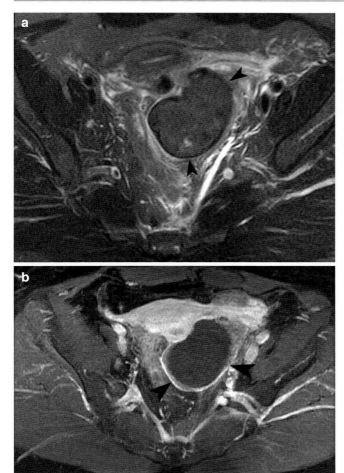

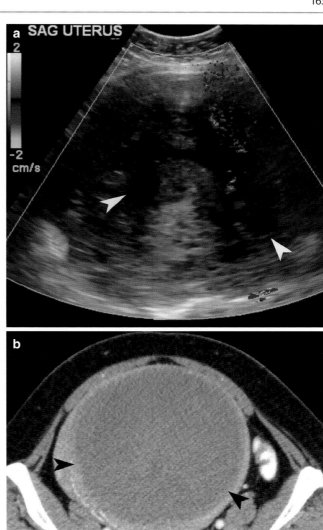

Fig. 13.11 Degenerating uterine fibroid. (**a**) Axial noncontrast T2-weighted MR image with fat saturation obtained in the pelvis demonstrates a hypointense mass with a peripheral rim of low signal intensity which is characteristic of a leiomyoma undergoing red degeneration (*arrowheads*). (**b**) Axial postcontrast T1-weighted MR imaging with fat saturation confirms that there is no contrast enhancement within the subserosal leiomyoma undergoing degeneration (*arrowheads*)

3. Ovarian torsion is most common in women of reproductive age and almost always occurs in the setting of an ovarian abnormality such as a mass or cyst.

4. Although a less convenient and more expensive modality, the sensitivity and specificity for MRI is high with advanced anatomical delineation for most acute pelvic processes.

Fig. 13.12 Degenerating fibroid. (**a**) Pelvic ultrasound with color flow demonstrates a large heterogeneous mass with irregular cystic areas (*arrowheads*) within the degenerating fibroid. (**b**) Axial contrast-enhanced CT demonstrates a large, necrotic, well-circumscribed uterine leiomyoma, which does not enhance (*arrowheads*)

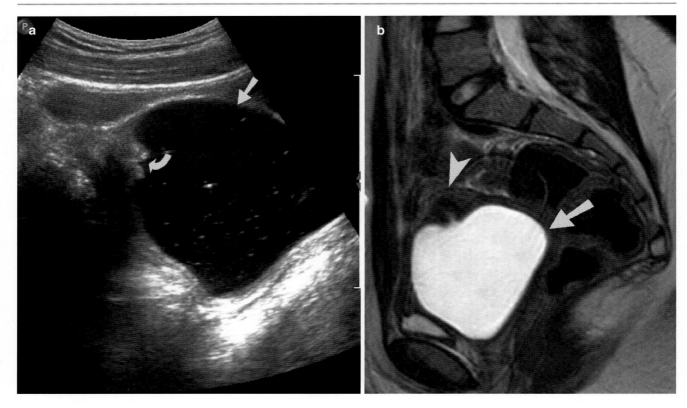

Fig. 13.13 Hematocolpos due to imperforate hymen. (**a**) Transabdominal ultrasound shows a large hypoechoic fluid collection with floating internal echogenic debris within a markedly distended vaginal cavity (*arrow*). The cervix can be seen along the superior aspect of the fluid collection (*curved arrow*). (**b**) Sagittal T2-weighted images of the pelvis demonstrate a large, T2 hyperintense fluid collection within the distended vaginal cavity (*arrow*). The uterus (*arrowhead*) can be seen displaced superiorly by the distended, fluid-filled vagina

References

1. Levine D, Brown DL, Andreotti RF, et al. Management of asymptomatic ovarian and other adnexal cysts imaged at US Society of Radiologists in Ultrasound consensus conference statement. Ultrasound Q. 2010;26(3):121–31.
2. Bottomley C, Bourne T. Diagnosis and management of ovarian cyst accidents. Best Pract Res Clin Obstet Gynaecol. 2009;23(5):711–24.
3. Tamai K, Koyama T, Saga T, et al. MR features of physiologic and benign conditions of the ovary. Eur Radiol. 2006;16(12):2700–11.
4. Horrow MM. Ultrasound of pelvic inflammatory disease. Ultrasound Q. 2004;20(4):171–9.
5. Timor-Tritsch IE, Lerner JP, Monteagudo A, Murphy KE, Heller DS. Transvaginal sonographic markers of tubal inflammatory disease. Ultrasound Obstet Gynecol. 1998;12(1):56–66.
6. Lambert MJ, Villa M. Gynecologic ultrasound in emergency medicine. Emerg Med Clin North Am. 2004;22(3):683–96.
7. Sam JW, Jacobs JE, Birnbaum BA. Spectrum of CT findings in acute pyogenic pelvic inflammatory disease. Radiographics. 2002;22(6):1327–34.
8. Kim SH, Kim SH, Yang DM, Kim KA. Unusual causes of tubo-ovarian abscess: CT and MR imaging findings. Radiographics. 2004;24(6):1575–89.
9. Singh AK, Desai H, Novelline RA. Emergency MRI of acute pelvic pain: MR protocol with no oral contrast. Emerg Radiol. 2009;16(2):133–41.
10. Kilickesmez O, Tasdelen N, Yetimoglu B, et al. Diffusion-weighted imaging of adnexal torsion. Emerg Radiol. 2009;16(5):399–401.
11. Woodward PJ, Sohaey R, Mezzetti Jr TP. Endometriosis: radiologic-pathologic correlation. Radiographics. 2001;21(1):193–216; questionnaire 288–94.
12. Chamie LP, Blasbalg R, Pereira RMA, Warmbrand G, Serafini PC. Findings of pelvic endometriosis at transvaginal US, MR imaging, and laparoscopy. Radiographics. 2011;31(4):E77–100.
13. Marcal L, Nothaft MA, Coelho F, Choi H. Deep pelvic endometriosis: MR imaging. Abdom Imaging. 2010;35(6):708–15.
14. Bennett GL, Slywotzky CM, Cantera M, Hecht EM. Unusual manifestations and complications of endometriosis – spectrum of imaging findings: pictorial review. AJR Am J Roentgenol. 2010;194(6 Suppl):WS34–46.
15. Chang HC, Bhatt S, Dogra VS. Pearls and pitfalls in diagnosis of ovarian torsion. Radiographics. 2008;28(5):1355–68.
16. Chiou S-Y, Lev-Toaff AS, Masuda E, Feld RI, Bergin D. Adnexal torsion: new clinical and imaging observations by sonography, computed tomography, and magnetic resonance imaging. J Ultrasound Med. 2007;26(10):1289–301.
17. Galinier P, Carfagna L, Delsol M, et al. Ovarian torsion. Management and ovarian prognosis: a report of 45 cases. J Pediatr Surg. 2009;44(9):1759–65.
18. Hiller N, Appelbaum L, Simanovsky N, et al. CT features of adnexal torsion. AJR Am J Roentgenol. 2007;189(1):124–9.
19. Patel MD, Dubinsky TJ. Reimaging the female pelvis with ultrasound after CT. Ultrasound Q. 2007;23(3):177–87.

20. Vijayaraghavan SB. Sonographic whirlpool sign in ovarian torsion. J Ultrasound Med. 2004;23(12):1643–9; quiz 1650–1.

21. Rha SE, Byun JY, Jung SE, et al. CT and MR imaging features of adnexal torsion. Radiographics. 2002;22(2):283–94.

22. Johansen TEB. The role of imaging in urinary tract infections. World J Urol. 2004;22(5):392–8.

23. Blatt AH, Titus J, Chan L. Ultrasound measurement of bladder wall thickness in the assessment of voiding dysfunction. J Urol. 2008;179(6):2275–8; discussion 2278–9.

24. Chang C-B, Chang C-C. Emphysematous cystitis: a rare cause of gross hematuria. J Emerg Med. 2011;40(5):506–8.

25. Bennett GL, Slywotzky CM, Giovanniello G. Gynecologic causes of acute pelvic pain: spectrum of CT findings. Radiographics. 2002; 22(4):785–801.

26. Wilde S, Scott-Barrett S. Radiological appearances of uterine fibroids. Indian J Radiol Imaging. 2009;19:222–31.

27. Dykes T, Siegel C, Dodson W. Imaging of congenital uterine anomalies: review and self-assessment module. AJR Am J Roentgenol. 2007;189(3):S1–10.

28. Kim TH, Lee HH, Chung SH. Presenting features of pyometra including an increase in iatrogenic causes. J Low Genit Tract Dis. 2011;15(4):316–7.

Emergency Radionuclide Imaging of the Thorax and Abdomen

14

Paul F. von Herrmann and M. Elizabeth Oates

Introduction

Nuclear medicine (NM) utilizes a variety of unsealed radioactive compounds, known as radiopharmaceuticals or radiotracers. Given in small (tracer) quantities, radiopharmaceuticals typically consist of two components: a radionuclide (also known as a radioisotope) and a molecular or cellular carrier; the latter determines the biologic distribution upon administration to a patient. The most common routes of administration in clinical practice are intravenous (IV) and oral.

Based on its respective radionuclide, a radiopharmaceutical emits specific gamma rays, which can be detected and processed into medical images by gamma cameras, which is termed scintigraphy. The resulting scintigraphic images depict the biodistribution of the administered radioactivity within the patient's body, thereby reflecting normal or abnormal physiological function combined with a low-resolution anatomical representation of the organs/organ systems under investigation. The physiological data are complementary to the anatomical data and, in certain conditions, prove more beneficial than the anatomical data alone.

In the emergency setting, appropriate triage and timely diagnosis are of utmost importance. Emergency physicians have come to rely more and more heavily on medical imaging for diagnosis and management; decisions to admit or discharge often hinge on the radiological diagnosis. NM examinations are generally underutilized in the emergency setting for a number of fundamental reasons. Emergency physicians tend to be less familiar with the NM options and are less experienced with their respective appropriateness and advantages. Common logistical challenges include limited availability and longer duration compared to other types of imaging examinations. Specifically, there may be difficulty obtaining radiopharmaceuticals during evenings, nights, and weekends. In many institutions, NM personnel are typically only on-site during regular working hours; at some institutions, the NM technologists are "on call" while in others, there is no availability during the off-hours. This lack of ready access is likely one of the major determinants that leads emergency physicians to request fewer NM examinations. Even when available, however, scintigraphic examinations generally require more time than radiography (X-ray) or computed tomography (CT).

Nevertheless, NM can play important primary and secondary roles in diagnosis and management in the emergency setting. Within the radiological armamentarium, selected scintigraphic examinations offer significant value because those negative examinations exclude diagnoses with high certainty, while positive examinations direct appropriate management. Currently, the most common radionuclide imaging examinations of the thorax and abdomen in the emergency setting are ventilation/perfusion (V/Q) lung scintigraphy, myocardial perfusion imaging (MPI), hepatobiliary scintigraphy (HBS), and gastrointestinal (GI) bleeding scintigraphy (Table 14.1). This chapter will review their appropriate utilization, highlight their advantages and disadvantages, and illustrate each by way of representative case examples.

Acute Pulmonary Embolism: Ventilation/Perfusion (V/Q) Lung Scintigraphy

Pulmonary embolism (PE) is a potentially fatal complication of deep venous thrombosis. In acute PE, thrombus dislodges from the vein, migrates to the pulmonary vasculature, and lodges in a main pulmonary artery or segmental branch. Thromboemboli reduce the cross-sectional area of the pulmonary arterial vascular bed, thus potentially resulting in hypoxia and hemodynamic compromise. Diagnosing acute PE can be very difficult clinically due to nonspecific symptoms and confounding clinical presentations mimicking other acute thoracic and abdominal conditions.

P.F. von Herrmann, MD (✉) • M.E. Oates, MD
Department of Radiology, University of Kentucky,
800 Rose Street, HX-307B, Lexington, KY 40536-0293, USA
e-mail: pvo222@email.uky.edu

A. Singh (ed.), *Emergency Radiology*,
DOI 10.1007/978-1-4419-9592-6_14, © Springer Science+Business Media New York 2013

Table 14.1 Common clinical indications for emergency radionuclide imaging of the thorax and abdomen

Clinical indication	Examination	Radiopharmaceuticals	Typical time to completion	Sensitivity	Specificity	Positive predictive value	Negative predictive value	References
Acute pulmonary embolism	V/Q lung scintigraphy	*Ventilation:* ^{133}Xe gas, inhaled, or ^{99m}Tc DTPA aerosol, inhaled *Perfusion:* ^{99m}Tc MAA, IV	30–60 min	70–85 % for high-probability interpretation	96–98 % for normal/very low-probability interpretation	96–99 % for high-probability interpretation with high clinical suspicion	97–98 % for normal/very low-probability interpretation	[1–3]
Acute coronary syndrome	Myocardial perfusion imaging	^{99m}Tc sestamibi IV or ^{99m}Tc tetrofosmin IV	1–2 h	90–100 %	63–71 %	15–22 %	97–99 %	[3–8]
Acute biliary conditions: cystic duct obstruction (acute cholecystitis) and common bile duct obstruction	Hepatobiliary scintigraphy	^{99m}Tc IDA analog, IV	1–4 h	88–100 %	93–100 %	85–90 %	95–99 %	[9–11]
Acute biliary conditions: bile duct injury			1–2 h	100 %	90–100 %	91–100 %	100 %	[12]
Gastrointestinal bleeding	GI bleeding scintigraphy	^{99m}Tc RBCs, IV	1–2 h	78–97 %	70–100 % for diagnosis, 88–97 % for localization	75–77 %	76–93 %	[13–16]

Table 14.2 Typical ventilation/perfusion (V/Q) lung scintigraphy technical protocol

1. Obtain contemporaneous chest radiography in posterior-anterior (PA) and lateral projections
2. Patient inhales 20 mCi (740 MBq) of ^{133}Xe gas or 3 mCi (111 MBq) of aerosolized ^{99m}Tc diethylenetriaminepentaacetic acid (DTPA)
3. Acquire ventilation images in posterior (^{133}Xe gas) or anterior, posterior, bilateral anterior oblique, and bilateral posterior oblique (^{99m}Tc DTPA aerosol) projections
4. Administer 4 mCi (148 MBq) of ^{99m}Tc macroaggregated albumin (MAA) IV
5. Acquire perfusion images in anterior, posterior, bilateral anterior oblique, and bilateral posterior oblique projections

Both CT angiography (CTA) and ventilation/perfusion (V/Q) lung scintigraphy are well-accepted modalities for the imaging evaluation of suspected acute PE. Nowadays, CTA is performed in the vast majority of patients. However, V/Q scintigraphy remains relevant because radionuclide imaging of the lungs provides physiological information regarding not only regional pulmonary arterial perfusion but also bronchoalveolar ventilation. V/Q scintigraphy also spares the patient exposure to potentially nephrotoxic iodinated contrast and results in lower radiation dosimetry [3].

Although V/Q lung scintigraphy protocols vary by institution, ventilation images, using one of two commercially available radiopharmaceuticals, are typically acquired first. The perfusion phase using a standard radiopharmaceutical follows (Table 14.2). Perfusion imaging is based on the principle of capillary blockade. The radioactive MAA particles are larger than the capillaries and lodge in the precapillary arterioles; thus, their biodistribution reflects pulmonary arterial blood flow to both lungs. On these scintigraphic images, pulmonary segments with normal perfusion demonstrate uniform perfusion throughout (Fig. 14.1), while those with decreased perfusion demonstrate lower radioactivity than normal segments (Figs. 14.2 and 14.3). Classically, underlying lung disease presents as mildly to markedly abnormal perfusion that is "matched" by abnormal ventilation (Fig. 14.2). Acute PE affects perfusion only while ventilation should be preserved, resulting in the so-called V/Q mismatch pattern (Fig. 14.3). The PIOPED II criteria can be used to interpret V/Q lung scintigraphy (Table 14.3) [2].

In selecting the optimal radiological approach for suspected acute PE, the emergency physician should take into account multiple factors, not the least of which include sensitivity and specificity of the different imaging examinations, technical availability, and patient safety. First, for a patient with acute symptomatology, conventional chest radiography remains first-line. Patients with significantly abnormal chest radiographs should be directed to CTA and are not well suited for V/Q lung scintigraphy because there is greater likelihood of a nondiagnostic interpretation due to

confounding underlying pulmonary conditions such as chronic obstructive lung disease, pneumonia, pleural effusion, or atelectasis [17]. Concomitantly, there can be considerable interobserver variability of V/Q interpretations, especially in low and intermediate categories. CTA has the distinct advantage of evaluating the entire chest and upper abdomen and can delineate alternate thoracic or abdominal pathologies.

Second, in most institutions today, CTA is available around the clock with an on-site CT technologist who can perform the examination in a timely manner. During the standard workday, V/Q lung scintigraphy can be performed relatively quickly; however, during the off-hours, the NM technologist usually needs to travel into the hospital, and the radiopharmaceuticals may need to be prepared in-house or delivered from an outside pharmacy, all requiring additional time.

Third, there is much concern about radiation dosimetry, and the risks related to iodinated contrast are well established [3]. With CTA, there is higher radiation exposure to the patient, particularly to the female breast. The tissue dose to the breasts of nonpregnant women can be 10–60 mGy (1–6 rad) and is probably higher in pregnancy. Conversely, the breast dose from V/Q lung scintigraphy can be much lower than 0.31 mGy (0.031 rad) or almost 200 times less than CTA, and during the first trimester of pregnancy, the fetal dose can be halved using a modified reduced dose V/Q lung scintigraphy protocol [3]. Thus, for selected patients with special medical considerations such as pregnancy, breast-feeding, poor renal function, or IV contrast allergy, V/Q lung scintigraphy may represent the most appropriate imaging examination.

In summary, V/Q lung scintigraphy can be considered as a primary imaging approach in patients with suspected acute PE when there is:

1. Normal chest radiography
2. No concurrent cardiopulmonary process
3. Available NM facilities and personnel
4. Relative contraindication to CTA regarding radiation exposure or use of iodinated contrast

Acute Coronary Syndrome: Myocardial Perfusion Imaging

Acute coronary syndrome (ACS) accounts for approximately 10 % of all emergency department visits, making it one of the most commonly encountered medical emergencies. ACS refers to a spectrum of clinical presentations ranging from ST-segment elevation myocardial infarction to unstable angina. Clinical presentation, electrocardiography (ECG), and cardiac biomarkers, such as troponin, guide initial risk stratification. Troponin has become the favored biomarker for determination of myocardial necrosis because of

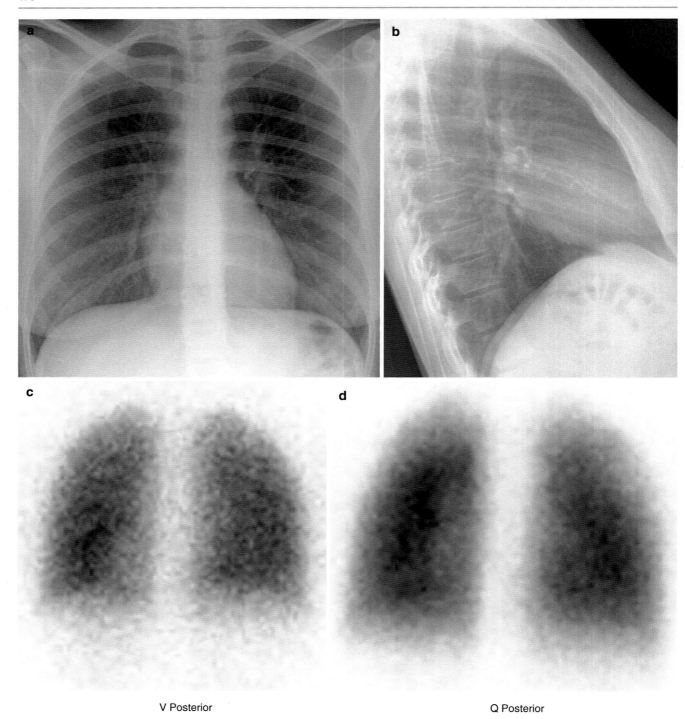

Fig. 14.1 Normal. Normal posterior-anterior (**a**) and lateral (**b**) chest radiographs. Normal ventilation (**c**) and perfusion (**d**) scintigraphy performed with ^{133} Xe gas (ventilation) and ^{99m}Tc MAA (perfusion)

the high sensitivity and specificity. However, myocardial biomarkers can only diagnose infarction and cannot identify ischemia in the absence of necrosis; also, laboratory evidence lags behind the physiological event. By convention, patients are stratified into three risk groups: high risk, moderate risk, and low risk.

The majority of patients with chest pain have no history of coronary artery disease and no ischemic ECG changes. Risk of ACS in such patients is low; however, it is not zero. Identification of high-risk patients within this cohort can be difficult clinically. Thus, many patients without ischemia are admitted for observation and further testing.

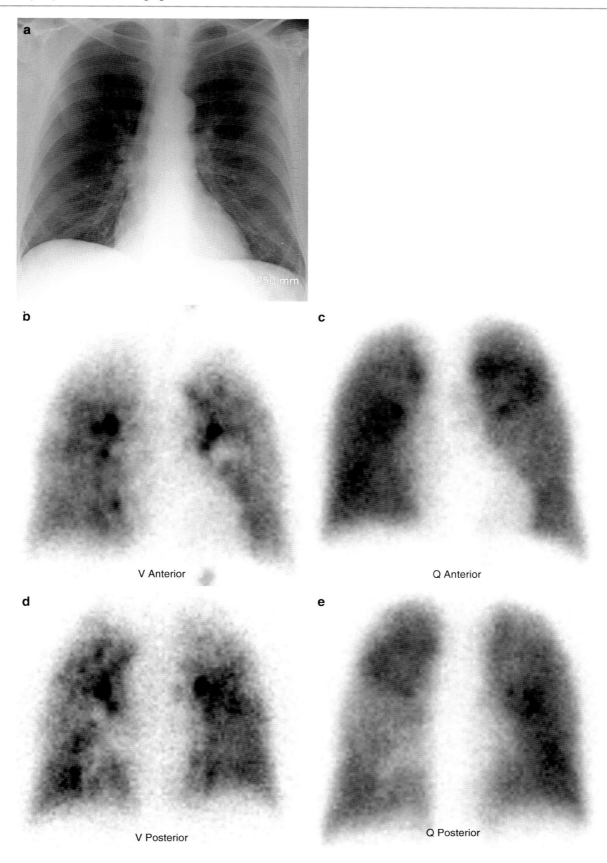

Fig. 14.2 Multiple matched V/Q abnormalities related to underlying airways disease. Normal chest radiograph (**a**). Heterogeneous ^{99m}Tc DTPA ventilation (*left panel*: **b**, **d**, **f**, **h**) and heterogeneous ^{99m}Tc MAA perfusion (*right panel*: **c**, **e**, **g**, **i**)

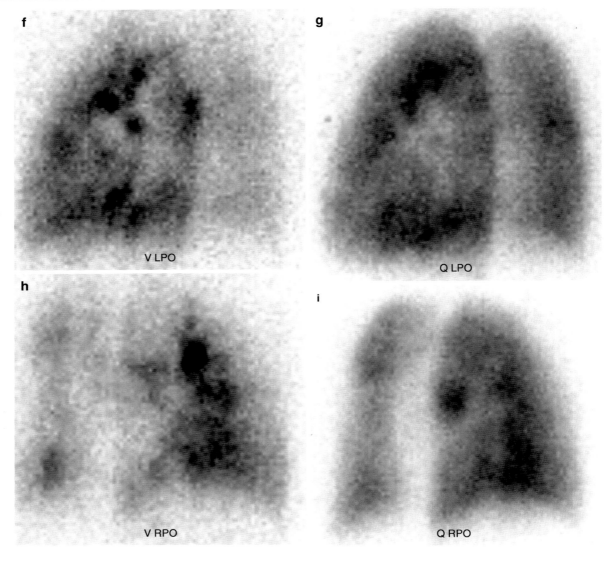

Fig. 14.2 (continued)

Conversely, despite a low threshold for admission, a significant minority of patients with atypical symptoms of ACS who actually have acute myocardial infarction are initially triaged as low risk and are unintentionally discharged home [18].

Myocardial perfusion imaging (MPI) can be effectively used as a triage tool in patients with chest pain of unclear etiology. MPI typically utilizes one of two available ^{99m}Tc radiopharmaceuticals, ^{99m}Tc sestamibi and ^{99m}Tc tetrofosmin (Table 14.4). The biodistribution within the left ventricular myocardium is generally proportional to coronary arterial blood flow at the time of IV administration; these tracers do not redistribute for several hours. Normally, there is uniform myocardial perfusion (Fig. 14.4). If a patient with ACS is injected at rest while experiencing coronary-related chest pain, the distribution of the perfusion agent will be altered and will demonstrate diminished regional perfusion corresponding to the vascular territory involved (Fig. 14.5). However, acute or prior myocardial infarction may produce a similar perfusion defect on rest MPI; therefore, differentiation between ischemia and infarction is not possible with rest MPI alone.

Rest MPI in symptomatic patients has reported sensitivities of 90–100 % with negative predictive values (NPV) of greater than 99 % for identifying patients without cardiac events [19]. The high sensitivity of rest MPI is dependent on the presence of chest pain during tracer injection; that is, MPI in patients injected after cessation of chest pain does not yield the same sensitivity, and that subgroup should undergo stress testing. Thus, the high NPV of rest MPI in patients with chest pain allows the emergency physician to establish confidently the absence of myocardial ischemia or infarction as the etiology of the symptomatology. Specifically, negative rest MPI directs disposition of patients who might otherwise have a prolonged hospital stay, and, conversely, positive rest MPI identifies high-risk patients who might be categorized incorrectly as low risk and might have a delayed diagnosis of ACS.

Incorporation of MPI into the acute chest pain diagnostic algorithm is beneficial. The ERASE trial [20] demonstrated that MPI in the emergency setting reduced unnecessary admissions without increasing inappropriate discharges. MPI as a triage tool is most effective when used on low-risk patients who are experiencing active chest pain (i.e., hemodynamically stable, no ECG changes, no prior coronary disease).

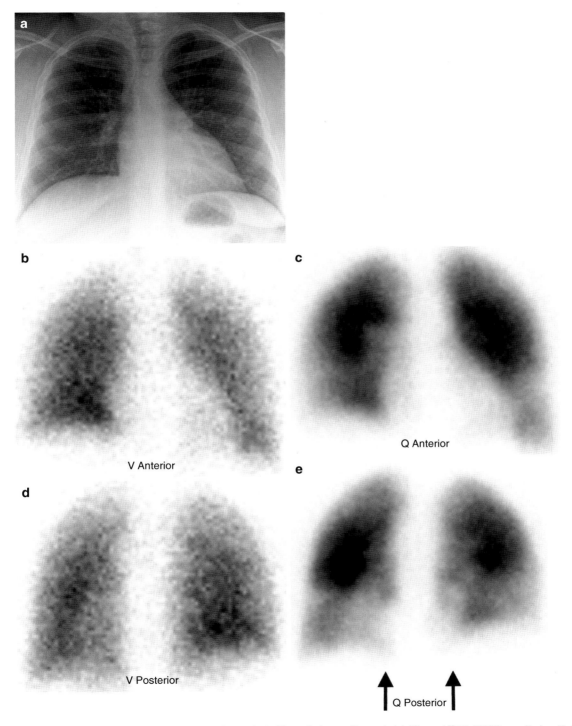

Fig. 14.3 High probability for acute PE (multiple V/Q mismatches). Normal chest radiograph (**a**). Normal ^{99m}Tc DTPA ventilation (*left panel*: **b**, **d**, **f**, **h**) and abnormal ^{99m}Tc MAA perfusion (*right panel*: **c**, **e**, **g**, **i**) with multiple bilateral lower lobe segmental perfusion defects (*arrows*)

Fig. 14.3 (continued)

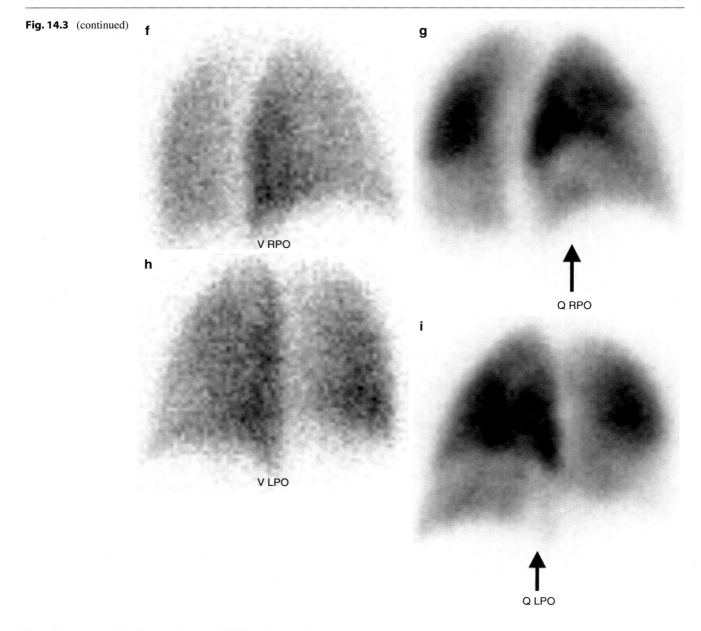

Together, concordantly negative rest MPI and negative bio-markers identify patients who can safely be discharged, or, alternatively, undergo early stress testing with or without hospital admission depending on those results. MPI is the only commonly available imaging technique that provides a direct and accurate assessment of myocardium at risk [19]. The greatest benefit of MPI lies in its high NPV, which assists the emergency physician in effectively excluding ACS in low-risk patients, lowering costs, shortening length of hospital stay, and decreasing morbidity [7, 21, 22].

In summary, in conjunction with biomarkers such as troponin, MPI can be used as a triage tool to establish the absence of myocardial ischemia or infarction as the etiology of active chest pain in patients who meet the following criteria:

1. Hemodynamically stable
2. Chest pain of unclear etiology
3. Considered low risk for ACS
4. No ischemic ECG changes

Acute Biliary Conditions: Hepatobiliary Scintigraphy

Cystic Duct Obstruction (Acute Cholecystitis) and Common Bile Duct Obstruction

Greater than 95 % of acute cholecystitis is caused by complete obstruction of the cystic duct, typically related to one or multiple gallstones. The blockage results in potentially fatal

Table 14.3 Simplified criteria for interpretation of V/Q lung scintigraphy for diagnosis of acute PE

Interpretation	Patterns on V/Q lung scintigraphy
PE absent: "normal"	No perfusion defects
PE absent: "very low probability"	Nonsegmental perfusion defects (e.g., cardiomegaly, enlarged hila, elevated hemidiaphragm)
	Perfusion defect smaller than corresponding X-ray abnormality
	Two or more V/Q matches with corresponding normal chest X-ray and otherwise relatively normal perfusion
	Three or fewer small segmental perfusion defects
	Triple-matched V/Q/X-ray abnormality in upper/mid-lung
	Stripe sign (i.e., preserved perfusion to pleural surface)
	Large pleural effusion with otherwise normal perfusion
Nondiagnostic for PE: "low probability" or "intermediate probability"	All other patterns, including triple-matched V/Q/X-ray abnormality in lower lung
PE present: "high probability"	Two or more segmental V/Q mismatches

Adapted from Sostman et al. [2]

Table 14.4 Typical rest with chest pain myocardial perfusion imaging (MPI) technical protocol

1. Administer 25 mCi (925 MBq) of ^{99m}Tc sestamibi or ^{99m}Tc tetrofosmin IV while patient has chest pain at rest
2. Wait 15–30 min
3. Perform single-photon emission computed tomography (SPECT) imaging
4. Evaluate rest-only images

pathophysiologic changes including lymphatic and venous obstruction, mucosal congestion and edema, acute inflammatory leukocyte infiltration, hemorrhage and necrosis, and, finally, complications of gangrene, perforation, and abscess [23]. Therefore, early diagnosis and appropriate management are essential to reduce mortality and morbidity.

Hepatobiliary scintigraphy (HBS), colloquially known as HIDA scanning or cholescintigraphy (Table 14.5), provides a physiologic map of hepatocellular function and bile flow. Given IV, the ^{99m}Tc iminodiacetic acid (IDA) analogs are extracted by the liver and are rapidly secreted into the bile. Normally, radioactive bile enters the biliary system including the gallbladder and passes into the small bowel within 1 h (Fig. 14.6).

In acute cholecystitis, there is a high likelihood that the cystic duct is obstructed. Thus, the hallmark finding of acute cholecystitis on HBS is nonvisualization of the gallbladder yet prompt visualization of the common bile duct and duodenum (Fig. 14.7). Complicated acute cholecystitis is supported by the pericholecystic rim sign, which is manifested by increased hepatic radiotracer activity adjacent to the gallbladder fossa. The rim sign is seen in approximately 20 % of HBS with a nonvisualized gallbladder and is strongly associated with complicated acute cholecystitis; furthermore, approximately 40 % have a gangrenous or perforated gallbladder (Fig. 14.7). Delayed gallbladder visualization suggests chronic cholecystitis with resistance to bile flow within the cystic duct without true obstruction (Fig. 14.8). Causes of false-positive and false-negative interpretations of HBS for acute cholecystitis are listed in Table 14.6.

Sensitivity and specificity for the accurate HBS diagnosis of acute cholecystitis increase with time. For conventional HBS, the false-positive rate decreases from 10 % when imaging is completed at 1 h to less than 1 % when imaging is continued to 4 h, and the specificity improves from 88 to 99 % [23]. Consequently, delayed imaging became the standard methodology used to differentiate acute cholecystitis from chronic cholecystitis, the latter condition demonstrating delayed gallbladder visualization. The administration of IV morphine sulfate during HBS shortens the duration and increases the specificity for acute cholecystitis [24]. By constricting the sphincter of Oddi, morphine sulfate raises pressure within the common bile duct, thereby diverting bile through a patent cystic duct and facilitating gallbladder visualization (Fig. 14.8). The small bowel must be visualized to apply the morphine augmentation protocol. It is also important to ascertain what pain medications have been given to the patient in the emergency department to ensure that additional opiates are not administered inadvertently. Morphine-augmented cholescintigraphy has a high accuracy and is as accurate as delayed imaging [24–26].

When compared to ultrasonography for the diagnosis of acute cholecystitis, HBS has superior sensitivity (88 % vs. 50 %), specificity (93 % vs. 88 %), positive predictive value (85 % vs. 64 %), negative predictive value (95 % vs. 80 %), and accuracy (92 % vs. 77 %) [10]. However, as discussed earlier in this chapter, logistical challenges limit availability of NM during off-hours and impact on the clinical application of this excellent scintigraphic technique. Thus, right upper quadrant ultrasonography reigns as the first-line modality for acute cholecystitis; additionally, it can provide information regarding alternate non-biliary diagnoses.

When bile fails to flow from the liver, the differential diagnosis includes acute high-grade/complete common bile duct obstruction, often related to distally impacted gallstones, versus underlying hepatocellular dysfunction. HBS can continue up to 24 h; however, the clinical context may direct management after only a few hours of imaging. The classic HBS finding of common bile duct obstruction is a persistent liver ("hepatogram") without excretion into the bile ducts (Fig. 14.9) [23]. Up to 72 h might be required for

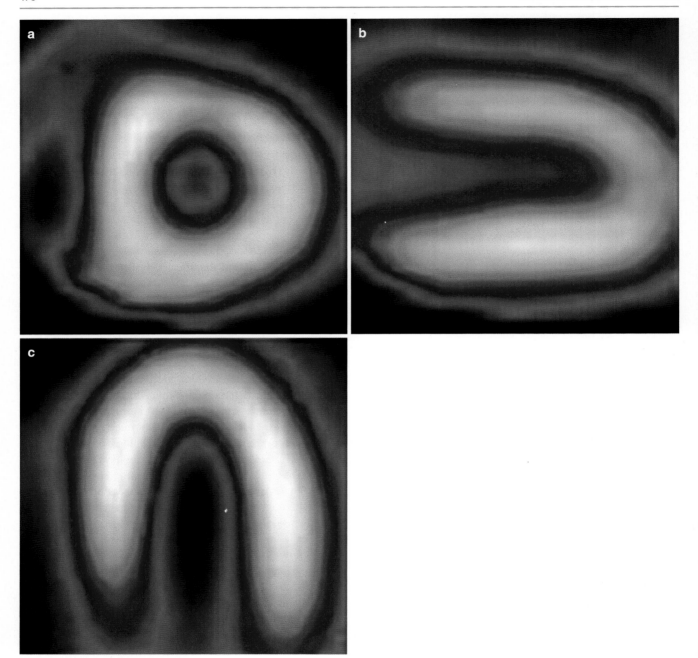

Fig. 14.4 Normal rest MPI. Uniform ^{99m}Tc sestamibi activity throughout the left ventricular myocardium. (**a**) Short-axis, (**b**) vertical long-axis, and (**c**) horizontal long-axis images

the common bile duct to dilate with a distal obstruction; thus, ultrasonography may be normal early on. It should be noted that the patency of the cystic duct cannot be established by HBS when bile flow from the liver is so severely impaired.

Bile Duct Injury

Bile duct injuries commonly occur after blunt abdominal trauma and are secondary to a shearing injury of the hepatobiliary system. A bile duct injury may lead to bile peritonitis,

which may require days or weeks to develop; clinical diagnosis may be elusive. While CT and ultrasonography can identify and localize intra-abdominal fluid collections, they cannot characterize them as containing bile.

HBS is the noninvasive standard for diagnosis of bile leak [27]. As discussed earlier in this chapter, HBS uses ^{99m}Tc IDA analogs. For evaluating bile leaks, the technical protocol is modified (Table 14.7). HBS can detect free or localized bile collections (bilomas) as well as provide information on the rate and extent of the leak. Leaks may be slow or fast, active or intermittent. If radioactive bile

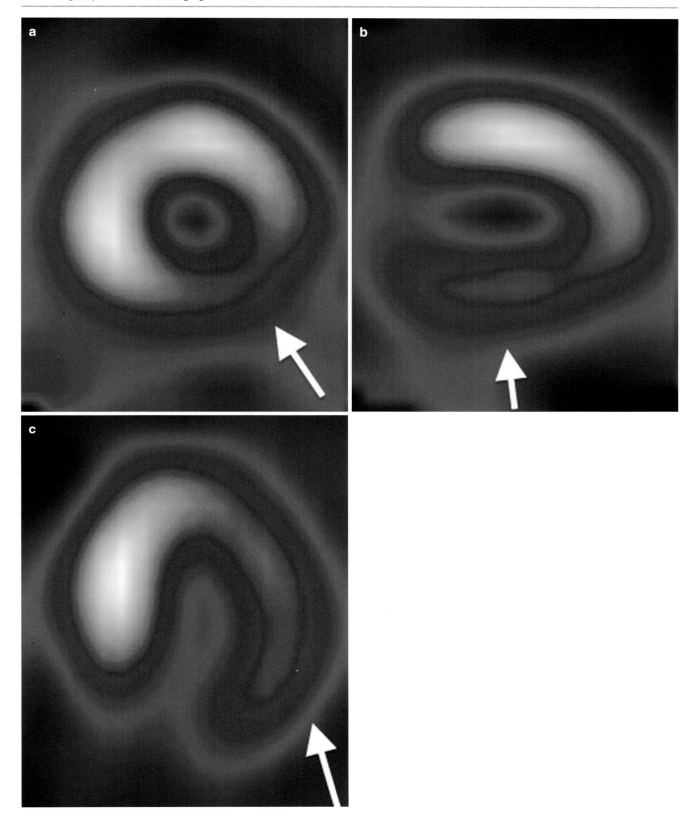

Fig. 14.5 Abnormal rest MPI. High-grade occlusion of left circumflex coronary artery as etiology of active chest pain during ⁹⁹ᵐTc sestamibi administration IV. Large, moderately severe perfusion defect in the inferior-lateral wall extending from apex to base (*arrows*). (**a**) Short-axis, (**b**) vertical long-axis, and (**c**) horizontal long-axis images

Table 14.5 Typical hepatobiliary scintigraphy technical protocol for acute cholecystitis or common bile duct obstruction

1. Fasting for 4 h; if fasting longer than 24 h, administer sincalide (synthetic CCK, 0.02 ucg/kg, IV) to prepare gallbladder

2. Administer 4 mCi (148 MBq) of ^{99m}Tc IDA analog IV

3. Acquire anterior images dynamically at 1 frame/min for 60 min or until gallbladder and small bowel are visualized

4. If common bile duct and small bowel are visualized, without gallbladder visualization, administer morphine sulfate (0.04 mg/kg IV)

5. Acquire anterior, left anterior oblique, and right lateral images 30 min later

6. If neither gallbladder nor small bowel is visualized, morphine sulfate is contraindicated

7. Acquire delayed images in multiple projections for an additional 2–4 h or up to 24 h in selected patients

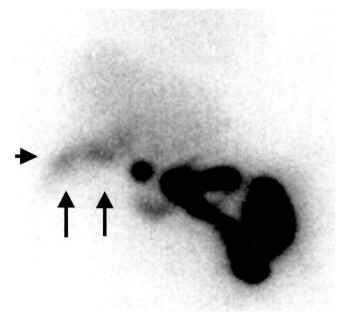

Fig. 14.7 Acute gangrenous cholecystitis. Anterior image at 2 h after IV ^{99m}Tc IDA analog. Nonvisualization of gallbladder with pericholecystic rim sign (*arrows*)

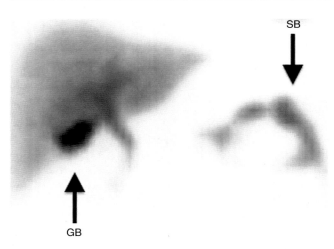

Fig. 14.6 Normal. Anterior image 20 min after ^{99m}Tc IDA analog IV. Visualization of gallbladder (*GB*) and small bowel (*SB*)

extravasates outside of the normal biliary and gastrointestinal tracts, there is an active bile leak (Fig. 14.10). Management may be conservative or may progress to percutaneous drainage, endoscopic retrograde cholangiography, or laparotomy.

In the emergency setting, particularly after blunt or penetrating trauma, HBS may be appropriate to identify an active bile leak or to characterize an abnormal fluid collection visualized on CT. For example, a liver laceration with significant bile duct injury may require different initial management compared to one without bile duct injury [28].

In summary, by providing a physiologic map of the biliary system, HBS should be strongly considered and utilized whenever available in the acute emergency setting to:

1. Establish patency of the entire hepatobiliary-small bowel axis

2. Provide a more specific diagnosis of acute cholecystitis as compared to ultrasonography

3. Evaluate for high-grade common bile duct obstruction

4. Detect an active bile leak, particularly after trauma

Gastrointestinal Hemorrhage: GI Bleeding Scintigraphy

Acute GI hemorrhage can be a life-threatening event and requires prompt diagnosis and appropriate intervention. Upper GI hemorrhage is defined as bleeding that originates proximal to the ligament of Treitz, whereas lower GI hemorrhage occurs distal to this landmark. Upper GI hemorrhage typically presents with either hematemesis or melanotic stools, whereas lower GI hemorrhage usually presents with bright red blood per rectum.

Endoscopy is a well-tolerated and generally successful first-line approach for patients with suspected upper GI hemorrhage; esophageal, gastric, or duodenal bleeding sites can be visualized and treated directly. Suspected lower GI hemorrhage presents different challenges. Prompt localization of the bleeding site is crucial to patient management; time to diagnosis is an important determinant of outcome in high-risk lower GI hemorrhage [29]. Endoscopy is an option, but is more limited in an unprepared colon that might be filled with blood from a proximal source, and the small bowel cannot be examined. Two diagnostic imaging modalities are available to identify and localize the lower GI source: ^{99m}Tc RBC scintigraphy and angiography. Despite the well-documented sensitivity, only 10–15 % of patients presenting with lower GI hemorrhage are evaluated with scintigraphy [14].

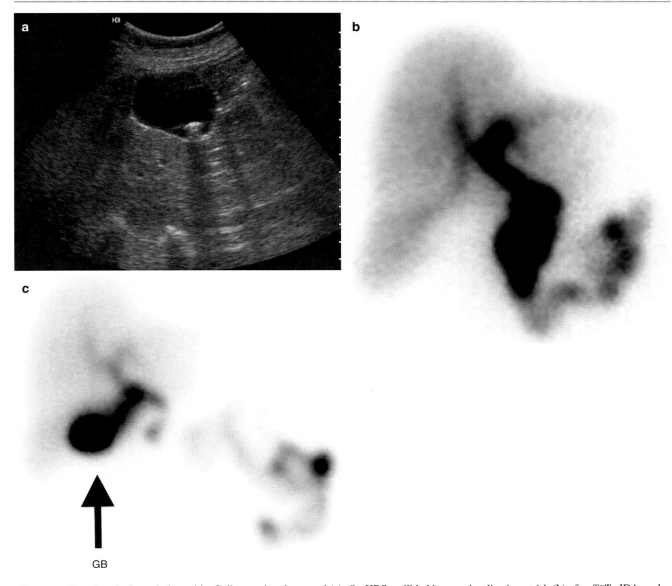

Fig. 14.8 Chronic calculous cholecystitis. Gallstones by ultrasound (**a**). On HBS, gallbladder nonvisualization at 1 h (**b**) after ^{99m}Tc IDA analog IV, but visualization (*GB*) at 20 min following morphine sulfate IV (**c**)

Table 14.6 False-positives and false-negatives on HBS for acute cholecystitis

Causes of false-positive interpretations (nonvisualized gallbladder)	Causes of false-negative interpretations (visualized gallbladder)
Recent meal (<4 h)	Acalculous cholecystitis
Prolonged fasting (>24 h)	Perforated acute cholecystitis
Hyperalimentation	Accessory cystic duct
Chronic cholecystitis	Duodenal diverticulum (misinterpretation)
Hepatic insufficiency	
Cystic duct cholangiocarcinoma	
Alcoholism	
Pancreatitis	

Dynamic GI bleeding scintigraphy utilizes ^{99m}Tc red blood cells (RBCs) (Table 14.8) and can effectively identify and localize slow or rapid, active or intermittent lower GI bleeding. Radiolabeled RBCs that extravasate from the normal circulatory system (referred to as the blood pool) are relatively easily identified because of a high target-to-background ratio. The extravasated radiolabeled RBCs will move in the bowel lumen over time, aiding in pinpointing the site of origin (Fig. 14.11).

RBC scintigraphy offers several advantages over angiography in localizing bleeding sites. First, bleeding rates as low as 0.1–0.3 mL/min are detectable with scintigraphy [30]; angiography requires rates at least tenfold higher. High

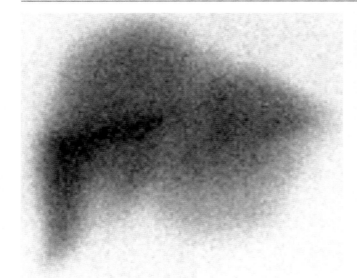

Fig. 14.9 Complete common bile duct obstruction. On HBS, uniform liver activity without biliary activity at 5 h after ^{99m}Tc IDA analog IV

Table 14.7 Typical hepatobiliary scintigraphy technical protocol for bile leak

1. Administer 4 mCi (148 MBq) of ^{99m}Tc IDA analog IV
2. Acquire anterior images dynamically at 1 frame/min for 60 min or until liver is cleared or bile leak is identified
3. Acquire anterior and posterior, right and left anterior oblique, and/or right lateral planar images up to 24 h, as needed

sensitivity (93 %) and specificity (95 %) have been reported for scintigraphy [15]. Second, RBC scintigraphy allows examination of the entire lower GI tract continuously for whatever period of time is needed and tolerated by the patient's clinical condition. Third, there are fewer complications compared with more invasive angiography, and the radiation exposure is significantly lower. Last, RBC scintigraphy can direct angiographic confirmation, expediting intervention [31].

As a noninvasive modality with high sensitivity, scintigraphy has been assessed as an important prognostic tool in GI hemorrhage. Negative results predict good clinical outcome [30]; positive results predict greater hospital morbidity and mortality [29, 32]. Positive results are accurate in localizing the bleeding site in approximately 75 % [30]. False-positives include horseshoe kidney, hepatic hemangiomata, ischemic bowel, uterine leiomyomata, and aneurysmal vasculature [33].

In summary, RBC scintigraphy should be considered as the primary imaging approach in patients presenting with GI bleeding under the following conditions:
1. Hemodynamically stable.
2. Localization of the source is desired to direct intervention.

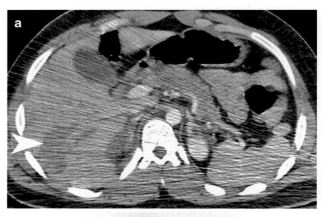

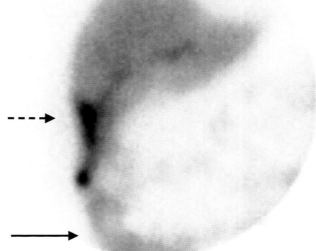

Fig. 14.10 Active bile leak. Liver laceration in right lobe (*arrowhead*) on CT (**a**) after blunt trauma. On hepatobiliary image at 30 min after ^{99m}Tc IDA analog IV (**b**), free leakage of bile (*dashed arrow*) into the right paracolic gutter (*long arrow*) and throughout the peritoneal cavity without expected intraluminal small bowel activity

Table 14.8 Typical dynamic red blood cell scintigraphy technical protocol

1. Remove blood for radiolabeling
2. Radiolabel red blood cells by in vitro method
3. Administer 25 mCi (925 MBq) of ^{99m}Tc red blood cells IV
4. Acquire anterior images dynamically at 1 frame every 10–60 s for 60–90 min
5. Review images in cinematic mode

Teaching Points

- Ventilation/perfusion (V/Q) lung scintigraphy should be considered as the primary imaging approach in patients with suspected acute PE and normal chest radiography, no concurrent cardiopulmonary process, relative contraindications

Fig. 14.11 Active bleed in proximal transverse colon. Selected images at 6 min (**a**), 38 min (**b**), and 50 min (**c**) after ^{99m}Tc RBCs IV. Active extravasation into right upper quadrant (**a**, *arrow*) with movement into the mid-abdomen (**b**, *arrow*) and further movement distally into the descending colon and sigmoid colon (**c**, *arrow*) over time

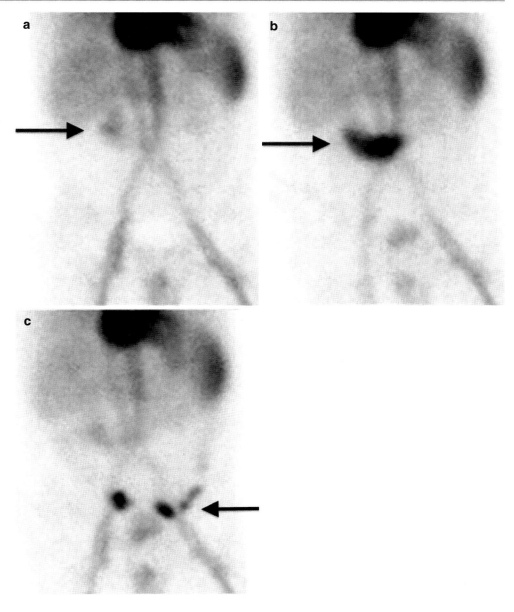

to iodinated contrast for CTA, or concerns related to radiation dosimetry.

• Rest myocardial perfusion imaging (MPI) is most effective as a triage tool when applied to low-risk patients who present with active chest pain; negative rest MPI and concordantly negative biomarkers identify patients who can safely be discharged or, alternatively, undergo early stress testing to determine need for admission.

• Hepatobiliary scintigraphy (HBS) provides a physiologic map of bile flow, uncovering normal or obstructive patterns, and boasts superior diagnostic capabilities as compared to ultrasonography for the diagnosis of acute cholecystitis. HBS can detect subtle bile duct injuries, particularly in the setting of blunt trauma.

• Dynamic ^{99m}Tc red blood cell (RBC) scintigraphy can pinpoint the source of active or intermittent lower gastrointestinal hemorrhage and directs angiographic or surgical intervention.

References

1. Mansi L, Rambaldi PF, Cuccurullo V, Varetto T. Nuclear medicine in emergency. Q J Nucl Med Mol Imaging. 2005;49:171–91.
2. Sostman HD, Miniati M, Gottschalk A, Matta F, Stein PD, Pistolesi M. Sensitivity and specificity of perfusion scintigraphy combined with chest radiography for acute pulmonary embolism in PIOPED II. J Nucl Med. 2008;49:1741–8.
3. Amini B, Patel CB, Lewin MR, Kim T, Fisher RE. Diagnostic nuclear medicine in the ED. Am J Emerg Med. 2011;29:91–101.

4. Forberg JL, Hilmersson CE, Carlsson M, Arheden H, Bjork J, Hjalte K, et al. Negative predictive value and potential cost savings of acute nuclear myocardial perfusion imaging in low risk patients with suspected acute coronary syndrome: a prospective single blinded study. BMC Emerg Med. 2009;9:12.

5. Gallagher MJ, Ross MA, Raff GL, Goldstein JA, O'Neill WW, O'Neil B. The diagnostic accuracy of 64-slice computed tomography coronary angiography compared with stress nuclear imaging in emergency department low-risk chest pain patients. Ann Emerg Med. 2007;49:125–36.

6. Kontos MC, Jesse RL, Anderson FP, Schmidt KL, Ornato JP, Tatum JL. Comparison of myocardial perfusion imaging and cardiac troponin I in patients admitted to the emergency department with chest pain. Circulation. 1999;99:2073–8.

7. Kontos MC, Schmidt KL, McCue M, Rossiter LF, Jurgensen M, Nicholson CS, et al. A comprehensive strategy for the evaluation and triage of the chest pain patient: a cost comparison study. J Nucl Cardiol. 2003;10:284–90.

8. Schaeffer MW, Brennan TD, Hughes JA, Gibler WB, Gerson MC. Resting radionuclide myocardial perfusion imaging in a chest pain center including an overnight delayed image acquisition protocol. J Nucl Med Technol. 2007;35:242–5.

9. Alobaidi M, Gupta R, Jafri SZ, Fink-Bennet DM. Current trends in imaging evaluation of acute cholecystitis. Emerg Radiol. 2004;10:256–8.

10. Chatziioannou SN, Moore WH, Ford PV, Dhekne RD. Hepatobiliary scintigraphy is superior to abdominal ultrasonography in suspected acute cholecystitis. Surgery. 2000;127:609–13.

11. Flancbaum L, Choban PS, Sinha R, Jonasson O. Morphine cholescintigraphy in the evaluation of hospitalized patients with suspected acute cholecystitis. Ann Surg. 1994;220:25–31.

12. Wahl WL, Brandt MM, Hemmila MR, Arbabi S. Diagnosis and management of bile leaks after blunt liver injury. Surgery. 2005;138:742–7; discussion 747–748.

13. Brunnler T, Klebl F, Mundorff S, Eilles C, Reng M, von Korn H, et al. Significance of scintigraphy for the localisation of obscure gastrointestinal bleedings. World J Gastroenterol. 2008;14:5015–9.

14. Currie GM, Kiat H, Wheat JM. Scintigraphic evaluation of acute lower gastrointestinal hemorrhage: current status and future directions. J Clin Gastroenterol. 2011;45:92–9.

15. Maurer A. Gastrointestinal bleeding. In: Murray IPCEP, Ell PJ, editors. Nuclear medicine in clinical diagnosis and treatment. 2nd ed. Edinburgh: Churchill Livingstone; 1998. p. 67–74.

16. Ng DA, Opelka FG, Beck DE, Milburn JM, Witherspoon LR, Hicks TC, et al. Predictive value of technetium tc 99m-labeled red blood cell scintigraphy for positive angiogram in massive lower gastrointestinal hemorrhage. Dis Colon Rectum. 1997;40:471–7.

17. Freeman LM, Stein EG, Sprayregen S, Chamarthy M, Haramati LB. The current and continuing important role of ventilation-perfusion scintigraphy in evaluating patients with suspected pulmonary embolism. Semin Nucl Med. 2008;38:432–40.

18. Kontos MC, Tatum JL. Imaging in the evaluation of the patient with suspected acute coronary syndrome. Semin Nucl Med. 2003;33:246–58.

19. Kontos MC. Myocardial perfusion imaging in the acute care setting: does it still have a role? J Nucl Cardiol. 2011;18:342–50.

20. Udelson JE, Beshansky JR, Ballin DS, Feldman JA, Griffith JL, Handler J, et al. Myocardial perfusion imaging for evaluation and triage of patients with suspected acute cardiac ischemia: a randomized controlled trial. JAMA. 2002;288:2693–700.

21. McGuire DK, O'Shea JC, Dyke CK, Kandzari DE, East MA, Tolleson TR. Highlights from the American college of cardiology 49th annual scientific sessions: march 12 to 15, 2000. Am Heart J. 2000;140:181–8.

22. Radensky PW, Hilton TC, Fulmer H, McLaughlin BA, Stowers SA. Potential cost effectiveness of initial myocardial perfusion imaging for assessment of emergency department patients with chest pain. Am J Cardiol. 1997;79:595–9.

23. Ziessman HA. Interventions used with cholescintigraphy for the diagnosis of hepatobiliary disease. Semin Nucl Med. 2009;39:174–85.

24. Fink-Bennett D, Balon H, Robbins T, Tsai D. Morphine-augmented cholescintigraphy: its efficacy in detecting acute cholecystitis. J Nucl Med. 1991;32:1231–3.

25. Fig LM, Wahl RL, Stewart RE, Shapiro B. Morphine-augmented Hepatobiliary scintigraphy in the severely ill: caution is in order. Radiology. 1990;175:467–73.

26. Kistler AM, Ziessman HA, Gooch D, Bitterman P. Morphine-augmented cholescintigraphy in acute cholecystitis. A satisfactory alternative to delayed imaging. Clin Nucl Med. 1991;16:404–6.

27. Fleming KW, Lucey BC, Soto JA, Oates ME. Posttraumatic bile leaks: role of diagnostic imaging and impact on patient outcome. Emerg Radiol. 2006;12:103–7.

28. Mittal BR, Sunil HV, Bhattacharya A, Singh B. Hepatobiliary scintigraphy in management of bile leaks in patients with blunt abdominal trauma. ANZ J Surg. 2008;78:597–600.

29. O'Neill BB, Gosnell JE, Lull RJ, Schecter WP, Koch J, Halvorsen RA, et al. Cinematic nuclear scintigraphy reliably directs surgical intervention for patients with gastrointestinal bleeding. Arch Surg. 2000;135:1076–81; discussion 1081–1072.

30. Mellinger JD, Bittner JG, Edwards MA, Bates W, Williams HT. Imaging of gastrointestinal bleeding. Surg Clin North Am. 2011;91:93–108.

31. Gunderman R, Leef J, Ong K, Reba R, Metz C. Scintigraphic screening prior to visceral arteriography in acute lower gastrointestinal bleeding. J Nucl Med. 1998;39:1081–3.

32. Kouraklis G, Misiakos E, Karatzas G, Gogas J, Skalkeas G. Diagnostic approach and management of active lower gastrointestinal hemorrhage. Int Surg. 1995;80:138–40.

33. Howarth DM. The role of nuclear medicine in the detection of acute gastrointestinal bleeding. Semin Nucl Med. 2006;36:133–46.

Ajay Singh

Foreign Body in the Pharynx and Esophagus

The most common foreign bodies in the pharynx and esophagus include coins, fish bones, batteries, tooth fragment, buttons, and plastic pieces. Although most small foreign bodies will pass through the gastrointestinal tract without producing symptoms, those which cause symptoms most commonly lodge above the cricopharyngeus.

Investigation of a patient with pain after eating fish leads to demonstration of fish bone in 21 % of the cases, most commonly in the oropharynx [1]. The most common site of impaction of fish bone is the base of the tongue. If no fish bone is demonstrated, the symptoms will usually resolve spontaneously. The complications of fish bone include perforation and sepsis. The most definitive test for evaluation of foreign body in the pharynx is rigid endoscopy. The density of the fish bone depends on a type of fish eaten by the patient. Fish such as salmon, trout, skate, and herring have lower radiopaque bone density and are difficult to see on radiographic assessment.

The radiographic findings seen on lateral view of the neck include prevertebral soft tissue swelling, soft tissue air, and demonstration of radiopaque bone (Figs. 15.1 and 15.2). It is important to include at least the sixth cervical vertebra, so as to evaluate the cricopharyngeus for foreign body. The plain radiograph may be obtained by asking the patient to sing "E," which raises the larynx and brings more of the upper esophagus into the field of view.

Radiopaque coins are the most commonly ingested foreign body in the pediatric patient. In patients with symptoms

related to the esophageal coin, immediate removal with endoscopy is recommended, while in asymptomatic patients with esophageal coin, conservative management for 12–24 h is recommended, with the hope of spontaneous passage of the coin [2]. The management of esophageal coin in asymptomatic patients where the coin is located below the thoracic inlet includes next radiograph. If the follow-up x-ray demonstrates persistent esophageal coin, then endoscopic removal is required [3].

Infections

Oral cavity infections are most often related to periodontal diseases. Periodontal infection originates from gingivitis and leads to periodontal pocket of infection, seen as radiolucency around the root of the teeth. Infections from periodontal disease can extend into the submandibular or sublingual space, depending on whether the roots of the teeth extend above or below the mylohyoid muscle insertion. Cortical destruction is more common on the lingual aspect of the mandible than the buccal aspect because of the thinner cortex on the lingual aspect. Odontogenic infection from incisors, canines, and first premolar tends to involve the lingual space. The second and third mandibular molar roots extend below mylohyoid muscle insertion and therefore tend to involve the submandibular space.

Infection in buccal space arises from maxillary incisor, canine, premolar, and first molar. Masticator space infections arise from the second maxillary molar. Infection from the third maxillary molar tends to involve the parapharyngeal space.

On contrast-enhanced CT scan study, bony erosions can be identified around the root of the affected teeth, with extension of the abscess in to the soft tissues of the floor of mouth (Fig. 15.3) [4].

A. Singh, MD
Department of Radiology,
Massachusetts General Hospital, Harvard Medical School,
10 Museum Way, # 524, Boston, MA 02141, USA
e-mail: asingh1@partners.org

A. Singh (ed.), *Emergency Radiology*,
DOI 10.1007/978-1-4419-9592-6_15, © Springer Science+Business Media New York 2013

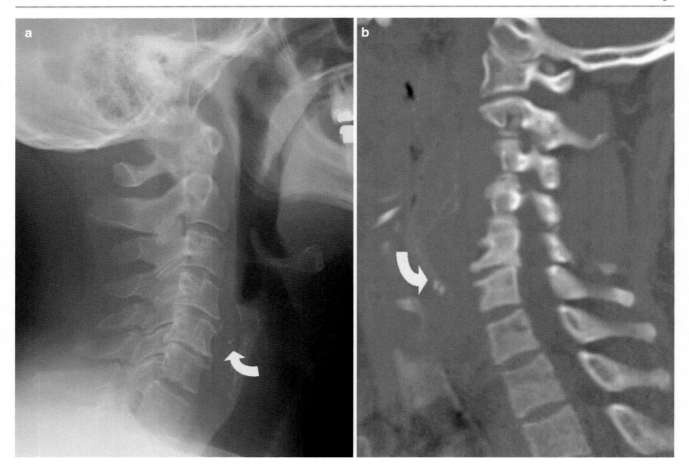

Fig. 15.1 Fish bone in the hypopharynx. (**a, b**) Lateral view of the neck and sagittal CT reformation demonstrating fish bone (*curved arrow*) in the prevertebral soft tissue, at the level of the C5 vertebra

Sialadenitis

Sialadenitis refers to viral or bacterial infection of salivary gland, most commonly affecting the parotid gland. The frequency of viral infection (mumps) has drastically decreased due to the widespread use of immunization. The viral causes of sialadenitis include mumps virus (most common), HIV, coxsackie, parainfluenza virus, and herpes virus. Bacterial infection can be caused by obstruction of Wharton's duct (submandibular gland) or Stensen's duct (parotid gland) by sialolithiases. The most common organisms causing sialadenitis include *Staphylococcus aureus*, *Streptococcus viridans*, *Haemophilus influenzae*, *Streptococcus pyogenes*, *Pseudomonas aeruginosa*, and *Escherichia coli*. Sjögren syndrome most commonly is associated with parotid sialadenitis, keratoconjunctivitis sicca, and xerostomia.

Salivary gland duct obstruction secondary to sialolithiases most commonly involves the submandibular gland. The stones are most commonly composed of calcium phosphate or calcium carbonate and are usually radiopaque enough to be visible on plain radiography. Eighty to ninety-five percent of submandibular gland sialolithiases are radiopaque and therefore seen on plain radiography [5]. Sialography is the imaging modality of choice for demonstration of the salivary gland ducts.

The salivary gland can be imaged using plain radiography, sialography, ultrasonography, and CT scan. CT allows excellent comparison with contralateral salivary gland, demonstrating sialolithiases, distinguishing intrinsic from extrinsic inflammatory process, and defining abscess/phlegmon formation. Sialadenitis is typically seen on CT as salivary gland enlargement, surrounding inflammatory changes and ductal dilatation with calculi (Fig. 15.4) [6].

Fig. 15.2 Foreign body in the hypopharynx. (**a**) AP and lateral radiographs of the neck demonstrating radiopaque coin (*curved arrow*) lodged in the prevertebral soft tissues, above the cricopharyngeus. (**b**) Sagittal CT reformation of the neck demonstrates a plastic foreign body (*arrowhead*) in the prevertebral soft tissues, lodged just proximal to the cricopharyngeus muscle. (**c**) AP radiograph of the neck demonstrates radiopaque bottle cap (*arrowhead*) lodged in the hypopharynx soft tissues, above the cricopharyngeus

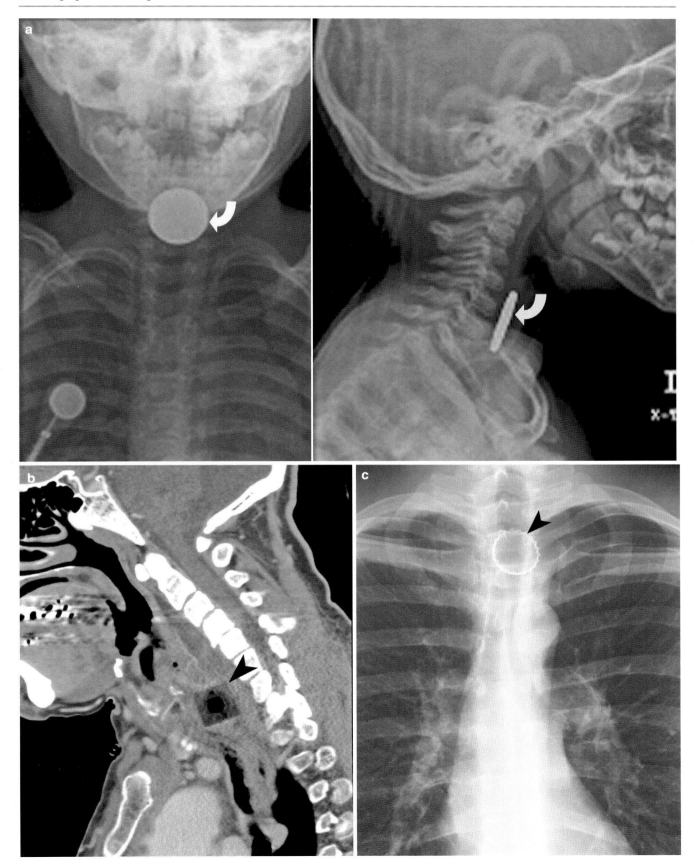

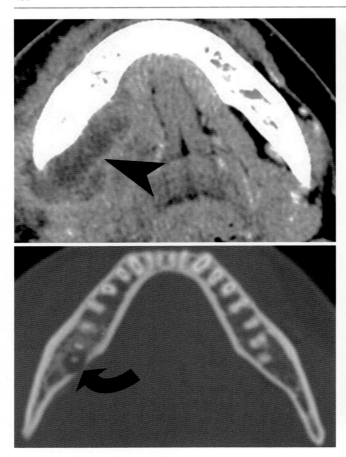

Fig. 15.3 Periodontal abscess. Contrast-enhanced CT scan study of the mandible demonstrates periodontal abscess (*curved arrow*) with extension of the abscess into the right submandibular triangle (*arrowhead*)

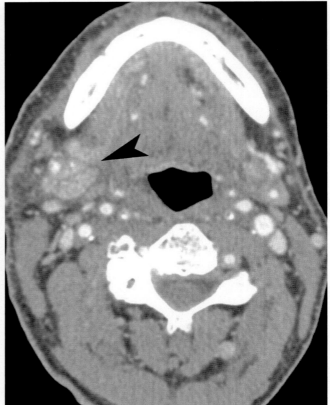

Fig. 15.4 Sialadenitis. Contrast-enhanced CT scan study of the floor of the mouth demonstrates unilateral enlargement of the right submandibular gland (*arrowhead*) with surrounding edema

Danger Space and Retropharyngeal Space Abscess

Danger space is located posterior to the retropharyngeal space and is bounded anteriorly by the alar fascia and posteriorly by the prevertebral fascia. The clinical significance of danger space infection is that the infection can directly spread to the posterior mediastinum, on either side of midline.

The retropharyngeal space is located between the buccopharyngeal fascia (visceral fascia surrounding the pharynx) and alar fascia. It is bounded laterally by the parapharyngeal space and carotid sheath. Inferiorly it extends to the level of the tracheal bifurcation, and superiorly it extends to the base of skull.

The plain radiographic findings include prevertebral soft tissue thickening, which is indicated by retrotracheal space (at C6) more than 14 mm in children and 22 mm in adults. Contrast-enhanced CT is the definitive test for demonstration of the size, location, and extent of the abscess in the deep spaces of the neck. It is not possible to distinguish retropharyngeal space from danger space abscess, unless the abscess is seen extending below the T4 vertebra (Fig. 15.5).

Retropharyngeal Abscess

It is most commonly seen before the age of 6 years and is most often caused by *Staphylococcus*, *Streptococcus*, and *Haemophilus*. It most often arises secondary to suppurative changes in retropharyngeal lymph nodes draining tonsillitis,

Fig. 15.5 Danger space abscess (**a**, **b**) and retropharyngeal abscess (**c**). (**a**) Sagittal information on the neck and chest demonstrates air containing abscess cavity (*arrowheads*) located posterior to the esophagus and extending from the neck into the mediastinum. (**b**) Plain radiograph of the neck also demonstrates the containing abscess cavity (*arrowheads*) in the prevertebral soft tissues. (**c**) Sagittal CT reformation demonstrates low-density retropharyngeal abscess (*curved arrow*) in the prevertebral soft tissues

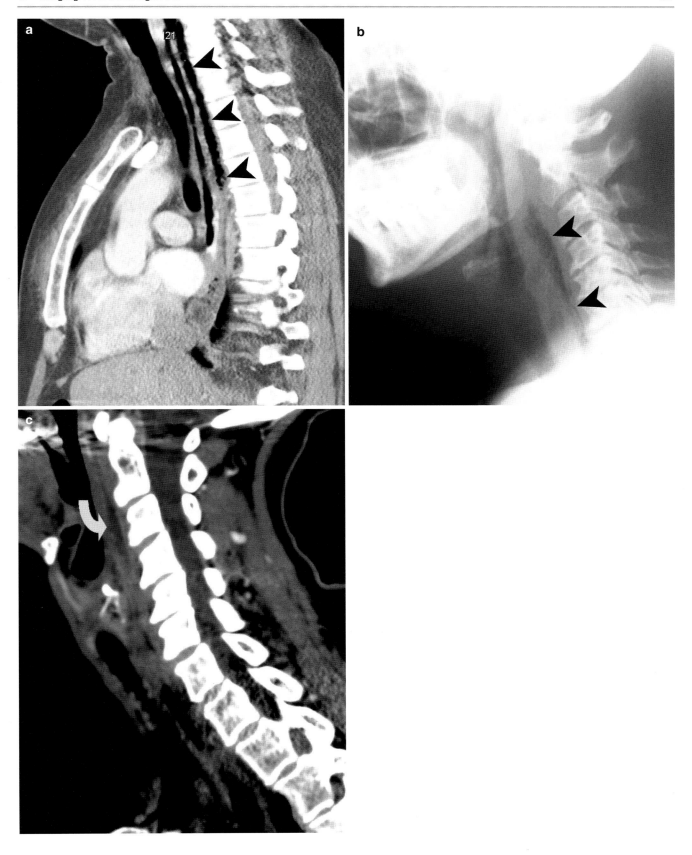

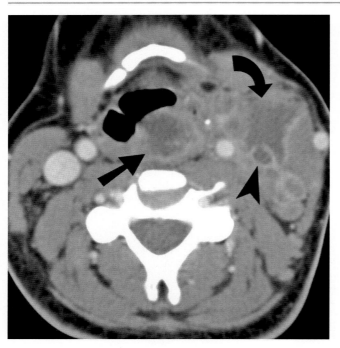

Fig. 15.6 Lemierre syndrome. Contrast enhanced CT scan study of the neck demonstrates retropharyngeal abscess (*straight arrow*) with extension on the left side to produce left internal jugular vein (*arrowhead*) thrombophlebitis. The septic thrombus in the left internal jugular vein is also producing abscess (*curved arrow*) in the soft tissues of the left anterior triangle of the neck

pharyngitis, or otitis media [7]. These suppurative lymph nodes can rupture and result in retropharyngeal abscess. The retropharyngeal abscess may also be caused by spine surgery, discitis, vertebral osteomyelitis, or pharyngeal perforation.

Contrast-enhanced CT is the imaging modality of choice and can show prevertebral soft tissue swelling and loculated abscess with enhancing wall (Fig. 15.8b). It can also show other findings such as discitis/osteomyelitis, airway compromise, thrombophlebitis, and epidural abscess.

Lemierre's Syndrome

Lemierre's syndrome, also called postanginal sepsis or necrobacillosis, is characterized by thrombophlebitis in the neck, most often due to *Fusobacterium necrophorum* infection [8]. Other species of *Fusobacterium* species are

responsible for 11 %, and other gram-negative organisms are responsible in 8 % of cases of Lemierre's syndrome [9]. It most commonly affects young adults after a complicated pharyngitis with parapharyngeal or peritonsillar abscess formation. These abscesses provide optimal surroundings for the growth of the anaerobic bacteria, which proliferate to involve the adjacent internal jugular vein. The thrombophlebitis of the internal jugular vein can cause embolization of the infected clot to the lungs and septicemia.

The imaging findings of septic thrombophlebitis and associated abscess can be demonstrated on US or CT study. The acute internal jugular vein thrombus can be seen on contrast-enhanced CT as low-density filling defect with distension of the vein (Fig. 15.6). Contrast-enhanced CT can also demonstrate the septic microemboli to the lungs indicated by multiple peripheral round- or wedge-shaped nodules and lung abscess formation. Other pulmonary findings include consolidation, pleural effusion, and empyema.

Tonsillitis and Peritonsillar Abscess

Peritonsillar abscess is a complication of acute tonsillitis, due to extension of infection through the tonsillar capsule, to the potential space between the capsule and the superior constrictor muscle. It represents the most common deep soft tissue infection of the neck, most commonly caused by *Staphylococcus*, *Streptococcus*, *Haemophilus*, *pneumococcus*, *Fusobacterium*, and *Peptostreptococcus*.

Imaging is most often performed in cases of complicated tonsillitis, where peritonsillar infection is suspected. The imaging findings include palatine tonsillar enlargement, striated enhancement, peritonsillar liquefaction, and loculated abscess formation (Fig. 15.7). The definitive treatment of peritonsillar abscess is surgical incision and drainage in the emergency room after intravenous antibiotics.

Adenoidal Hypertrophy

Adenoidal hypertrophy is common in the 6-month to 6-year age group. Clinical examination and flexible nasopharyngoscopy can be performed to evaluate the adenoidal size. Nasal endoscopy may be complementary to lateral radiograph of

Fig. 15.7 Tonsillitis and peritonsillar abscess. (**a**) Lateral radiograph of neck demonstrates enlargement of the pharyngeal tonsils (*arrowheads*) in the lateral wall of the oropharynx. (**b–d**). Contrast-enhanced T1-weighted MRI and noncontrast CT (axial and coronal) demonstrate bilateral palatine tonsillar enlargement (*bifid arrow*). (**e**) Contrast-enhanced CT scan study of the upper neck demonstrates left peritonsillar abscess (*curved arrow*), producing mass effect on the oropharyngeal airway. (**f**) Contrast-enhanced T1-weighted MRI of the upper neck demonstrates left peritonsillar abscess (*arrowhead*) with mass effect on the oropharyngeal airway

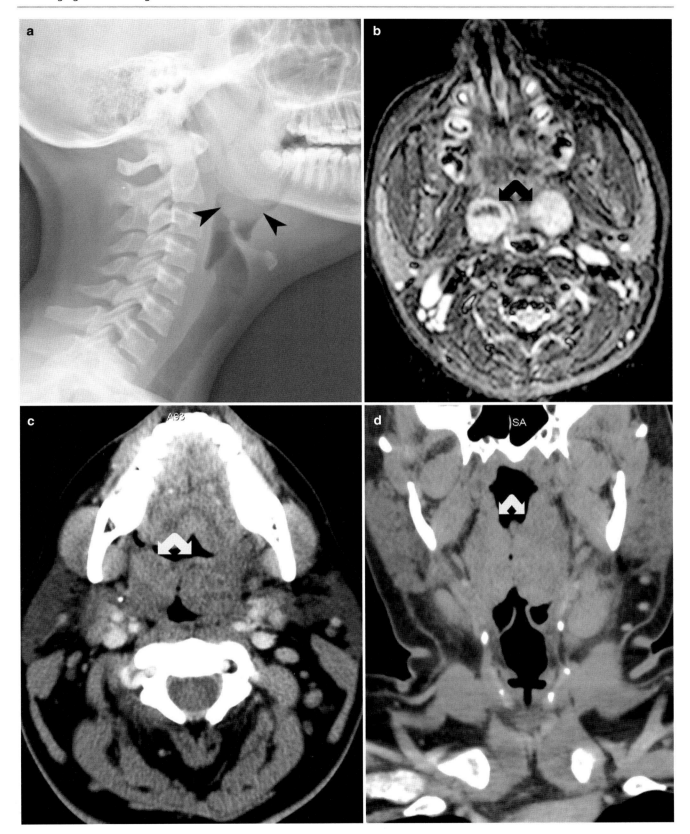

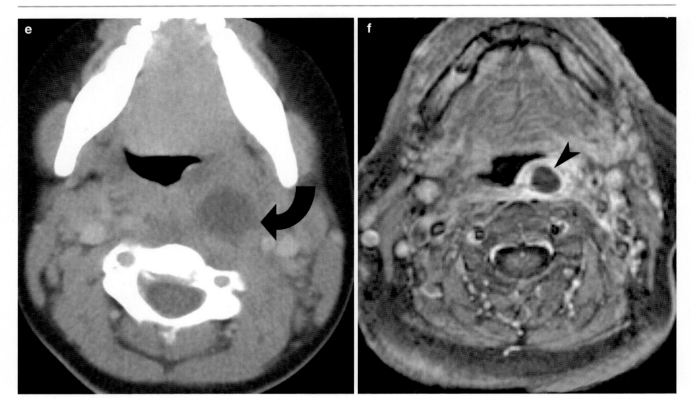

Fig. 15.7 (continued)

the neck in evaluation of the adenoids [10]. Although its role is controversial, lateral radiograph of the neck was shown to be a reliable diagnostic test in the evaluation of hypertrophied adenoids (Fig. 15.8a) [10, 11].

Croup

Croup is a viral infection of the airways and is typically characterized by acute laryngotracheobronchitis. It is most commonly caused by parainfluenza or respiratory syncytial virus. It is most commonly seen in the age group of 6 months to 3 years. It is associated with reactive subglottic edema which extends from true vocal cords to the conus elasticus, which can be seen on high-KV radiographs of the neck.

Normal AP radiograph of the neck shows shouldering in the subglottic larynx (Fig. 15.9a). The patients with croup will most often have subglottic edema, indicated by the steeple sign. The steeple sign is characterized by inverted V-shaped configuration of the subglottic larynx with loss of subglottic shouldering or convexity (Fig. 15.9b). The lateral

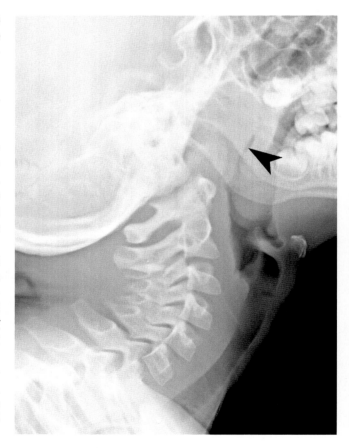

Fig. 15.8 Adenoidal hypertrophy. Lateral radiograph of the neck demonstrates gross adenoidal hypertrophy (*arrowhead*) along the posterior wall of the nasopharynx with severe compromise of the nasopharyngeal airway

Fig. 15.9 Steeple sign. (**a**) Normal AP radiograph of the neck demonstrates normal shouldering (*straight arrow*) seen in the subglottic laryngeal airway. (**b**) AP radiograph of the neck in a patient with croup demonstrates steeple-shaped narrowing (*straight arrow*) of the subglottic laryngeal airway

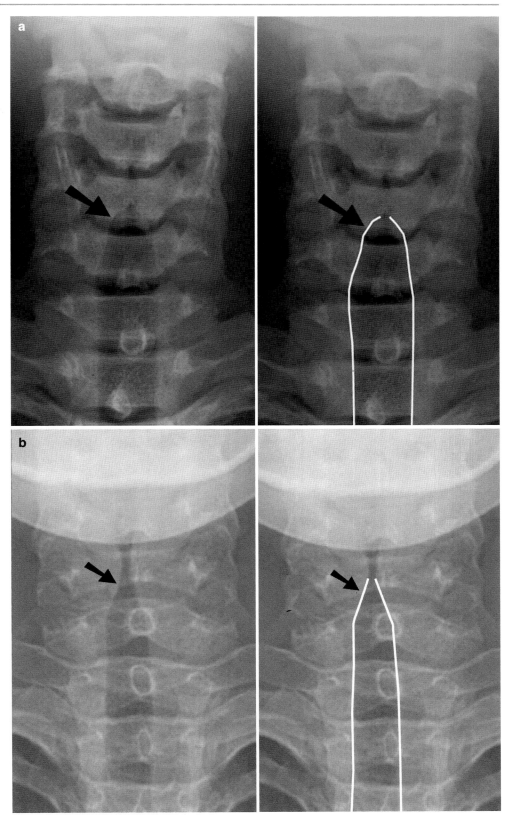

radiograph may also show distension of hypopharynx, secondary to the subglottic narrowing which measures 1–1.5 cm in length [12].

Croup is a self-limited disease with excellent prognosis with conservative management.

Epiglottitis

Epiglottitis is life threatening which can cause rapid airway compromise, especially in children. Unlike croup, epiglottitis is seen in older children, most often at the group of 6–7 years. *H. influenzae* epiglottitis is more rapidly progressive than other kinds of epiglottitis and therefore has high risk of upper airway occlusion. Imaging may be performed when the clinical diagnosis is not certain. The lateral radiograph of the neck shows thumb-like enlargement of the epiglottis and thickened aryepiglottic folds (Fig. 15.10). Contrast-enhanced CT can show enlargement of the epiglottitis, mucosal enhancement, and adjacent cellulitis/abscess formation.

Thyroglossal Duct Cyst

Thyroglossal duct cyst is the most common congenital anomaly of the neck and is caused by incomplete regression of the thyroglossal duct. It is most commonly seen in the first decade of life. These epithelial-lined cysts are commonly midline (except infrahyoid cysts) in position and are located in close proximity to the hyoid bone. Infrahyoid location is the most common (65 %) location of the thyroglossal duct cysts. The infrahyoid cysts which are not midline in location are most often located within 2 cm of midline. The complications of thyroglossal duct cysts include infection and malignant transformation (papillary carcinoma of thyroid).

The thyroglossal duct cysts can be imaged with ultrasound, CT, or MRI. On ultrasound imaging, four patterns of thyroglossal duct cyst have been described by Ahujaa et al. These four patterns include anechoic (28 %), homogeneously hypoechoic with internal debris (18 %), pseudosolid (28 %), and heterogeneous (28 %). The majority showed posterior enhancement (88 %), midline (63 %), and infrahyoid in location (83 %) [13].

The CT findings include a well-defined low-attenuation cystic lesion with thin wall, most commonly in infrahyoid location (Fig. 15.11). The cystic lesion has a low signal intensity on T1 and high signal intensity on T2-weighted images. The differential diagnosis of TDC in adults includes dermoid cyst, branchial cleft cyst, lymphadenopathy, thymic cyst, lymphangioma, and cystic thyroid nodule.

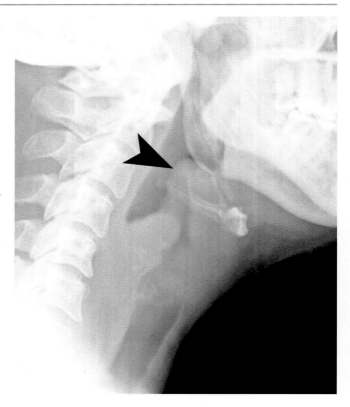

Fig. 15.10 Epiglottitis. Lateral radiograph of the neck demonstrates gross enlargement of the epiglottis (*arrowhead*) as well as the aryepiglottic fold, resulting in narrowing of the supraglottic laryngeal airway

Branchial Cleft Cyst

The second branchial cleft accounts for 95 % of the anomalies and is located in relation to the proximal third of the sternocleidomastoid muscle (Table 15.1). They are most commonly seen in 10–40-year age group as a painless cystic mass in the upper neck. On CT, it is typically seen as a cystic lesion with thin wall, in relation to the anterior border of the sternocleidomastoid, at the level of the angle of mandible (Fig. 15.12). Infected cyst may show wall thickening and enhancement. The differential diagnosis of paramedian cystic mass of the neck includes dermoid, laryngocele, plunging ranula, lymphangioma, thymic cyst (Fig. 15.13), and necrotic lymph node.

Temporal Fracture

CT is the imaging modality of choice for the evaluation of temporal bone fracture and ossicular disruption. Temporal bone fractures are classified as either longitudinal or transverse, depending on whether the fracture plane is parallel to the long

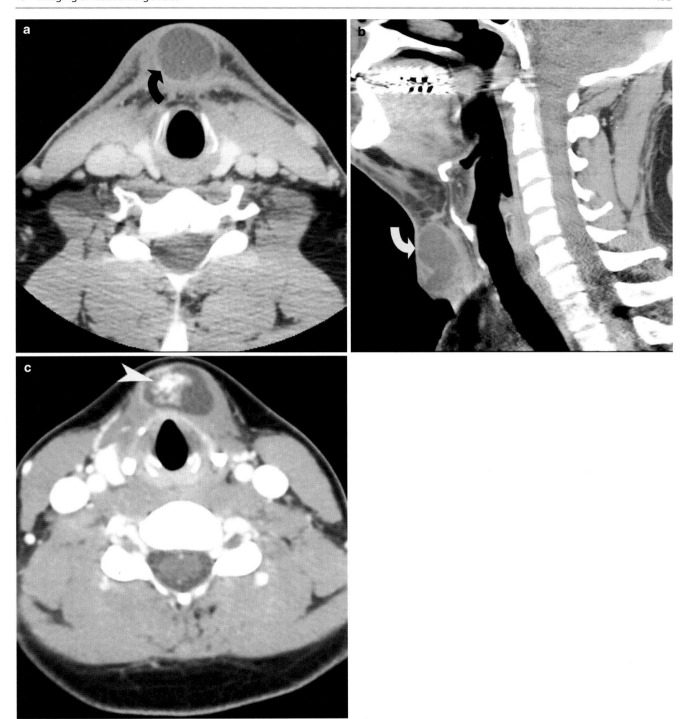

Fig. 15.11 Thyroglossal duct cyst. (**a, b**) Axial CT and sagittal C2 formation demonstrates well-defined infrahyoid cystic lesion with enhancing wall (*curved arrows*). (**c**) Contrast-enhanced CT scan study of the upper neck demonstrates midline thyroglossal duct cyst and infrahilar location. The enhancing irregular lesion with calcification identified within the cyst represents papillary thyroid carcinoma (*arrowhead*)

axis or perpendicular to the long axis of the petrous temporal bone. The injuries associated with petrous temporal bone fracture include seventh cranial nerve injury, CSF leak, sensorineural deafness, conductive deafness, and brain contusion.

Table 15.1 Branchial cleft cyst locations

Branchial cleft cyst	Location
First	External auditory canal (type 1) and submandibular gland (type 2)
Second	Anterior border of upper 3rd of sternocleidomastoid muscle
Third	Larynx and pyriform sinus
Fourth	Various locations, including thyroid gland and mediastinum

Transverse fractures of the temporal bone are often the result of trauma to the occipital or craniocervical junction. The transversely oriented fracture can cause sensorineural deafness because of the involvement of the vestibulocochlear apparatus (Fig. 15.14a). This fracture can also be associated with injury to the seventh cranial nerve, along its labyrinthine course.

The longitudinal fractures are the most common type of petrous temporal fractures (Fig. 15.14b). It is often the result of direct trauma to the temporal region and is therefore associated with fractures of the squamous temporal bone. The fracture line may pass through the facial nerve canal and

may also cause disruption of the ossicular chain, resulting in conductive deafness. Incudostapedial joint disarticulation is the most common posttraumatic abnormality of the middle ear ossicles (Fig. 15.15). Reconstruction of the ossicular chain is performed when there is conductive hearing loss of more than 30 dB that persists 6 months after trauma [14].

Hyoid Fracture

The hyoid bone consists of body, two greater cornua directed posteriorly, and two lesser cornua project superiorly. Hyoid bone fractures are clinically important because of its proximity to the airway and associated soft tissue injuries (Fig. 15.16). These fractures tend to involve the central part of the bone. Majority of isolated hyoid bone fractures are due to strangulation. Therefore, hyoid bone fracture in cases of suspected homicide strongly suggests strangulation injury [15]. Fractured hyoids are more likely in older patients where they are fused. The fractured hyoid bones tend to be longer in the anterior-posterior plane and more steeply sloping when compared with unfractured hyoids [15].

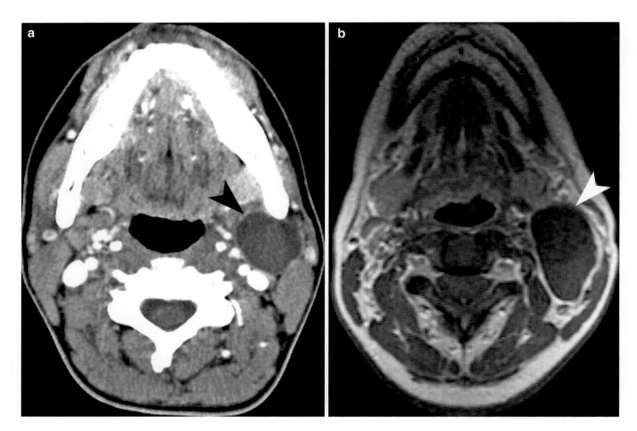

Fig. 15.12 Branchial cleft cyst. (**a**) Contrast-enhanced CT scan study of the upper neck demonstrates a second branchial cleft cyst (*arrowhead*) located in tear medial to the sternocleidomastoid muscle, at the level of the angle of the mandible. (**b**, **c**) Noncontrast T1-weighted and T2-weighted sequence of the upper neck demonstrates a well-defined second branchial cleft cyst (*arrowheads*) on the *left side*

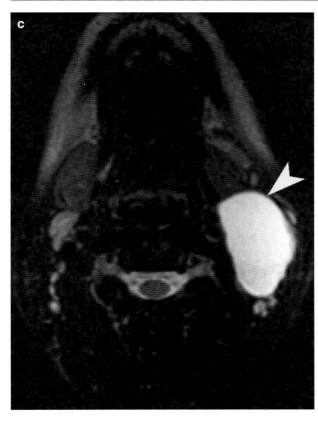

Fig. 15.12 (continued)

Cholesteatoma

Majority of cholesteatomas are acquired and are believed to arise secondary to middle ear infection, from the tympanic membrane. It is made up to densely packed squamous keratinized squamous epithelial cells which are continuously collecting inside the shell formed by the epithelial cells. The shell is formed by tympanic membrane retraction with obstruction of the neck by keratin.

CT is the imaging modality of choice and most often demonstrates the cholesteatoma in the Prussak's space with erosion of the scutum and medial displacement of the ossicles (Fig. 15.17). This classic appearance of cholesteatoma arises from the pars tensa and constitutes more than 80 % of the cholesteatomas. The less common (less than 20 %) pars tensa cholesteatomas extend medial to the incus and displace the ossicles laterally.

MRI does not allow the anatomical precision as CT study but may allow better tissue characterization for scar, granulation tissue, cholesteatoma (hyperintense on DWI), and cholesterol granuloma (T1 hyperintense). On MRI, cholesteatoma is T1 hypointense and T2 hyperintense, with hyperintensity on diffusion-weighted sequence.

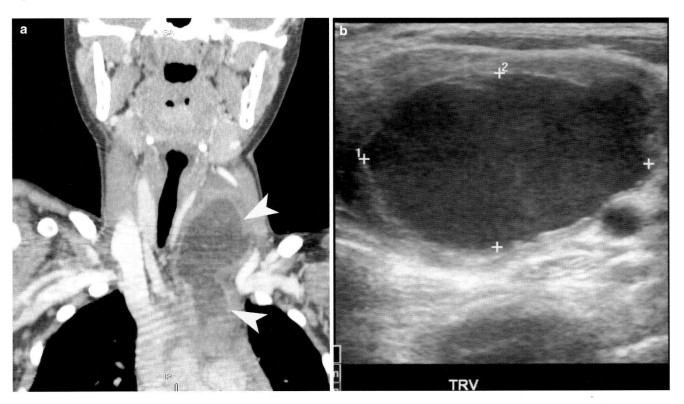

Fig. 15.13 Infected thymic cyst. (**a**) Coronal CT reformation demonstrates a large left-sided thymic cyst (*arrowheads*) extending from the left superior mediastinum to the left supraclavicular neck. (**b**) Ultrasound of the infected thymic cyst demonstrates low-level internal echoes within the cyst

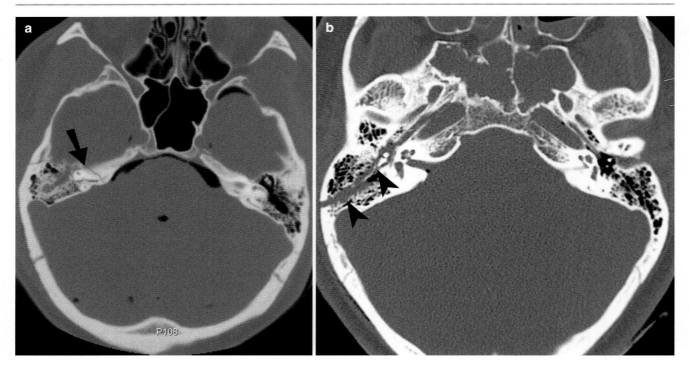

Fig. 15.14 Petrous temporal fracture. (**a**) Axial CT scan study of the petrous temporal bone demonstrates transversely oriented fracture (*straight arrow*) of the right petrous temporal bone. There is pneumocephalus identified due to communication of the mastoid air cells with the extra-axial spaces. (**b**) Axial CT scan study of the petrous temporal bone demonstrates a longitudinally oriented fracture line (*arrowheads*) through the right petrous temporal bone

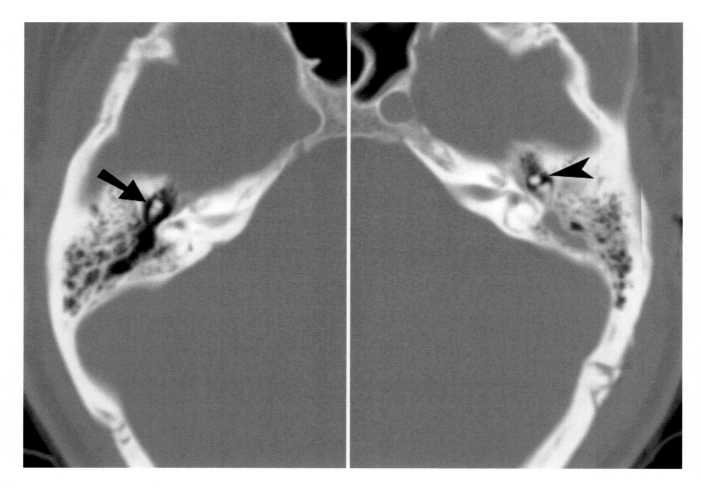

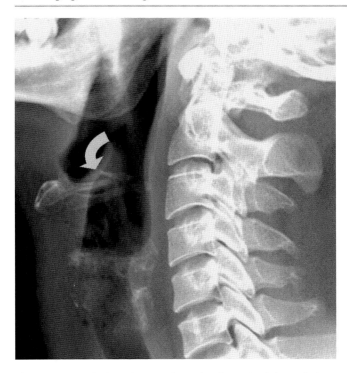

Fig. 15.16 Hyoid bone fracture. Lateral radiograph of the neck demonstrates fracture of the greater cornua (*curved arrow*)

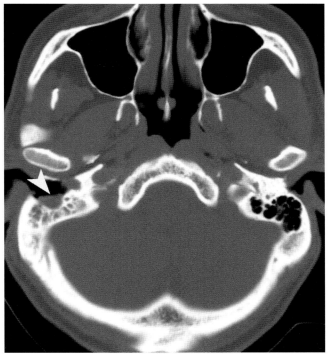

Fig. 15.17 Cholesteatoma. Soft tissue density cholesteatoma (*arrowhead*) is identified on the right side with associated destruction of the bony walls and opacification of the mastoid air cells

Petrous Apicitis

Petrous apicitis refers to the infection of the petrous temporal apex, resulting in osteomyelitis. It can be seen as a complication of mastoiditis or middle ear infection and is less commonly seen in today's practice because of the early use of antibiotics. *Pseudomonas* is most often responsible for petrous apicitis.

The classic clinical presentation includes headache, sixth cranial nerve palsy, and otorrhea. This is described as Gradenigo syndrome and is characterized abducent nerve paralysis as it passes through the Dorello's canal. The complications of petrous apicitis include dural venous sinus thrombosis, extradural abscess, meningitis, as well as brain abscess formation.

CT scan study is the imaging modality of choice and is characterized by presence of bony erosion with ill-defined margins and peripheral enhancement. MRI is more sensitive for evaluation of the extension of inflammation to the dura and intracranial extension. The MRI findings include hyperintensity on T2-weighted images due to the presence of fluid as well as granulation tissue and post-gadolinium enhancement due to the presence of inflammation (Fig. 15.18) [16].

Mastoiditis

Mastoiditis refers to infection of the mastoid air cells of the temporal bone. Because of their close anatomical relationship with the middle ear, mastoiditis is often caused by extension of the otitis media. Mastoiditis can progress from infection of the mucosa lining of the mastoid air cells to osteomyelitis and formation of abscess cavity which in turn may extend outside the confines of the mastoid cortex. The complications of acute mastoiditis include dural sinus thrombosis, osteomyelitis, brain abscess, subdural abscess, and epidural abscess.

Acute mastoiditis is most commonly seen in young children and is often secondary to acute otitis media. The CT findings include opacification of the mastoid air cells, which in later stages can be associated with bony destruction, bony dehiscence, and abscess formation. Bezold's abscess refers to dehiscence of mastoid wall with extension of inflammation into the soft tissues of the neck and abscess formation (Fig. 15.19).

Fig. 15.15 Ossicular disruption. Axial noncontrast CT scan study of the petrous temporal bone demonstrates normal orientation of the right middle ear ossicles (*straight arrow*). The CT scan study demonstrates left-sided incudostapedial ossicular disruption (*arrowhead*), indicated by presence of air between the malleus and incus

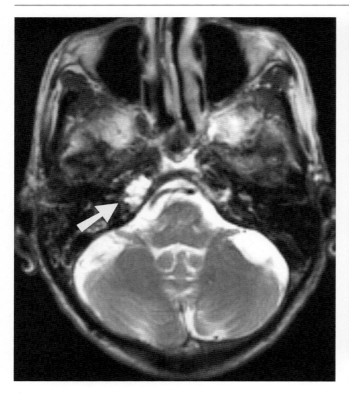

Fig. 15.18 Petrous apicitis. T2-weighted MRI petrous temporal bone demonstrates high signal intensity (*straight arrow*) in the right petrous apex

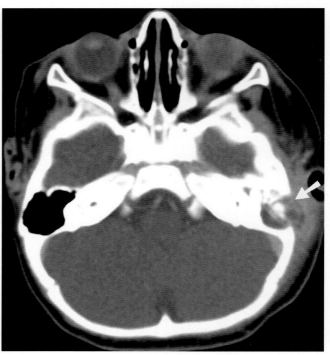

Fig. 15.19 Mastoiditis and Bezold's abscess. Axial contrast-enhanced CT scan study of the petrous temporal bone demonstrates destruction of the left mastoid air cells with extension of abscess (*straight arrow*) into the soft tissues over the left mastoid process

Teaching Points

1. Unlike retropharyngeal abscess, danger space abscess can extend below T4 vertebra.
2. Lemierre's syndrome is characterized by thrombophlebitis in the neck, most often due to *Fusobacterium necrophorum* infection.
3. Eighty to ninety-five percent of submandibular gland sialolithiases are radiopaque and therefore seen on plain radiography.

References

1. Knight LC, Lesser THJ. Fish bones in the throat. Arch Emerg Med. 1989;6:13–6.
2. Waltzman ML. Management of esophageal coins. Curr Opin Pediatr. 2006;18(5):571–4.
3. Sharieff GQ, Brousseau TJ, Bradshaw JA, Shad JA. Acute esophageal coin ingestions: is immediate removal necessary? Pediatr Radiol. 2003;33(12):859–63.
4. Capps EF, Kinsella JJ, Gupta M, Bhatki AM, Opatowsky MJ. Emergency imaging assessment of acute, nontraumatic conditions of the head and neck. Radiographics. 2010;30:1335–52.
5. Isacsson G, Isberg A, Haverling M, et al. Salivary calculi and chronic sialoadenitis of the submandibular gland: a radiographic

and histologic study. Oral Surg Oral Med Oral Pathol. 1984;58(5):622–7.
6. Zenk J, Iro H, Klintworth N, Lell M. Diagnostic imaging in sialadenitis. Oral Maxillofac Surg Clin North Am. 2009;21(3):275–92.
7. Shefelbine SE, Mancuso AA, Gajewski BJ, Ojiri H, Stringer S, Sedwick JD. Pediatric retropharyngeal lymphadenitis: differentiation from retropharyngeal abscess and treatment implications. Otolaryngol Head Neck Surg. 2007;136(2):182–8.
8. Screaton NJ, Ravenel JG, Lehner PJ, Heitzman ER, Flower CD. Lemierre syndrome: forgotten but not extinct – report of four cases. Radiology. 1999;213(2):369–74.
9. Sinave CP, Hardy GJ, Fardy PW. The Lemierre syndrome: suppurative thrombophlebitis of the internal jugular vein secondary to oropharyngeal infection. Medicine. 1989;68:85–94.
10. Saedi B, Sadeghi M, Mojtahed M, Mahboubi H. Diagnostic efficacy of different methods in the assessment of adenoid hypertrophy. Am J Otolaryngol. 2011;32(2):147–51.
11. Mary Kurien M, Lepcha A, Mathew J, Ali A, Jeyaseelan L. X-Rays in the evaluation of adenoid hypertrophy: It's role in the endoscopic era. Indian J Otolaryngol Head Neck Surg. 2005;57(1):45–7.
12. Mozhdeh SM. The steeple sign. Radiology. 2000;216:428–9.
13. Ahujaa AT, Kinga AD, Kinga W, Metrewelia C. Thyroglossal duct cysts: sonographic appearances in adults. AJNR Am J Neuroradiol. 1999;20:579–82.
14. Lee D, Honrado C, Har-El G, Goldsmith A. Pediatric temporal bone fractures. Laryngoscope. 1998;108:816–21.
15. Pollanen MS, Chiasson DA. Fracture of the hyoid bone in strangulation: comparison of fractured and unfractured hyoids from victims of strangulation. J Forensic Sci. 1996;41(1):110–3.
16. Lee YH YH, Lee NJ, Kim JH, Song JJ. CT, MRI and gallium SPECT in the diagnosis and treatment of petrous apicitis presenting as multiple cranial neuropathies. Br J Radiol. 2005;78:948–51.

Imaging of Acute Head Emergencies

Majid Khan, Sneha Patel, and Ajay Singh

Introduction

In the management of acute intracranial emergencies, triage of patients is key, and therefore, the proper diagnosis on early imaging can go a long way in directing the appropriate workup and management.

Pseudo-subarachnoid Hemorrhage

Increased density in the subarachnoid spaces at the basal cisterns is typically seen in patients with diffuse subarachnoid hemorrhage. However, it is imperative to examine the brain parenchyma for signs of increased cerebral edema, as the increased density in the subarachnoid space may well be engorged dural, arterial, and venous vessels from brain swelling (Fig. 16.1). Other CT mimics of subarachnoid hemorrhage include intrathecal contrast injection, infectious meningitis, and leakage of intravascular contrast into the subarachnoid spaces.

The pathologic cause of the increased cisternal density is not definitively known, but is postulated to be secondary to a combination of factors, including displacement of normally hypodense cerebrospinal fluid, engorgement of the superficial vasculature, and the edematous and hypodense adjacent brain [1].

Carbon Monoxide Poisoning

Patients found unresponsive and brought for acute neuroimaging can have a whole host of imaging findings, some subtle and others obvious. Carbon monoxide poisoning is one potentially subtle imaging finding which, if detected early, can significantly improve the clinical prognosis of the patient.

Carbon monoxide poisoning is a typically symmetric anoxic encephalopathy, with a much higher affinity for hemoglobin than oxygen. Cerebral injury has a predilection for the globi pallidi (Fig. 16.2) [2]. The cerebral white matter may or may not be also involved, depending on the duration of exposure. If diagnosed within 6 h on initial injury, long-term neuropsychiatric morbidity can be curtailed. Standard treatments include hyperbaric oxygen and 100 % oxygen.

Differential considerations include Creutzfeldt-Jakob disease, Wilson's disease, and Leigh syndrome, all entities which can affect the globi pallidi, although all of these have more widespread gray matter involvement than CO poisoning.

Central Nervous System Infections

Cerebral abscesses are typically located at the corticomedullary junction and have thin, regular capsule formation that appears hypointense on T2-weighted images. The causes of brain abscess include bacterial, fungal, or tuberculosis. The disease evolves from an early cerebritis and extensive T2 signal intensity abnormality to liquefaction and capsule formation.

The medial temporal lobe involvement by focal process can be from arterial ischemia, which originates from the PCA territory; pyogenic infection, which can arise from otogenic infection; and herpes encephalitis, which has a predilection

M. Khan, MD
Department of Radiology, Oakland University,
William Beaumont School of Medicine,
William Beaumont Hospital,
Royal Oak, MI, USA

S. Patel, MD
Department of Diagnostic Radiology,
William Beaumont Hospital,
Royal Oak, MI, USA

A. Singh, MD (✉)
Department of Radiology,
Massachusetts General Hospital, Harvard Medical School,
10 Museum Way, # 524, Boston, MA 02141, USA
e-mail: asingh1@partners.org

A. Singh (ed.), *Emergency Radiology*,
DOI 10.1007/978-1-4419-9592-6_16, © Springer Science+Business Media New York 2013

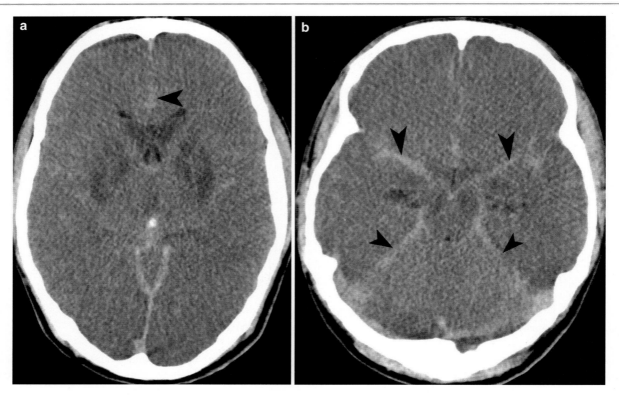

Fig. 16.1 (**a**, **b**) Cerebral edema. Noncontrast axial CT image of the brain shows diffuse hypodensity in the brain parenchyma, with loss of the gray-white interface compatible with brain edema. Extra-axial high attenuation (*arrowheads*) has the appearance of subarachnoid hemorrhage but is simply secondary to brain swelling

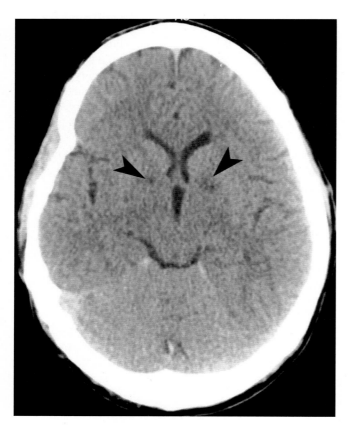

for the hippocampal formation [3]. If the focal abnormality involves the lateral temporal lobe, MCA territory arterial ischemia should be considered. If the edema involves the entire temporal lobe, one has to consider tumor. If otogenic infection is left untreated, there can be dural breech, leading to empyema, cerebritis, and abscess formation (Fig. 16.3).

Parasitic infection, such as neurocysticercosis, paragonimiasis, and echinococcus infection, should be considered when there is history of travel to an endemic region. Neurocysticercosis is the most common parasitic infection involving the central nervous system in developing countries and is endemic to Mexico, South America, Africa, Eastern Europe, and Asia. The neurocysticercosis involving the central nervous system is of four types:

• Meningeal
• Parenchymal
• Ventricular
• Mixed

While the meningeal cysts form mostly in the basal meninges, parenchymal cysts are usually found in the

Fig. 16.2 Carbon monoxide poisoning. Noncontrast axial CT image of the brain shows subtle areas of decreased attenuation in bilateral globi pallidi (*arrowheads*), compatible with ischemic injury in the setting of carbon monoxide poisoning

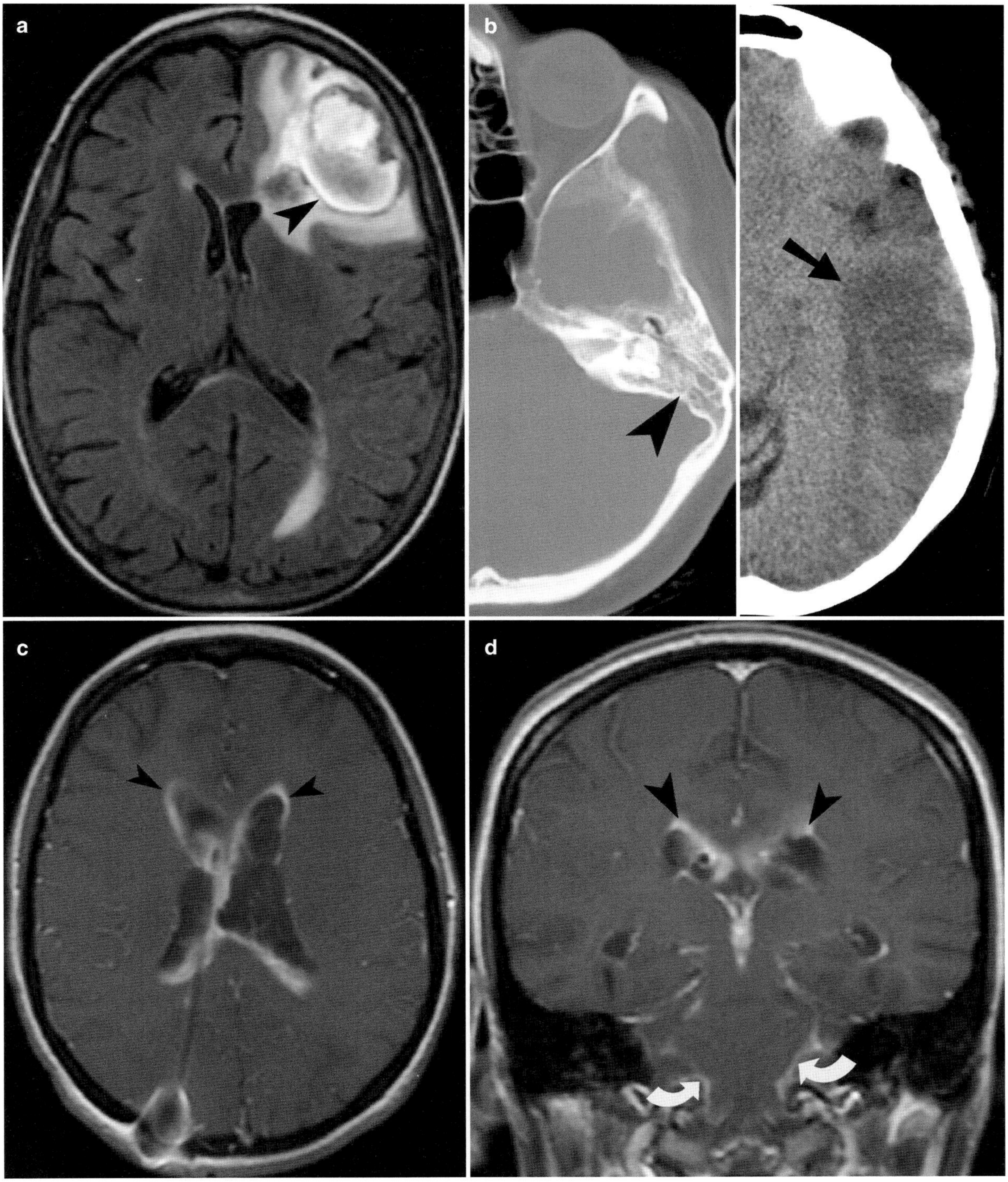

Fig. 16.3 Intracranial infection: brain abscess, ventriculitis, meningitis, and neurocysticercosis. (**a**) FLAIR sequence demonstrates left frontal brain abscess (*arrowhead*) from fungal infection with surrounding edema. The wall of the abscess is thinner on the medial aspect, a feature of brain abscess which is the result of limited vascular supply on the medial aspect. (**b**) Noncontrast axial CT image of the brain shows confluent decreased attenuation (*arrowhead*) in the left temporal lobe, from a combination of abscess and edema (*arrow*). Bone windows at the same level shows fluid in mastoid air cells (*arrowhead*). (**c, d**) Contrast-enhanced T1-weighted MRI shows extensive ependymal enhancement of the ventricular wall (*arrowheads*). There is also enhancement of the basal cisterns (*curved arrows*). The defect seen in the right parietal bone is from a ventriculostomy catheter which had become infected and was taken out. (**e, f**) T1-weighted sequence demonstrates multiple spherical parenchymal neurocysticercosis (*arrowheads*) containing scolex, at the gray-white matter junction. Postgadolinium T1-weighted (**f**) sequence shows rim enhancement of the multiple cystic lesions in the supratentorial compartment

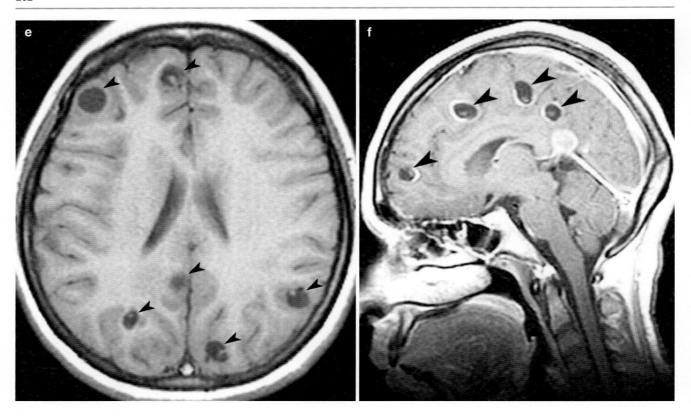

Fig. 16.3 (continued)

cerebral cortex. The white matter is rarely involved. Ventricular cysts are seen in 15 % of patients with neurocysticercosis, most commonly involving the fourth ventricle. In approximately nine fifths of cases of ventricular disease, there is associated parenchymal involvement.

Parenchymal neurocysticercosis is typically seen as 1 cm (range, 4–20 mm) diameter spherical shape lesion with a 2–3 mm mural nodule produced by the scolex. The presence of surrounding edema and enhancement of capsule indicates that the parasite is in degenerative or colloidal state. On T1-weighted sequence, the fluid in the cystic lesion is hypointense to white matter and hyperintense to cerebrospinal fluid. On T2-weighted sequence the cystic fluid is markedly hyperintense. There is usually no enhancement in the earlier vesicular stage, when the larva is still viable and the cyst is antigenically inert. In nodular calcified stage, cystic lesion is calcified and does not show any enhancement.

Herpes Encephalitis

Herpes simplex virus infection is ubiquitous in the general population, usually contracted initially via oronasopharyngeal contact. The virus then lies dormant within the trigeminal ganglion. HSV encephalitis is the most common viral infection in the central nervous system. What precipitates viral reactivation in the CNS is not known, although some patients have been found to have a viral prodrome prior to full manifestation [4]. Patients usually present with fever and a gradual onset of altered mental status, over the course of a few days. Infrequently are there focal neurological signs.

Fortunately, there are many imaging features for HSV encephalitis that are characteristic. The limbic system is a characteristic location (Fig. 16.4). It can be bilateral, usually asymmetric. Enhancement is typically gyriform. Restricted diffusion is often seen in the limbic system. Hemorrhage is a late feature. If a patient has these features, a presumptive diagnosis of herpes encephalitis should lead the clinical team to start IV acyclovir, as prompt antiviral therapy has been shown to improve outcomes.

The differential possibilities include infarction, especially if the symptoms are very acute in onset; postictal states can cause swelling and patchy areas of enhancements, mimicking HSV encephalitis, especially if the focus is in the temporal lobes, and limbic encephalitis, especially if the onset of symptoms is more gradual, such as over the course of months rather than days in herpetic encephalitis.

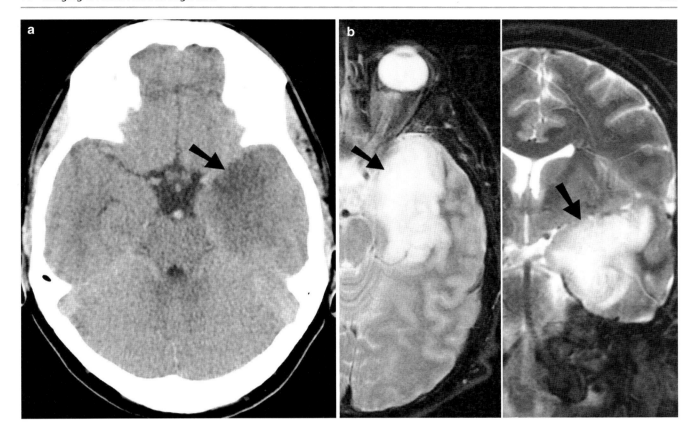

Fig. 16.4 Herpes encephalitis. (**a**) Noncontrast axial CT image of the brain shows decreased attenuation in the medial left temporal lobe (*arrow*). (**b**) Axial and coronal T2-weighted images show edema (*arrows*) in the medial temporal lobe, with contrast-enhanced T1-weighted images demonstrating patchy areas of enhancement

Tension Pneumocephalus

Tension pneumocephalus, a serious and potentially life-threatening condition, is due to increased air pressure in the subdural space causing mass effect on the frontal lobes and leading to neurological deterioration. The pathogenesis is described as a ball and valve mechanism. There is communication of the extracranial and intracranial spaces with ingress of air intracranially due to lower intracranial pressure and that the egress of air is blocked by an obstruction. Most cases occur due to head trauma but tension pneumocephalus can also occur due to skull base surgery, paranasal sinus surgery, CSF shunting, evacuation of a subdural hematoma, or posterior fossa surgery.

Patients with tension pneumocephalus often have headache and, most importantly, a diminishing level of consciousness. Imaging findings are characteristic, but not pathognomonic: prominent bifrontal subdural air collections that cause a mass effect on both frontal lobes, with widening of the interhemispheric spaces between the frontal lobes (Mt. Fuji sign) (Fig. 16.5) [5, 6].

If a patient who has had recent surgery has this imaging appearance and is clinically deteriorating, a diagnosis of tension pneumocephalus should be highly considered. Treatments include burr hole placement, craniotomy, needle aspiration, and closure of dural defects.

Giant MCA Aneurysm

Giant intracranial aneurysms are aneurysms that have a diameter greater than 2.5 cm. Most giant aneurysms are saccular rather than fusiform [7]. They tend to occur at branch points, arising de novo in defects in the intima or arising from enlarging smaller aneurysms due to hemodynamic stress. While ruptured giant aneurysms have typical symptoms of the "worst headache of my life," unruptured giant aneurysms have a sinister clinical presentation, often presenting due to mass effect on the adjacent structures or due to thromboemboli. Any large hyperdense mass in the vicinity of the cisterns and subarachnoid spaces should at least raise the possibility of a cerebral aneurysm (Fig. 16.6). Aside from

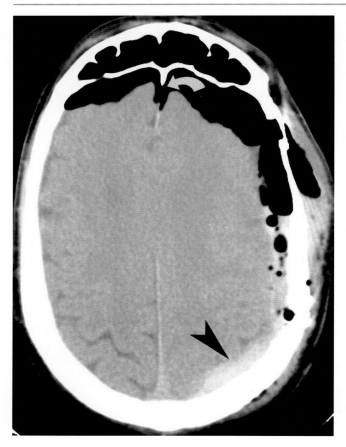

Fig. 16.5 Tension pneumocephalus. Noncontrast CT of the head shows prominent bifrontal subdural air collections with mass effect on both frontal lobes and widening of the interhemispheric space (Mt. Fuji sign) (*curved arrow*). A hyperdense left-sided subdural hematoma (*arrowhead*) is seen over the left parietal lobe

size, other imaging features of giant cerebral aneurysms are rim calcifications, a laminated and adjacent parenchymal hypodensity due to edema from pulsation.

Spontaneous Intracranial Hypotension

Spontaneous intracranial hypotension is characterized by low CSF pressure and postural headaches in the absence of prior trauma, surgery, or lumbar puncture [8]. It is usually due to an occult CSF leak from small meningeal defects. Clinical presentation is a new onset of headache with prompt and striking relief of pain in the supine position and recurrence of pain in the sitting or standing position. Headache may be associated with nausea, vomiting, vertigo, blurred vision, photophobia, neck stiffness, and occipitocervical pain with neck flexion. Imaging findings on CT or MR brain imaging include bilateral subdural hematomas, diffuse pachymeningeal enhancement, caudal displacement of the cerebellar tonsil and brainstem, decreased size of the ventricles and basal cisterns,

and enlargement of the pituitary gland (Fig. 16.7) [9]. The condition is generally self-limited but treatment of associated subdural hematoma or headaches may be needed. Persistent headaches may be treated with the use of autologous epidural blood patch if conservative measures fail.

Extra-axial Hemorrhages

Extra-axial hemorrhages are classified into three main compartments: epidural, subdural, and subarachnoid (Fig. 16.8) [10].

Traumatic subarachnoid hemorrhage is the most common extra-axial hemorrhage associated with head trauma. It is caused by traumatic injuries of veins and arteries at the base of the brain, and there is less hemorrhage compared to subarachnoid hemorrhage due to aneurysm rupture.

Subdural hematomas occur between the inner dural layer and the arachnoid. Approximately half are due to shearing of the bridging veins, and the other half are due to tear of the cortical arteries. The hemorrhage is crescentic in shape acutely and crosses sutures commonly but cannot cross the midline. Interhemispheric location in children suggests non-accidental trauma.

Epidural hematomas occur in the potential space between the calvarium and the outer dural layer. The most common cause is a temporal bone fracture and arterial laceration (usually the middle meningeal artery) with smaller percentage associated with dural venous sinus tear. The hemorrhage is biconvex in configuration and is limited by sutures due to the firm adherence of the dura to the inner table and its attachment to the sutures. In less than 50 % of cases, there is a lucid interval in which the patient is knocked out by the initial concussion and then lapses into unconsciousness again after recovery. Prompt recognition and treatment can significantly decrease morbidity and mortality associated with epidural hemorrhages.

Herniation Syndromes

The brain, CSF, and blood coexist in a rigid and non-expandable container: the cranium. When most other organs enlarge, there is generally some room for expansion; however, the brain, when it expands due to edema, tumor, or hemorrhage, has very little space in which to expand. If the intracranial pressure increases enough, it will cause the brain to herniate from one compartment to another (Fig. 16.9a–d) [11].

Subfalcine herniation, the most common type of herniation, occurs when the cingulate gyrus and pericallosal branches of the anterior cerebral artery herniate beneath the falx cerebri. There is effacement of the ipsilateral ventricle and enlargement of the contralateral ventricle due to

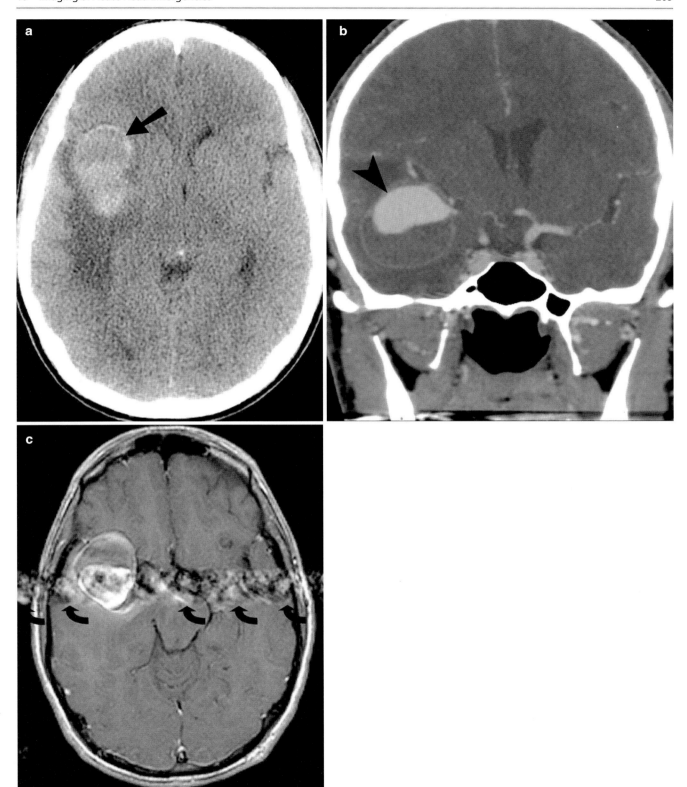

Fig. 16.6 MCA aneurysm. (**a**) Noncontrast axial CT image of the brain demonstrates a heterogeneously hyperdense lesion (*arrow*) in the right sylvian cistern with edema within the right temporal lobe. (**b**) Coronal CTA image shows a 4.5 cm diameter, partially thrombosed aneurysm (*arrowhead*) arising off the M2 segment of the right MCA. (**c**) Axial T1-weighted images with contrast show pulsation artifacts (*curved arrows*) in the phase-encoding direction, indicative of a high-flow process in the aneurysm

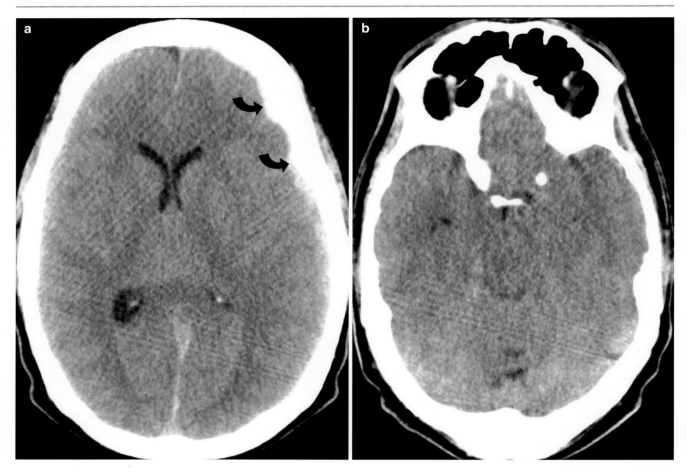

Fig. 16.7 Intracranial hypotension. (**a**) Unenhanced axial CT images of the brain demonstrate effacement of the basal cisterns, brainstem sagging, and left-sided subdural hematoma (*curved arrow*). (**b**)

Unenhanced sagittal T1 MRI image of the brain demonstrates sagging of the brainstem and descent of the cerebellar tonsils

continuous production of CSF by the choroid plexus. There are possible compression of the ipsilateral anterior cerebral artery or internal cerebral veins and risk of infarction.

Uncal herniation occurs when the medial temporal lobe tissue (uncus and hippocampus) is displaced medially through the free edge of the tentorium cerebelli and compresses the brainstem and adjacent structures (posterior cerebral artery, oculomotor nerve and anterior choroidal artery). There is compression of the ipsilateral oculomotor nerve, causing a fixed and dilated pupil, and ipsilateral posterior cerebral artery, causing an infarct in its distribution. Complications also include periaqueductal necrosis; midbrain (Duret) hemorrhages; hemorrhages in the tegmentum of the pons and midbrain, as a result of stretching of the upper branches of the basilar artery; and compression of the contralateral cerebral peduncle against the free edge of the tentorium, Kernohan-Woltman notch.

Tonsillar herniation occurs due to mass effect in the posterior fossa leading to obstruction of the fourth ventricle, hydrocephalus, and inferior displacement of the cerebellar tonsils and cerebellum through the foramen magnum. There

is compression of the medulla resulting in depression of the vital centers for respiration and cardiac rhythm control.

Less common herniations include central transtentorial herniation, due to end result of downward displacement of the cerebral hemispheres and basal nuclei with possible complete obliteration of the basal cisterns, and ascending transtentorial (superior vermian) herniation, caused by a slowly growing cerebellar or brainstem process forcing upward herniation of the vermis and cerebellar hemispheres through the tentorium.

Cerebral Contusions

Contusions represent acceleration/deceleration injuries to the brain involving the peripheral surfaces of the brain due to trauma. They are the second most common primary traumatic neuronal injury after diffuse axonal injury. The location of the contusions is characteristic, namely, the anterior and inferior surfaces of the temporal and frontal lobes (Fig. 16.9e, f) [12]. These parts of the brain are the

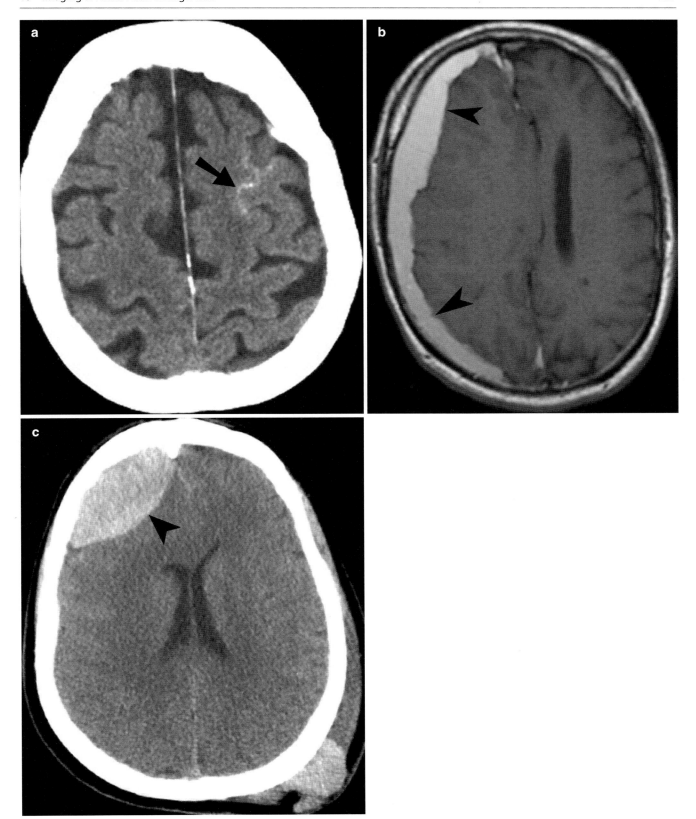

Fig. 16.8 Intracranial hemorrhage. (**a**) Noncontrast CT demonstrates subarachnoid hemorrhage (*arrow*) in the sulci over the left frontal convexity. (**b**) Unenhanced axial T1 MRI image of the brain demonstrates a hyperintense subdural fluid collection (*arrowheads*) along the right cerebral convexity consistent with a subacute subdural hematoma. (**c**) Noncontrast CT demonstrates a biconvex-shaped epidural hematoma (*arrowhead*) over the right frontal convexity produced by countercoup injury. It is producing mass effect over the right lateral ventricle

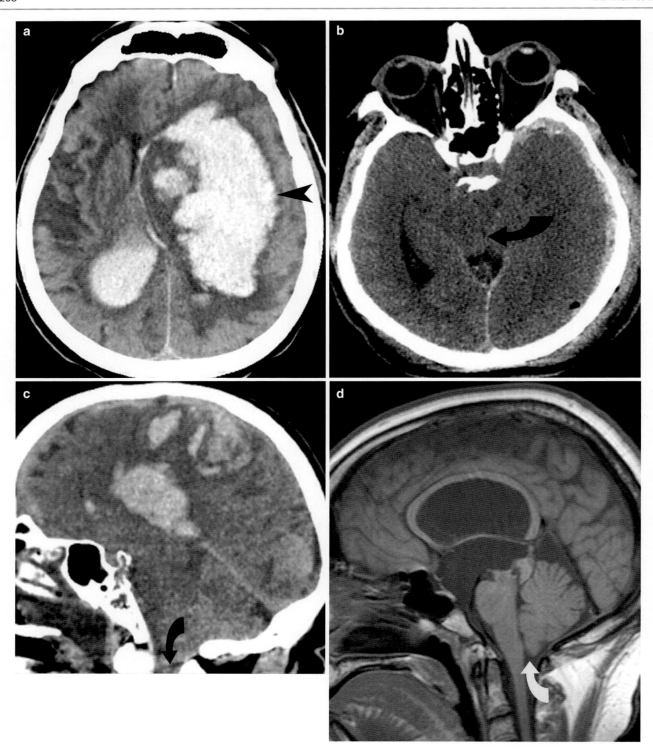

Fig. 16.9 Intraparenchymal hemorrhage. (**a**) Unenhanced axial CT image of the brain shows a large intraparenchymal hemorrhage (*arrowhead*) within the left cerebral hemisphere causing rightward subfalcine herniation. There is compression of the ipsilateral ventricle and dilatation of the contralateral ventricle and intraventricular hemorrhage. (**b**) Noncontrast CT in a patient with uncal herniation from left subdural hemorrhage demonstrates medial temporal lobe (uncus) (*curved arrow*) displaced medially through the free edge of the tentorium cerebelli and compressing the midbrain. (**c**, **d**) CT and MRI demonstrate tonsillar herniation (*curved arrows*) in two patients from parenchymal hemorrhage (**c**) and hydrocephalus (**d**). (**e**) Noncontrast axial CT images demonstrate intraparenchymal hemorrhage within the temporal and frontal lobes compatible with traumatic hemorrhagic contusions (*arrowheads*). Subarachnoid (*arrow*) and subdural blood is also seen, often coexistent with contusions. (**f**) Noncontrast CT of the head in a patient with gunshot injury demonstrates the entry wound (*arrowhead*), bullet track through the midbrain (*curved arrow*), and exit wound (*straight arrow*). There is pneumocephalus as well as subarachnoid hemorrhage

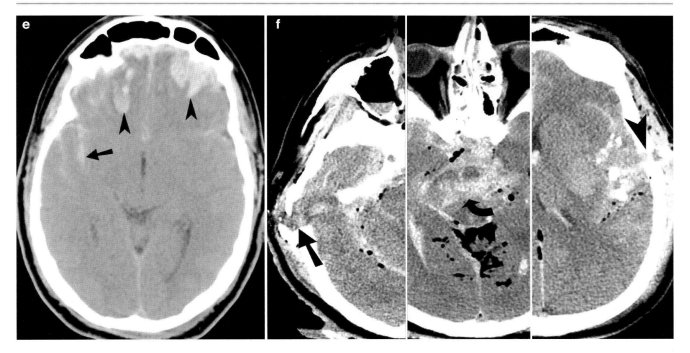

Fig. 16..9 (continued)

most mobile areas and have more fixed proximal portions and thus brush up against the irregular inner calvarial surfaces of the anterior and inferior frontal bone of the anterior cranial fossa and the greater sphenoid wing and temporal bone in the middle cranial fossa. Less frequently, contusions can occur in the parasagittal cerebral hemispheres, as the parenchyma contuses along the rigid interhemispheric falx.

It is important in the setting of contusions, both hemorrhagic and nonhemorrhagic, to get short-term follow-up, as new lesions may appear within the first few days, and existing injuries may become larger. An important differential to exclude is venous occlusive disease, as sinus thrombosis can often have a similar appearance and location. The treatment is to prevent secondary injury, such as hematoma formation, mass effect, or herniation – all or which may require surgical intervention.

Cortical Laminar Necrosis

Cortical laminar necrosis is important to know for two reasons: one, it is a hallmark of subacute injury, i.e., roughly 14–21 days after initial insult; two, the cortical hyperdensity (or hyperintensity on T1 MRI) is secondary to *hypoxic* ischemic injury rather than hemorrhagic injury. This patient was a 35-year-old female who earlier had a cesarean section and, approximately 3 months postpartum, presented to the emergency department with signs and symptoms of hypertensive

urgency. The patient's labile response to blood pressure correction led to a severe pressure drop, which precipitated worsening mental status changes. Subsequent head CT exams demonstrated patchy hypodensities in the parietal and occipital lobes. Three weeks after presentation, findings had progressed to laminar necrosis.

The differential diagnosis includes cerebritis, low-grade cortical neoplasm, and Sturge-Weber. Hyperdense gyri may or may not be present on CT, but the characteristic high signal intensity on T1 sequence is most sensitive (Fig. 16.10) [13]. Subacute infarcts are infrequently imaged, and so knowledge of the myriad imaging appearances, coupled with appropriate history, can often aid clinicians in treatment and prevent needless tests (i.e., neoplasm or infectious disease workups).

Overall, the presence of cortical laminar necrosis is indicative of a poor clinical prognosis. Interestingly, although incompletely understood, the hyperdensity and hyperintensity on CT and MRI are not due to blood or calcification, but felt to be due to reactive gliosis and fat-laden macrophages. To our knowledge, there is no association in the literature between CLN and hypertension or hypertensive crisis.

Cerebral Arterial Air Embolism

Aside from the airway, the paranasal sinuses, and the mastoid and petrous temporal bones, the head should not have air within it. Cerebral air emboli can be venous or arterial.

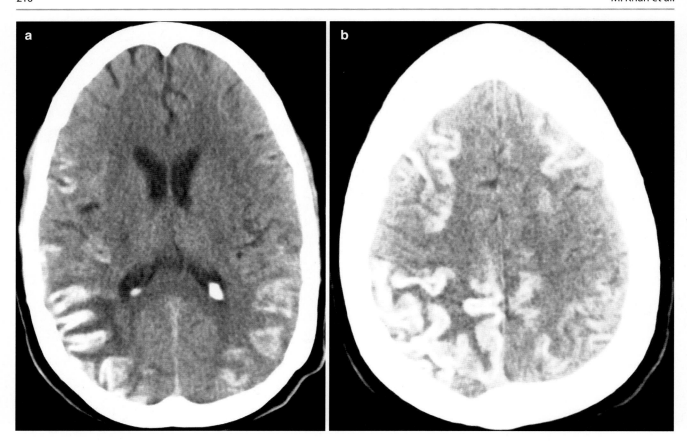

Fig. 16.10 Cortical laminar necrosis. (**a**, **b**) Noncontrast axial CT images of the brain demonstrate extensive, diffuse cortical gyral wavy hyperdensities, most consistent with cortical laminar necrosis. Although incompletely understood, the hyperdensity and hyperintensity on CT are not due to blood or calcification

Venous air emboli can occur due to central catheter placement or other instrumentation related to venous access such as from a CT injector. Intracranially, air is often seen in the cavernous sinus and superficial maxillofacial venous branches. If minimal, patients are often asymptomatic, but it is still worthwhile to alert the clinicians of the presence of venous air.

Arterial cerebral air embolism, however, is an infrequent but potentially devastating entity with serious sequelae. Arterial air emboli can cause an inflammatory response that can result from the air itself or due to a reduction in perfusion distal to the obstruction [14].

Arterial air emboli are often the result of trauma, surgery, or procedures such as lung biopsy. Air can reach the arterial system through the pulmonary vein (and ultimately the systemic circulation) via a biopsy needle or broncho-venous fistula of any cause, by way of the systemic venous side by traversing the pulmonary microvasculature (even without an arteriovenous communication) or through any form of right-to-left shunt. The air detected on CT scan can reabsorb rapidly and therefore will not be apparent on a follow-up study (Fig. 16.11).

Patients often present with generalized seizures and focal neurological deficits. Treatment is 100 % oxygen, aggressive fluid resuscitation, and hyperbaric oxygen therapy. Prompt diagnosis and clinician communication can initiate aggressive treatment and mitigate the extent of damage.

Obstructive Hydrocephalus

Obstructive hydrocephalus is caused by obstruction to the flow of CSF at the level of foramen of Monro, third ventricle, aqueduct of Sylvius, or fourth ventricle. The imaging findings of obstructive hydrocephalus include prominence of ventricular system above the occlusion. The most common site of obstruction is aqueduct of Sylvius and results in prominence of the lateral and third ventricle. Obstruction to the outflow of the fourth ventricle results in additional prominence of the fourth ventricle which loses its triangular configuration and appears round. The supratentorial cisterns, fissures, and sulci are much less prominent due to ventricular dilatation. Periventricular edema may occur due to transependymal spread of fluid (Fig. 16.12).

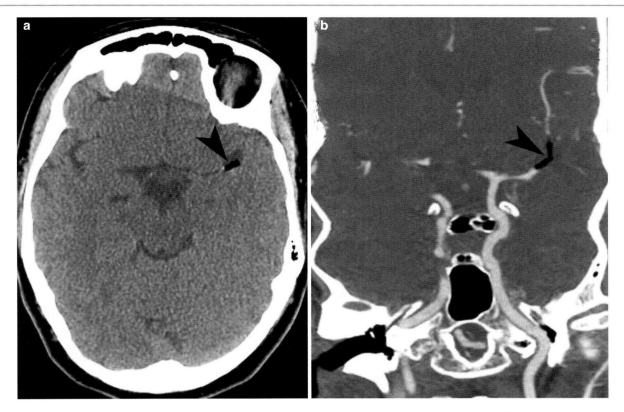

Fig. 16.11 Air embolism. (**a**, **b**) Noncontrast axial CT and CT angiogram of the brain demonstrate a focal area of intravascular air (*arrowhead*) within the M1 (sylvian) segment of the left middle cerebral artery, compatible with arterial air embolism

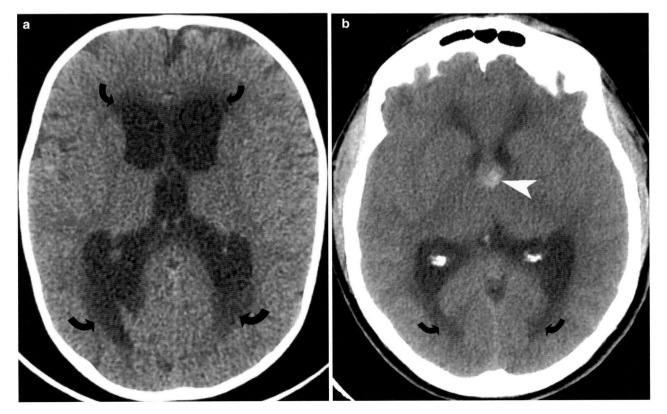

Fig. 16.12 Obstructive hydrocephalus. (**a**, **b**) Noncontrast CT of the head demonstrates acute obstructive hydrocephalus with transependymal edema (*curved arrows*), caused by posterior fossa hemorrhage (**a**) and colloid cyst at the foramen of Monro (*arrowhead*) (**b**). (**c**) T2-weighted MRI shows acute obstructive hydrocephalus with transependymal edema (*curved arrows*) around the lateral ventricles

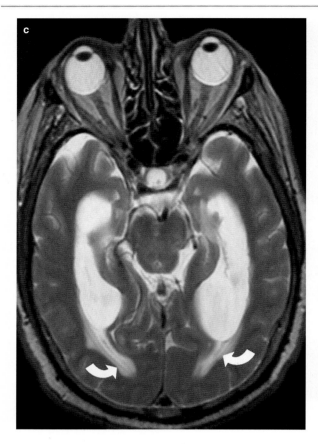

Fig. 16.12 (continued)

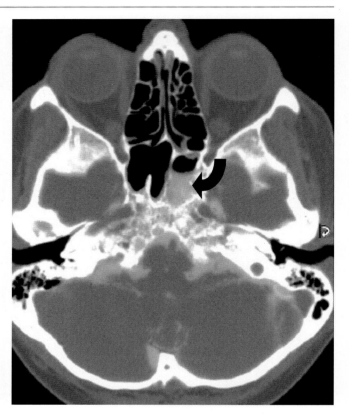

Fig. 16.14 Posttraumatic CSF leak. CT cisternogram study demonstrates radiopaque contrast leaking through dural and osseous defect in sphenoid sinus wall. The contrast is seen collecting in the left sphenoid sinus (*curved arrow*)

Acute Hypertensive Encephalopathy

It is seen in patients with severe hypertension and is believed to be due to abnormal cerebrovascular autoregulation. It is also called posterior reversible encephalopathy syndrome.

On CT imaging, there is bilateral cortical or subcortical low density, most commonly in the posterior circulation. The occipital lobes and posterior parietal lobes are most commonly involved by the process, which is more often patchy than confluent (Fig. 16.13). On MR imaging, the patchy lesions are bright on T2-weighted and FLAIR sequences. The differential diagnosis includes cerebral infarcts, progressive multifocal encephalopathy, demyelinating disease, and metabolic derangements (dialysis).

CSF Leak

Majority (90 %) of the cases are posttraumatic, often occurring through the floor of anterior cranial fossa and resulting in CSF rhinorrhea. Fracture of temporal bone may result in otorrhea, accounting for 20 % of the cases. Eighty percent of CSF leak occur within 48 h for the traumatic event and 95 % occur within 3 months.

CT cisternogram is the gold standard in demonstrating CSF leak from the base of skull. If the CSF leak is intermittent,

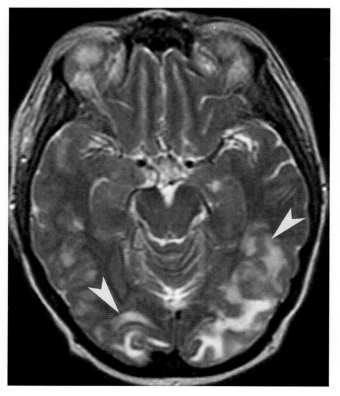

Fig. 16.13 Acute hypertensive encephalopathy. T2-weighted MR image demonstrates patchy and confluent hyperintensities (*arrowheads*) in both occipital lobes

Fig. 16.15 Brain death. Tc99m HMPAO study demonstrates hot nose sign (*arrowhead*) in this patient with no intracranial uptake (light bulb sign) of radiotracer

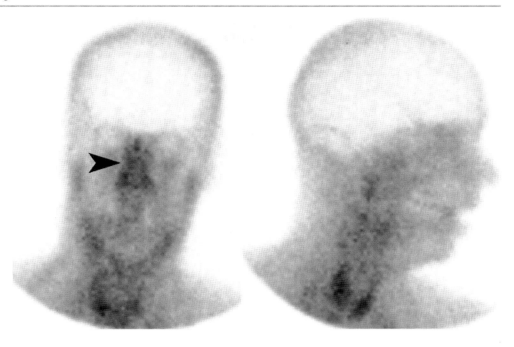

then the timing of the study is important in detecting the leak. A positive study will show contrast material leaking through the dural and osseous defect (Fig. 16.14). Since the anatomical site of defect is more difficult to see on radionuclide cisternograms (indium 111 diethylenetriaminepentaacetic acid), they are used as second-line imaging modality. The biological half-life of 2.8 days prolonged imaging for up to 3 days after radiotracer administration.

Brain Death

The best imaging test to confirm brain death is a neuralite study. Brain death is characterized by irreversible loss of brain function with marked brain swelling and obliteration of sulci. The intracranial pressure exceeds the vascular perfusion pressure and leads to irreversible ischemia. The EEG of a patient with brain death is isoelectric due to cessation of physiologic functions.

Normal brain shows uptake of Tc99m HMPAO, and Tc99m ECD does cross the blood–brain barrier, in proportion to the regional blood flow. On Tc99m ECD (neuralite) or Tc99m HMPAO (Ceretec) study, there is no flow to the intracranial supratentorial as well as infratentorial structures after brain death. These patients will typically show increased radiotracer in the nasal area (hot nose sign). The absence to radiotracer in the intracranial region produces a lightbulb sign (Fig. 16.15).

References

1. Given CA et al. Pseudo-subarachnoid hemorrhage: a potential imaging pitfall associated with diffuse cerebral edema. AJNR Am J Neuroradiol. 2003;24:254–6.
2. Sener RN. Acute carbon monoxide poisoning: diffusion MR imaging findings. AJNR Am J Neuroradiol. 2003;24:1475–7.
3. Paolini S et al. Gas-containing otogenic brain abscess. Surg Neurol. 2002;58(3–4):271–3.
4. Baringer JR. Herpes simplex infections of the nervous systems. Neurol Clin. 2008;26(3):657–74, viii.
5. Sinclair AG et al. Imaging of the post-operative cranium. Radiographics. 2010;30:461–82.
6. Michel SJ. The Mount Fuji sign. Radiology. 2004;232:449–50.
7. Mehta RI et al. Best cases from the AFIP: giant intracranial aneurysm. Radiographics. 2010;30:1133–8.
8. Jacobs MB, Wasserstein PH. Spontaneous intracranial hypotension: an uncommon and underrecognized cause of headache. West J Med. 1991;155:178–80.
9. Watanabe A, Horikoshi T, Uchida M, Koizumi H, Yagishita T, Kinouchi H. Diagnostic value of spinal MR imaging in spontaneous intracranial hypotension syndrome. AJNR Am J Neuroradiol. 2009;30:147–51.
10. Osborn AG, Salzman KL, Barkovich J. Trauma. In: Diagnostic imaging brain. 2nd ed. London: Amirys Publishing, Inc; 2005. p. I-2-3.
11. Coburn MW, Rodriguez FJ. Cerebral herniations. Appl Radiol. 1998;27:10–6.
12. Kim JJ et al. Imaging for the diagnosis and management of traumatic brain injury. Neurotherapeutics. 2011;8(1):39–53.
13. Kinoshita T et al. Curvilinear T1 hyperintense lesions representing cortical necrosis after cerebral infarction. Neuroradiology. 2005;47:647–51.
14. Yang MS et al. Iatrogenic and fatal air arterial embolism during CT scan. J Chin Med Assoc. 2011;74:188–91.

Imaging of Facial Fractures

Dennis Coughlin and Paul Jaffray

Introduction

Facial trauma is a common presentation to the emergency department, usually as a result of blunt trauma. The trauma can range from a simple, isolated nondisplaced fracture to complex displaced facial fractures. Multiple fracture patterns have been described that make it easier to efficiently detect, document, and communicate the diagnosis in patients with multiple fractures. Rene Le Fort made the earliest and most famous classification in 1901, and since that time multiple other fracture patterns have been described [1]. While these can be present in pure form, often they coexist, particularly in the setting of high-impact trauma.

Paralleling this development in facial trauma classification has been that of surgical fixation. After the advent of antibiotics, the most commonly used treatment of complex facial fractures is open reduction. A primary reason for improvement in surgical treatment of facial fractures is the introduction and refinement of the concept of functional units of the face. This concept was first described by Sicher and DuBrul in 1970 [2]. Through experience surgeons have learned that reducing these functional units leads to the best anatomical and functional outcome for facial fractures [3–5].

While physical exam is an essential component in the workup of a trauma patient, this is often difficult due to the patient's mental state, distracting injuries, and associated comorbidities. Imaging plays a central role in the workup of the trauma patient. This is particularly true with the advent of modern multidetector CT scans.

D. Coughlin, MD (✉) • P. Jaffray, MD
Department of Radiology,
University of Massachusetts Memorial Medical Center,
55 Lake Avenue North, Worcester, MA, USA
e-mail: dcoughlin25@gmail.com

Imaging of Craniofacial Trauma

Historically, initial assessment of facial trauma was performed with a facial radiograph series. Typical series included Caldwell, straight PA, Waters, Towne, lateral, and SMV views [6]. Radiographs are still being utilized, but their use has progressively diminished as CT technology continues to improve. In many institutions, the use of CT has largely replaced radiographs in the evaluation of the trauma patient. MRI is rarely used in the immediate workup of the trauma patient but can aid in evaluating complications.

Older generation CT scanners acquired axial images with subsequent patient repositioning required to obtain series in other planes. With improvement of imaging technology, helical acquisition on modern multi-slice CT scanners rapidly obtains a volume of data from which can be used to obtain reformations in any plane. Multiplanar imaging greatly aids in the detection and appropriate description of facial injuries.

Our CT trauma protocol for imaging of the head and maxillofacial region involves acquiring a data volume at 0.6 mm slice thickness from immediately below the mental protuberance to the skull vertex without intravenous contrast. Maxillofacial thin overlapping axial reconstructions as well as coronal and sagittal reformats, typically 2×1.5 mm, are generated using both bone and soft tissue algorithms. In addition, volume-rendered 3D images are generated.

Craniofacial Anatomy

Anatomically, the face is divided into upper, middle, and lower thirds (Fig. 17.1). The upper third is comprised of the frontal bone and extends to its zygomatic, maxillary, and nasal sutures. The middle third extends from the frontal bone to the upper teeth of the maxilla. The mandible represents the lower third. The "midface" is comprised of the maxilla, zygoma, nasal, lacrimal, vomer, inferior concha, and palatine bones. The frontal, sphenoid, and ethmoid bones form portions of both the cranium and face. The facial bones are

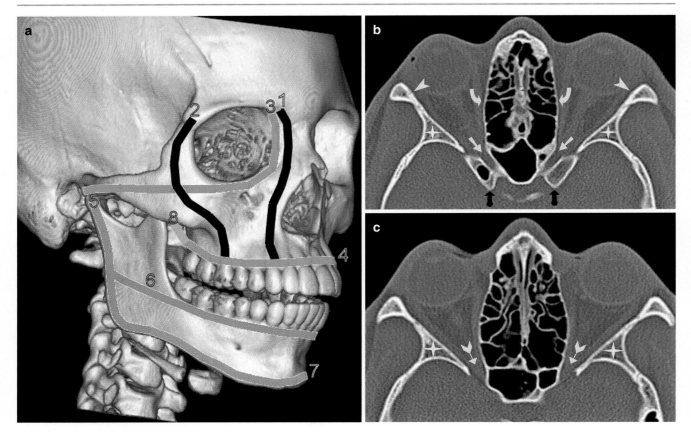

Fig. 17.1 Normal CT anatomy and facial buttresses. (**a**) 3D surface-rendered image demonstrating the four vertical and four transverse buttresses (*1* medial maxillary, *2* lateral maxillary, *3* upper transverse maxillary, *4* lower transverse maxillary, *5* posterior vertical, *6* upper transverse mandibular, *7* lower transverse mandibular, and *8* posterior maxillary). (**b**, **c**) Axial CT demonstrates the normal anatomy of the facial bones (*arrowhead* zygomatic arch, *curved arrow* laminae papyracea, *white straight arrow* optic canal, *black straight arrow* anterior clinoid process, *star* greater wing of sphenoid, and *white arrow* superior orbital fissure)

relatively weak owing to their multiple sinus cavities but are reinforced with a series of vertical and horizontal buttresses. They are able to withstand forces in the vertical direction but are much weaker in the horizontal and lateral directions. The goal of the surgeon is to restore alignment and integrity of these buttresses when they fracture. There are four vertical and four horizontal facial buttresses (variously termed struts of mastication, midfacial buttresses, or structural pillars).

The floor of the anterior cranial fossa (ACF) is formed by the cribriform plate of the ethmoid, the frontal bone, and the lesser wing of the sphenoid. The frontal bone forms the majority of the floor of the ACF and also comprises the majority of the orbital roof. The lesser wing of the sphenoid forms the posterior margin of the ACF. The floor of the middle cranial fossa (MCF) is formed by the greater wing of the sphenoid and the squamosal portion of the temporal bone [7].

Orbital Fractures

The orbit is shaped like a cone with the apex posterior and the base anterior. The apex of the orbit is at the convergence of the superior and inferior orbital fissures. The anterior orbital rim is composed of the frontal, maxillary, and zygomatic bones.

Fractures of the orbit can affect the orbital rim, orbital walls, or orbital apex. Orbital apex fractures are an important fracture to detect due to proximity to the optic nerve and are more commonly seen with complex injury. The most common isolated orbital fractures are the so-called blowout fractures that occur in the medial and inferior orbital walls.

Blowout Fracture

A blowout fracture is a fracture of the orbital wall that displaces outwardly. In 1957 Smith and Regan proposed a mechanism of increased intraorbital pressure secondary to a direct frontal blow to the globe [8]. The forces are transmitted through the orbital walls with fracturing of the weakest sections while the orbital rim remains intact [9]. The lamina papyracea is the thinnest bone but is reinforced with buttressing from the ethmoid air cells. The inferior orbital wall is made weaker by the presence of the infraorbital groove and is the most common site of a fracture. The fracture fragment

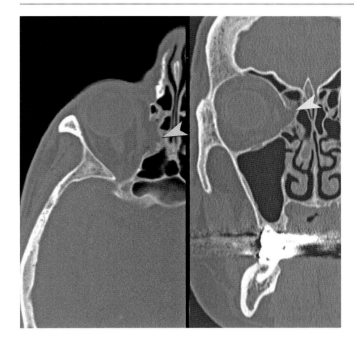

Fig. 17.2 Medial orbital wall blowout fracture. Axial and coronal CT images demonstrate a fracture (*arrowhead*) of the right medial orbital wall (lamina papyracea). Note the herniation of orbital fat through the defect in the right medial orbital wall

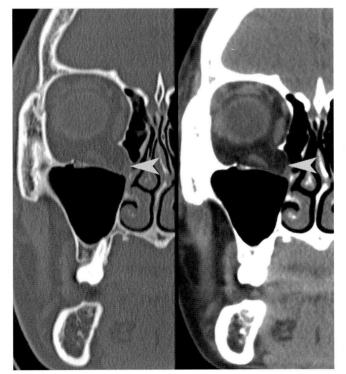

Fig. 17.3 Orbital floor lateral hinge blowout fracture. Coronal and sagittal images in bone and soft tissue algorithm demonstrating a right orbital floor blowout fracture. The displaced fragment hinges laterally at the infraorbital fissure. Note herniation of the orbital contents (*arrowhead*), including the inferior rectus muscle

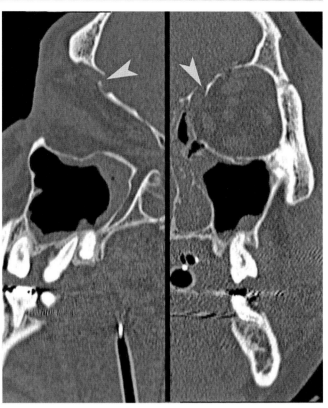

Fig. 17.4 Orbital roof blow-in fracture. Coronal and sagittal CT reformations demonstrate a "pure" orbital blow-in fracture (*arrowhead*) of the left orbital roof. The orbital rim is intact

can displace inferiorly into the maxillary sinus, resulting in herniation of intraorbital fat, and/or extraocular muscles. The "trapdoor" blowout fracture, which is more common in pediatric age group, occurs when the hinge fragment springs back into place often trapping the inferior rectus muscle. Entrapment of the inferior rectus muscle results in limitation of upward/outward gaze, while entrapment of the medial rectus muscle results in limitation in the lateral gaze.

The coronal and sagittal reformations are most useful for detecting orbital floor fracture. Axial and coronal images best detect fractures of the medial wall (Figs. 17.2 and 17.3). It is important to note the site of fracture, fracture displacement and/or fracture angulation, and the presence or absence of herniated orbital contents.

Blow-in Fractures

The blow-in fracture is an inwardly displaced fracture of the orbital wall and/or rim resulting in a reduced orbital volume. These are generally the result of high-energy trauma and are most commonly seen in association with other fractures [10, 11]. A "pure" blow-in fracture is one limited to the orbital walls while the orbital rim remains intact (Figs. 17.4

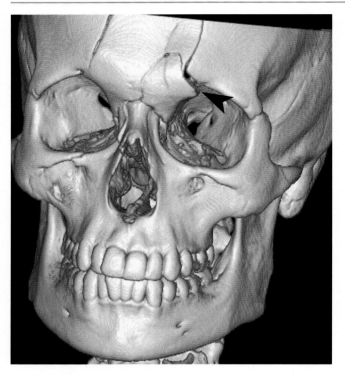

Fig. 17.5 Orbital rim blow-in fractures. Surface-rendered image demonstrating orbital rim blow-in fracture of the superomedial orbital rim associated with a frontal fracture (*arrowhead*)

and 17.5). "Impure" blow-in fractures, which are much more common, involve inward displacement of the orbital rim. Superior rim fractures, owing to their location and higher-impact forces, are usually more severe and associated with head injuries and frontal sinus fractures. Inferomedial blow-in rim fractures are the most common and seen with NOE fractures.

Fractures of the orbital apex may result in superior orbital fissure syndrome [12]. Symptoms include diplopia, ophthalmoplegia, ptosis, proptosis, and anesthesia in the ophthalmic nerve distribution. If there is associated blindness due to optic nerve injury (optic canal), it is termed orbital apex syndrome.

Zygoma Fractures

The zygoma (malar bone) is a dense solid bone that articulates with the frontal, maxillary, sphenoid, and temporal bones and forms the malar prominence (cheek), an important component of the facial contour. Since the zygoma is a solid bone, a direct blow to the cheek usually results in fractures of its relatively weaker articulation points. As the majority of the lateral orbital wall is formed by the zygoma, fractures to this region usually involve the orbit.

Zygomaticomaxillary Complex (ZMC) Fractures

While it is also called malar, tripod, tetrapod, and zygomatic complex fracture, the generally accepted and most commonly used term is zygomaticomaxillary complex (ZMC) fracture. It has a tendency to fracture at the weaker articulations with the frontal, sphenoid, maxillary, and temporal bones, resulting in disruption of the lateral maxillary and upper transverse maxillary buttresses [13].

While damage to the infraorbital nerve will result in loss of sensation to the eyelid and lateral nose, injury to the zygomatic nerve will result in sensory impairment to the lateral midface. Displaced fractures may result in flattening of the malar prominence and facial asymmetry.

Because of its complex articulation, the ZMC fragment can rotate in any plane along the fracture lines. The goal of imaging is to evaluate the extent of the fractures, the position and displacement of the ZMC fragment, and the status of the zygomatic arch (Figs. 17.6 and 17.7). The fractures may be associated with ocular injuries.

Isolated Fractures

A focused direct blow may result in an isolated arch fracture. The direction of the force usually results in a depressed V-shaped fracture with the apex directed toward the infratemporal fossa. Segmented fractures may result as well (Fig. 17.8). Complications result from impingement of the temporal muscle and injury to the zygomatic nerve.

Nasal Fractures

The bridge of the nose is formed by the paired nasal bones, the frontal process of the maxilla, and the nasal processes of the frontal bone. The ethmoid is comprised of multiple delicate buttressing bones and air cells and is bounded laterally by the orbits and maxillary sinuses. The nasal septum is formed by the vertical plate of the ethmoid and vomer posteriorly and cartilaginous septum anteriorly. The lateral nasal wall is formed by three longitudinal elevations called conchae (turbinates). The superior and middle turbinates are part of the ethmoid, while the inferior turbinate is a separate bone.

The nasal bones form a portion of the nasal bridge and, if fractured, may result in facial deformity. Injury can range from isolated nasal bone fractures to more complex patterns involving multiple bones (Fig. 17.9). Radiographs are still routinely ordered if there is suspicion of an isolated nasal fracture. On CT attention to the nasal septum is important to evaluate for the presence of a septal hematoma, which may lead to

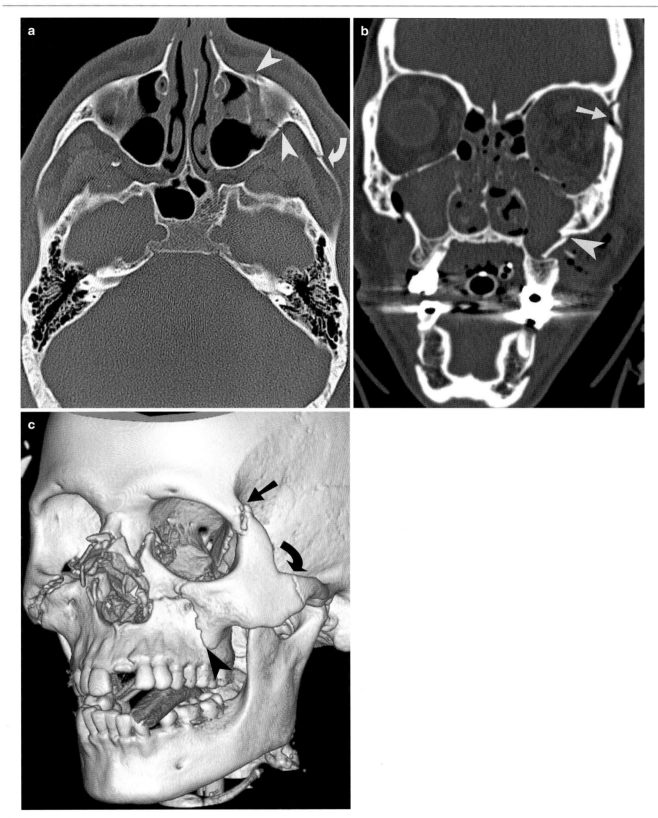

Fig. 17.6 ZMC fracture. (**a, b**) Axial and coronal CT demonstrates fractures of the anterior/posterolateral antral walls (*arrowheads*), orbital floor, lateral orbital rim, and zygomatic arch (*curved arrow*). (**c**) Surface-rendered image demonstrates fractures of the left zygomaticotemporal suture (*curved arrow*), zygomaticofrontal suture (*straight arrow*), and zygomaticomaxillary suture (*arrowhead*)

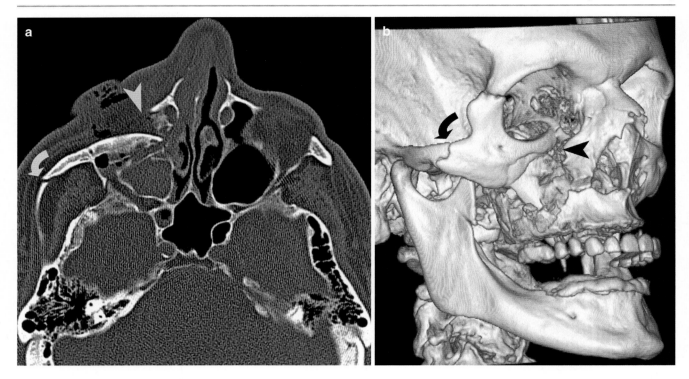

Fig. 17.7 Displaced and angulated ZMC fracture. (**a**, **b**) Axial image and surface-rendered image showing the zygoma complex posterolaterally displaced and internally rotated with displaced zygomaticomaxillary fracture (*arrowheads*) and zygomaticotemporal fracture (*curved arrows*). There is also fracture of the coronoid process of the mandible

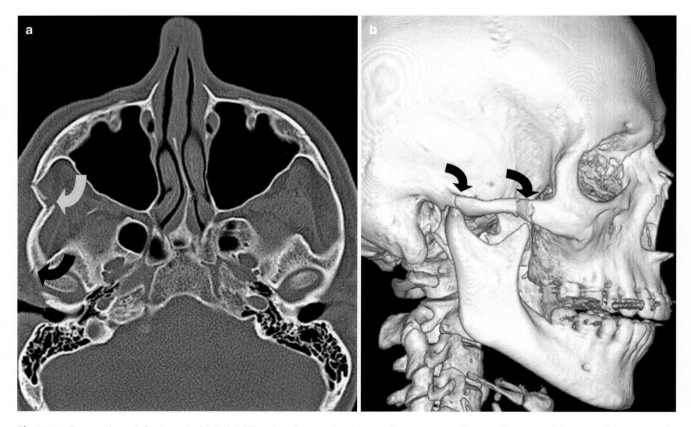

Fig. 17.8 Zygomatic arch fracture. (**a**, **b**) Axial CT and surface-rendered image demonstrates a depressed, segmental fracture of the zygomatic bone (*curved arrows*)

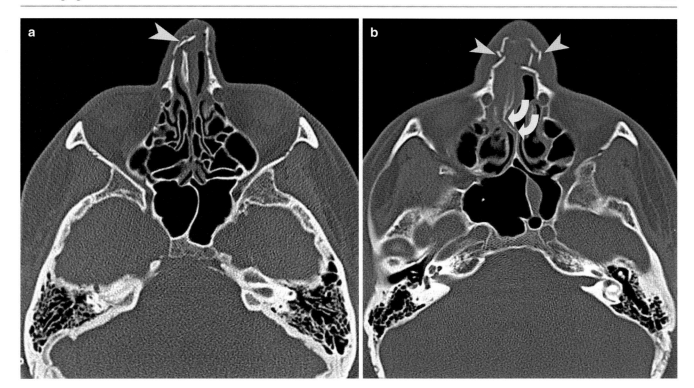

Fig. 17.9 Nasal fracture. (**a**) Axial CT demonstrates comminuted, displaced, and angulated right nasal bone fractures (*arrowhead*). (**b**) Axial CT demonstrates fractures that involve the nasal bones (*arrowheads*), frontal process of the maxilla, and nasal septum (*curved arrows*). Note posterior displacement with telescoping of the nasal septum

complications of ischemic necrosis or abscess formation. Associated anterior nasal spine fractures may be present.

Naso-Orbital-Ethmoid Fractures

A high-impact force to the central face may disrupt the medial maxillary and upper transverse maxillary buttresses, referred to as naso-orbital-ethmoid (NOE) fractures. A classification system developed by Markowitz and Manson is based on the degree of injury to the medial maxillary buttress at the insertion of the medial canthal ligament [14]. The posterior extension of the medial maxillary buttress is made up of thin delicate bones offering little support, which results in impaction and posterior telescoping of the midface. Depressed and displaced fractures may result in flattening of the nasal bridge and telecanthus.

Axial and coronal images provide the most information (Figs. 17.10 and 17.11). It is important to evaluate the medial maxillary buttress at the level of the lacrimal fossa, the site of medial canthal ligament attachment. Reconstruction of the attachment of the medial canthal ligament is essential to avoid telecanthus, enophthalmos, and dysfunction of the lacrimal system. It is also important to comment on the posterior extension of these buttresses – medial orbital walls and floor. Additional associated injuries may include nasofrontal duct injury, cribriform plate fracture, frontal sinus involvement, orbital apex involvement, and associated ocular injuries.

Frontal Fractures

The frontal bone progressively pneumatizes throughout childhood. The anterior table forms the forehead and the superior orbital rims. The posterior table forms the anterior wall of the anterior cranial fossa. This strong bone forms the transverse frontal buttress and provides the anchor for the vertical maxillary buttresses. Due to its strength, a large force is required to fracture the frontal bone [15]. The frontal sinus drains to the nose via the nasofrontal ducts. Injury to the nasofrontal duct can lead to later complications including mucocele or frontal sinusitis. Surgeons may obliterate the frontal sinus (cranialization) to prevent these complications [16, 17].

Depressed outer table fractures will result in forehead deformities although this may be masked by the edema. Fractures of the posterior table may result in dural tear and CSF rhinorrhea. Fractures of the cribriform plate may result in anosmia.

CT is important to evaluate the extent of the fracture and whether it involves the anterior table, posterior table, or both (Figs. 17.12 and 17.13). When evaluating posterior table fractures, one should look for displacement, depression, pneumocephalus (suggesting dural disruption), and intracranial injury.

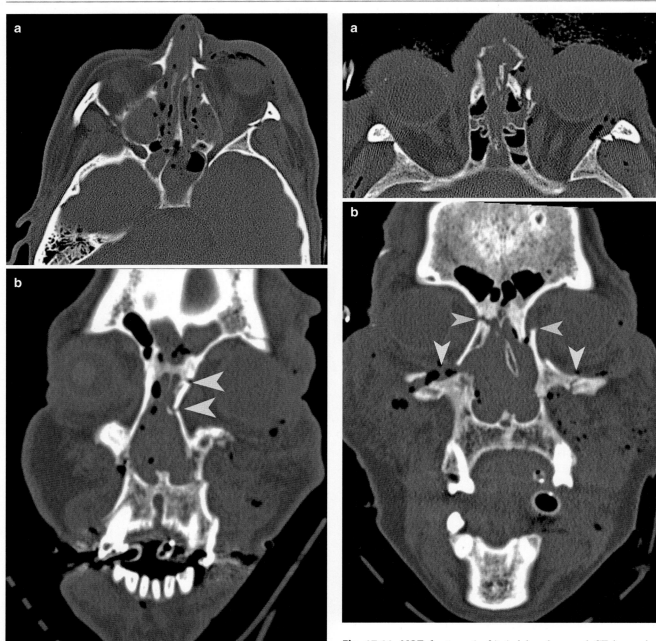

Fig. 17.10 Naso-orbital-ethmoid (NOE) fracture. (**a**) Axial CT image at the level of the lacrimal fossa demonstrates a comminuted fracture and disruption of the left medial maxillary buttress. (**b**) Coronal images at the level of the lacrimal fossa demonstrating disruption of the left medial maxillary buttress (*arrowheads*)

Fig. 17.11 NOE fracture. (**a**, **b**) Axial and coronal CT image in a patient with facial smash injury demonstrates NOE, Le Fort II (*arrowheads*), and bilateral ZMC fractures. The fractures have resulted in disruption of the medial maxillary, lateral maxillary, and upper transverse buttresses. There is posterior displacement of the central face and lateral displacement of the medial maxillary buttresses

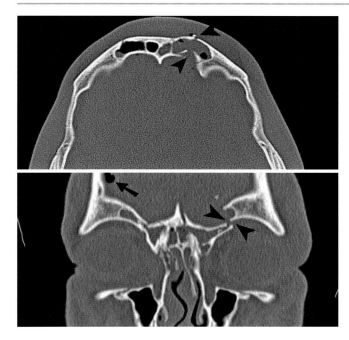

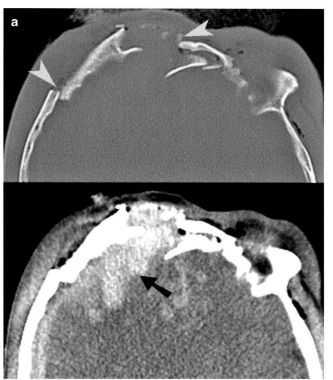

Fig. 17.12 Anterior and posterior table frontal fractures. Axial CT and surface-rendered images demonstrate comminuted fractures involving both the anterior and posterior tables (*arrowheads*). Pneumocephalus suggests dural disruption (*straight arrow*)

Maxillary Fractures

The maxilla, palatine and nasal bones form the majority of the midface. The anterior maxillary wall forms the flat portion of the face between the nose and cheek. The maxilla contains the maxillary antrum which is bordered by thin walls, resulting in predictable fracture patterns.

Le Fort Fractures

In 1901 Rene Le Fort published results of experiments performed on cadavers in which he demonstrated predictable fracture patterns of the midface [1]. Le Fort fractures are often seen in combination with other fractures [18].

Le Fort type I fractures result from trauma at a level immediately superior to the alveolar process of the maxilla. The horizontal fracture line extends through the anterior maxillary wall, medial antral wall, lateral antral wall, and pterygoid plates. There is depression of the lower transverse maxillary buttress, the hard palate. Type I fractures disrupt both medial and lateral maxillary buttresses (Fig. 17.14).

Le Fort type II fractures result from trauma at the level of the nasal bones with disruption of the (inferior) lateral and (superior) medial maxillary buttresses. These are also

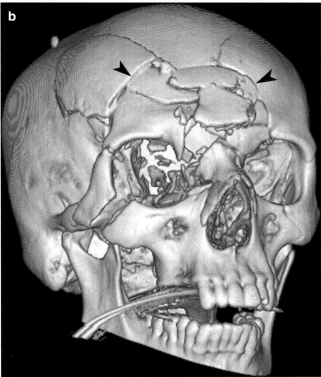

Fig. 17.13 Comminuted frontal fracture with intracranial injury. (**a**, **b**) Severely comminuted open frontal bone fractures (*arrowheads*) with associated intracranial subdural hemorrhage and frontal lobe contusion (*straight arrow*)

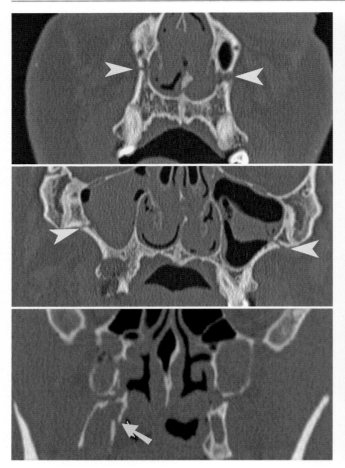

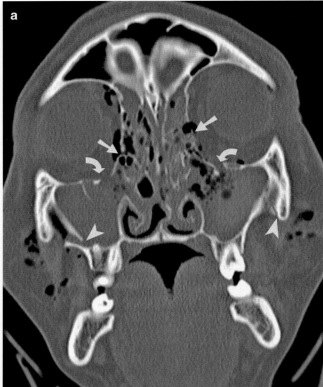

Fig. 17.14 Le Fort I fracture. Sequential coronal images from anterior to posterior showing a horizontal fracture through the medial maxillary buttresses (*arrowheads*), medial and lateral antral walls (*arrowheads*), and extending to the pterygoid plates (*straight arrow*)

referred to as pyramidal fractures, with the entire maxilla moving with respect to the skull base. Type II fractures extend across the nasal bridge, the inferomedial orbital rim, and zygomaticomaxillary suture and posteriorly through the maxillary sinus to the level of the pterygoid plates (Fig. 17.15).

Le Fort type III fractures result from a force delivered at the orbital level. The (superior) medial, (superior) lateral, and upper transverse maxillary buttresses are disrupted, resulting in craniofacial dissociation. The fracture line extends across the nasal bridge, zygomaticofrontal suture, zygomaticotemporal suture, and orbital walls, terminating posteriorly at the level of the pterygopalatine fossa, pterygoid process, or pterygoid plates. It is distinguished from the ZMC fracture by involvement of the medial orbital wall and posterior extension (Fig. 17.16).

Type I fractures may result in a free-floating palate. Type II injuries may demonstrate step deformities at the nasal bridge and infraorbital rim. Type III injuries may demonstrate craniofacial instability. With posterior displacement,

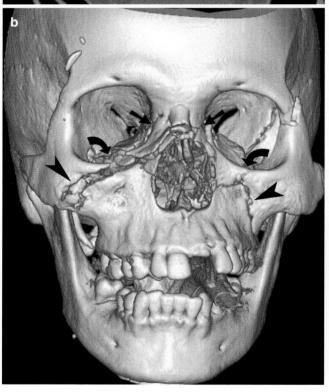

Fig. 17.15 LeFort II fracture. (**a**, **b**) Coronal CT reformation and surface rendered image demonstrate multiple comminuted pyramid shaped fracture of the mid face. There are fractures of medial orbital walls (*straight arrow*), orbital floor (*curved arrows*), and lateral antral wall (*arrowhead*).

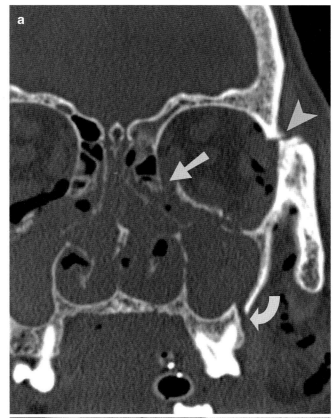

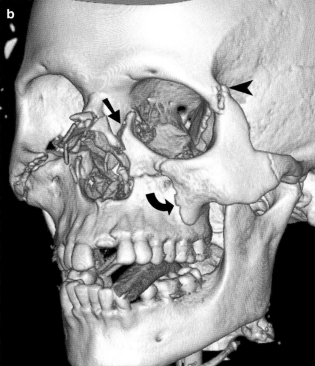

Type II and III injuries may demonstrate the characteristic "dish-face" deformity, a concave appearance of the face.

Type I injuries can be associated with dentoalveolar and mandible fractures. Type II and III injuries often demonstrate associated ZMC and NOE fractures. Type III injuries can be associated with skull fractures and intracranial injuries.

Dentoalveolar and Maxillary Sagittal Fractures

The hard palate is formed by the horizontal process of the maxilla and palatine bone. Fractures may affect the alveolus and/or palate in isolation or in combination with other more complex fractures [19, 20]. The World Health Organization (WHO) has developed an injury classification system of dentoalveolar fractures based upon fracture of the tooth, injury to the periodontal tissue, injury to the supporting bone, and injuries to the gingival or oral mucosa [21]. A classification system of maxillary sagittal fractures, developed by Hendrickson, is based on the fracture pattern through the palate [22].

Clinically, the presence of mobility of multiple teeth suggests a fracture of the alveolar process. Facial, chest, and abdominal radiographs may be helpful to evaluate for displaced, swallowed, or aspirated teeth and bone fragments. Panoramic radiographs can evaluate the teeth and the integrity of the periodontal ligament. When evaluating CT scans with dentoalveolar injury, it is important to note fractures of teeth, dental extrusion or intrusion, displacement, tooth socket fractures, tooth fragments lodged in soft tissues, and associated mandibular or other facial fractures.

Mandible Fractures

The mandible is formed by a horizontal U-shaped body and two vertical rami. The alveolar process arises from the body and contains the mandibular teeth. The superior portion of each ramus has two processes: a posterior condylar process and an anterior coronoid process, separated by the mandibular notch. The body and rami join at the angle of the mandible. The prominent position of the mandible in the lower third of the face makes it vulnerable to fracture. The mandible fractures can be divided into the following regions: symphyseal, parasymphyseal, alveolar, body, angle, ramus, condylar process, and coronoid processes. Condylar process

Fig. 17.16 Left Hemi-LeFort II and III fracture. (**a, b**) Coronal CT reformation and surface rendered image demonstrates fractures through the left medial orbital wall (*straight arrow*), orbital floor, lateral antral wall (*curved arrow*) and zygomaticofrontal suture (*arrowhead*). The posterior extension and involvement of the posteromedial orbital wall distinguishes these fractures from the ZMC fracture

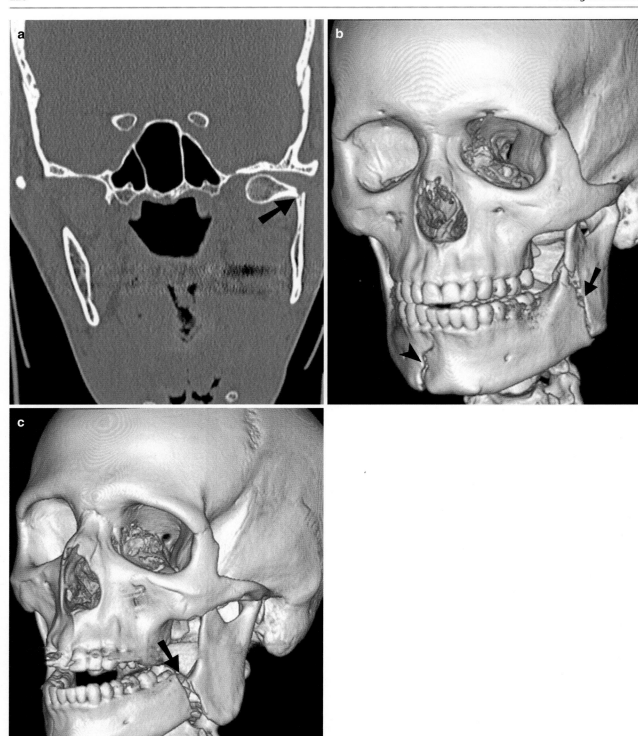

Fig. 17.17 Mandible fractures. (**a**) Coronal CT reformation shows angulated subcondylar fracture (*straight arrow*) with medial dislocation of the left mandible condylar head. (**b**) Surface-rendered CT image demonstrates right parasymphyseal (*arrowhead*) and left mandibular angle (*straight arrow*) fractures. (**c**) Surface-rendered CT image demonstrates displaced left mandibular angle fracture (*straight arrow*)

fractures are common, particularly the neck. In the setting of bilateral parasymphyseal fractures, the genioglossus, geniohyoid, and digastric muscles retract the symphysis posteriorly and inferiorly. The condylar head is often displaced medially in patients with condylar neck fractures due to the unopposed action of the lateral pterygoid muscle.

As with most current imaging of craniofacial trauma, MDCT acquisition with axial, coronal, sagittal, and 3D volume-rendered reformats allows complete evaluation of mandibular fractures as well as associated injuries (Fig. 17.17).

References

1. LeFort R. Etude experimentale sur les fractures de la machoire superieure. Rev Chir. 1901;23:208–27.
2. Sicher H, Debrul EL. Oral anatomy. 5th ed. St. Louis: Mosby; 1970. p. 78.
3. Gentry LR et al. High resolution of the CT analysis of the facial struts in trauma: 1 and 2: normal anatomy and osseous and soft-tissue complications. AJR Am J Roentgenol. 1983;140:523–41.
4. Manson P et al. Structural pillars of the facial skeleton: an approach to the management of Le Fort fractures. Plast Reconstr Surg. 1980;66(1):54–62.
5. Fonseca R et al. Oral and maxillofacial trauma. St. Louis: Elsevier/Saunders; 2005.
6. Dolan K et al. The radiology of facial fractures. Radiographics. 1984;4:575–663.
7. Moore K et al. Clinically oriented anatomy. 6th ed. Baltimore: Lippincott Williams & Wilkins; 2010.
8. Smith B, Regan WF. Blow-out fracture of the orbit, mechanism and correction of internal orbital fracture. Am J Ophthalmol. 1957;44:733–9.
9. Rhee J et al. Orbital blowout fractures: experimental evidence for the pure hydraulic theory. Arch Facial Plast Surg. 2002;4:98–101.
10. Chirico P et al. Orbital "blow-in" fractures: clinical and CT features. J Comput Assist Tomogr. 1989;13(6):1017–22.
11. Antonyshyn O et al. Blow-in fractures of the orbit. Plast Reconstr Surg. 1989;84(1):10–20.
12. Rohrich RJ et al. Superior orbital fissure syndrome: current management concepts. J Craniomaxillofac Trauma. 1995;1(2):44–8.
13. Hopper R et al. Diagnosis of midface fractures with CT: what the surgeon needs to know. Radiographics. 2006;26:783–93.
14. Markowitz B et al. Management of the medial canthal tendon in naso-ethmoid orbital fractures: the importance of the central fragments in classification and treatment. Plast Reconstr Surg. 1991;87(5):843–53.
15. Ioannides C et al. Fractures of the frontal sinus: classification and its implications for surgical treatment. Am J Otolaryngol. 1999;20(5):273–80.
16. Stanley R et al. Injuries of the nasofrontal orifices in frontal sinus fractures. Laryngoscope. 1987;97(6):728–31.
17. Gonty A et al. Management of frontal sinus fractures: a review of 33 cases. J Oral Maxillofac Surg. 1999;57:372–9.
18. Fraioli R et al. Facial fractures: beyond Le Fort. Otolaryngol Clin North Am. 2008;41:51–76.
19. Andreasen J, et al. Traumatic dental injuries: a manual. 3rd ed. Malden: Wiley-Blackwell; 2003. 18. p. 260–2.
20. Antoniades K et al. Sagittal fracture of the maxilla. J Craniomaxillofac Surg. 1990;18(6):260–2.
21. World Health Organization. Application of the International Classification of Diseases to Dentistry and Stomatology. IDC-DA. 3rd ed. Geneva: World Health Organization; 1995.
22. Hendrickson M et al. Palatal fractures: classification, patterns and treatment with rigid internal fixation. Plast Reconstr Surg. 1998;101:319–32.

Stroke and Its Imaging Evaluation

18

Sathish Kumar Dundamadappa, Melanie Ehinger, and Andrew Chen

Introduction

Stroke, defined as the sudden onset of persistent neurologic deficit, is a significant cause of morbidity and mortality in the USA. It is the third leading cause of death [1]. Ischemic infarction is by far the most common etiology comprising 88 % of stroke. Intracranial hemorrhage makes up an additional 10–15 %, with less common etiologies accounting for the remainder. Mortality rates vary with etiology, with a 38 and 8–12 % 30-day mortality seen in hemorrhagic and ischemic strokes, respectively.

Ischemic Stroke

Ischemia is by far the most common cause of stroke. Ischemic causes can be further subdivided into atherosclerotic, cardiogenic, hemodynamic, or cryptogenic sources. Atherosclerotic causes are the most common subtype as thrombi are formed in vessels with abnormal endothelium, usually directly at atherosclerotic plaque.

Emboli travel distally from the site of origin from the heart or intra-/extracranial vessels. Arterial emboli are often produced at the site of atherosclerotic plaque that dislodge and travel downstream creating an artery-to-artery embolism. Common sites for thromboembolic disease include the carotid bifurcation, carotid siphon, proximal portions of the anterior/middle cerebral arteries, subclavian artery, origin of the vertebral artery, distal vertebral artery, and basilar artery. Cardioembolic events may occur in the setting of relative

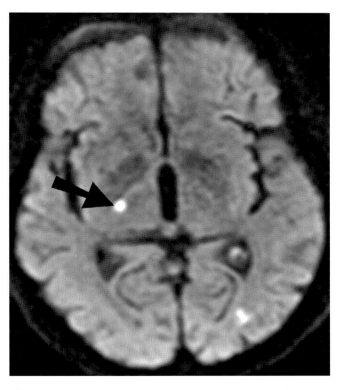

Fig. 18.1 Acute infarct. Diffusion-weighted images showing acute lacunar infarct (*arrow*) in posterior limb of right internal capsule

stasis of blood resulting in thrombus formation within the heart.

Occlusion of small perforating end arteries results in lacunar infarcts, which are infarcts less than 15 mm in diameter and frequently occur in the basal ganglia, internal capsule, pons, or corona radiata (Fig. 18.1). Occlusion of terminal branches causes cortical infarcts.

Less common etiologies, representing less than 5 % of acute stroke, include vasculopathies, immune-related diseases, hypercoagulable states, arterial dissection, global hypoperfusion, venous infarction, and mitochondrial disorders.

S.K. Dundamadappa, MD • M. Ehinger, MD • A. Chen, MD (✉)
Department of Radiology, University of Massachussetts,
55 Lake Avenue North, Worcester, MA 01655, USA
e-mail: andrew.chen@umassmemorial.org

Concept of Penumbra

Once vascular supply to the brain has been compromised, there is a window of opportunity for reversing ischemic symptoms depending upon the level to which the blood flow has dropped. Normal cerebral flow ranges between 60 and 100 ml/100 g/min, with varying degrees of hypoperfusion seen at lower flow rates. Brain parenchyma can compensate for a decrease in perfusion by increasing oxygen extraction to a cerebral blood flow (CBF) of approximately 20–23 ml/100 g/min. While blood flow of 10–20 ml/100 g/min may be reversible for a period of hours, more severe perfusion deficit (below 10 ml/100 g/min) may lead to infarction within minutes. Ischemic brain tissue can functionally be divided into three components – infarct core, penumbra, and oligemic region (Fig. 18.2). When a cerebral artery is occluded, a core of brain tissue with severe perfusion deficit dies rapidly while the surrounding brain tissue (ischemic penumbra) with moderately reduced blood flow that may have lose electrical activity. Tissue in the penumbra may be salvageable with reperfusion; otherwise, the tissue in penumbra will progress to infarction. Mildly reduced blood flow to the oligemic region surrounds the penumbra and is more likely to survive unless perfusion is further hemodynamically altered.

Imaging Workup of Acute Ischemic Stroke

In the past, imaging was primarily used to exclude hemorrhage and evaluate for surgically amenable lesions. The role of imaging has changed dramatically over the last decade and currently involves detection as well as extent of the infarct and penumbra.

Goals in acute stroke imaging are to assess the 4 "Ps" [2]:

Parenchyma: Assess early signs of acute stroke and rule out hemorrhage.

Pipes: Assess extracranial circulation and intracranial circulation for intravascular thrombus, occlusion, and severe stenosis.

Perfusion: Assess cerebral blood volume, cerebral blood flow, and mean transit time (MTT).

Penumbra: Assess tissue at risk of dying if ischemia continues without recanalization.

CT imaging, including noncontrast CT (NCCT), CT angiography (CTA), and CT perfusion (CTP), are the most often the initial imaging modalities in stroke evaluation. At our institution, NCCT followed by CTA is the initial study in stroke evaluation. CTP is performed in select cases to help stratify patients for treatment.

Noncontrast CT

Sensitivity of NCCT is 60–70 % in the first 3–6 h, and virtually all infarcts are seen by 24 h. Despite its relative insensitivity to acute infarcts in the emergency setting, NCCT remains the widely used initial imaging study in acute stroke. It is used to rule out intracranial hemorrhage and other stroke mimics.

CT signs of early ischemia include (Fig. 18.3):

Dense artery sign: Acute thrombus or embolus in a cerebral artery may produce linear hyperdensity in the vessel affected. Hyperdense MCA sign is associated with large MCA territory infarct and is seen in one-thirds of the hyperacute infarcts. MCA "dot" sign refers to hyperdensity in distal MCA and its branches in sylvian fissure.

Loss of gray-white differentiation: In MCA territory infarcts, there is often obscuration of lentiform nucleus (basal ganglia are more sensitive to ischemia due to their end-artery blood supply) and insular ribbon sign (insula is especially sensitive to ischemia due to its distance from collateral flow). Peripherally, acute infarction results in loss of definition of regions of cortex (cortical sign) in the affected vascular territory.

Hypodensity: This becomes more apparent and well circumscribed by 24 h. Variable amount of cerebral swelling develops after 24 h, usually peaks at 3–5 days. The degree of swelling depends on the restoration of flow.

The detection of early acute ischemic stroke on NCCT may be improved by using variable window width and center level settings to accentuate the contrast between normal and edematous tissue [3]. Multiplanar reformats may also help in identifying subtle infarcts (e.g., coronal reformats for superior cerebellar infarcts).

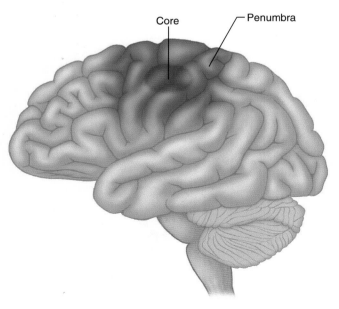

Core   Penumbra

Fig. 18.2 Schematic diagram shows an acute infarct and the surrounding penumbra

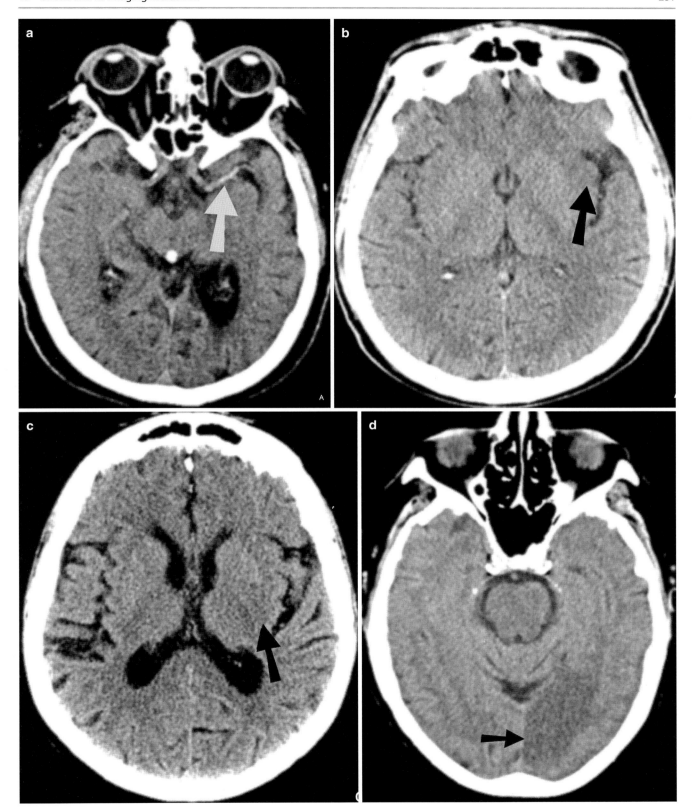

Fig. 18.3 CT signs of acute infarction. (**a**) Noncontrast CT showing hyperdense clot in the left M1 segment (*arrow*) of middle cerebral artery (hyperdense MCA sign). CTA (not shown) confirmed MCA occlusion. (**b**) Noncontrast CT shows loss of grey-white matter differentiation (*arrow*) at the insula (insular ribbon sign). (**c**) Noncontrast CT shows subte hypodensity in posterior aspect of left lentiform nucleus (*arrow*). (**d**) Noncontrast CT shows hypodensity involving both gray and white matter in left occipital lobe (PCA territory) (*arrow*)

CT Angiography

CTA is fast and noninvasive and allows for evaluation of etiology of acute ischemic stroke (such as thrombosis, occlusion, severe stenosis, and dissection). Both source images and 3D images should be reviewed. Though not very accurate, clot morphology like ulceration can also be assessed. When calcified plaques are present, the window can be widened for better evaluation.

CT Perfusion

CTP is a functional imaging technique that can be rapidly performed to evaluate ischemic but potentially salvageable penumbral tissue. CTP is based on the entry and washout of an intravenous iodinated bolus of contrast.

Severely diminished cerebral blood volume (CBV) has been demonstrated as a good correlate to the area of restricted diffusion on MRI and hence is considered a measure of the infarct core. Decreased cerebral blood flow (CBF) and increased mean transit time (MTT) are seen in areas of the brain either at risk for or undergoing infarct. Occasionally, increased CBV (luxury perfusion) may be seen in ischemic region due to autoregulatory vasodilatation and recruitment of collateral vessels. The combination of low CBF and normal/increased CBV represents an area at risk for ischemia (penumbra) but currently compensated by dilated collateral vessels (Fig. 18.4).

MR Imaging

MR imaging is more sensitive and specific than CT for detection of acute stroke. The most sensitive imaging sequence for detecting ischemia is diffusion-weighted MR imaging (DWI), with changes in acute infarction detected within minutes of onset of the symptoms. Cytotoxic edema of acute ischemia results in reduced water diffusion in the extracellular matrix. DWI detects this restriction of microscopic motion.

Acute infarct is seen as bright signal intensity on DWI due to restricted diffusion as well as secondary to increased water content (T2 effect), with corresponding decrease on apparent diffusion coefficient (ADC) sequence (Fig. 18.5a). DWI is positive in the acute phase with increasing intensity that peaks at 7 days. The time to normalization of DWI signal has been reported in literature to range from 14 to 72 days [4, 5]. ADC sequence initially has low signal intensity, with maximum hypointensity occurring at 24 h. Signal intensity then increases and normalizes between the 7th and 11th days [6].

Additional findings in acute infarct include the presence of lesion in arterial distribution, hyperintense signal on T2-weighted and fluid-attenuated inversion recovery sequence, subcortical white matter hypointensity on T2-weighted sequence (Fig. 18.5b), exaggerated intravascular enhancement, and findings of vascular occlusion (lack of normal flow void on long TE sequence and high arterial signal on FLAIR sequence related to slow flow/occlusion)

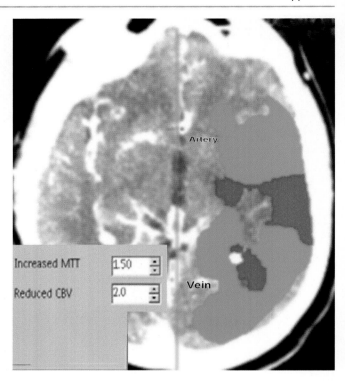

Fig. 18.4 Color-coded summary maps from CT perfusion study showing large penumbra (shown in *green*) in the left MCA territory. The red color indicates severely reduced cerebral blood volume

(Fig. 18.5c). However, T2 signal can be normal in the first 8 h after ictus. With time, infarcts become hyperintense on T2-weighted sequence, with maximum hyperintensity reached between 7 and 30 days.

MR Perfusion Imaging

MR perfusion imaging techniques include exogenous contrast-enhanced method or an endogenous method (arterial spin labeling). Exogenous dynamic susceptibility-weighted (T2*-weighted) sequence is the most commonly used technique in acute stroke evaluation. The technique involves tracking of the tissue signal loss caused by T2* effects of paramagnetic contrast agent to create a hemodynamic time–signal intensity curve. As in dynamic CT perfusion imaging, various parametric maps (CBV, MTT, CBF, TTP) are calculated from this curve by using a deconvolution technique. The core of infarct demonstrated by restricted diffusion is compared against CBF or MTT maps for mismatch which represents the penumbra, tissue at risk (Fig. 18.6).

Hemorrhagic Transformation

Hemorrhagic transformation of an infarct is a rare (3.6 %) complication in the acute phase. It is thought to be due to reperfusion of ischemic tissue during the first 2 weeks, occurring more commonly in larger infarcts and cardioembolic infarcts. Anticoagulant and thrombolytic agents increase the incidence of hemorrhagic transformation.

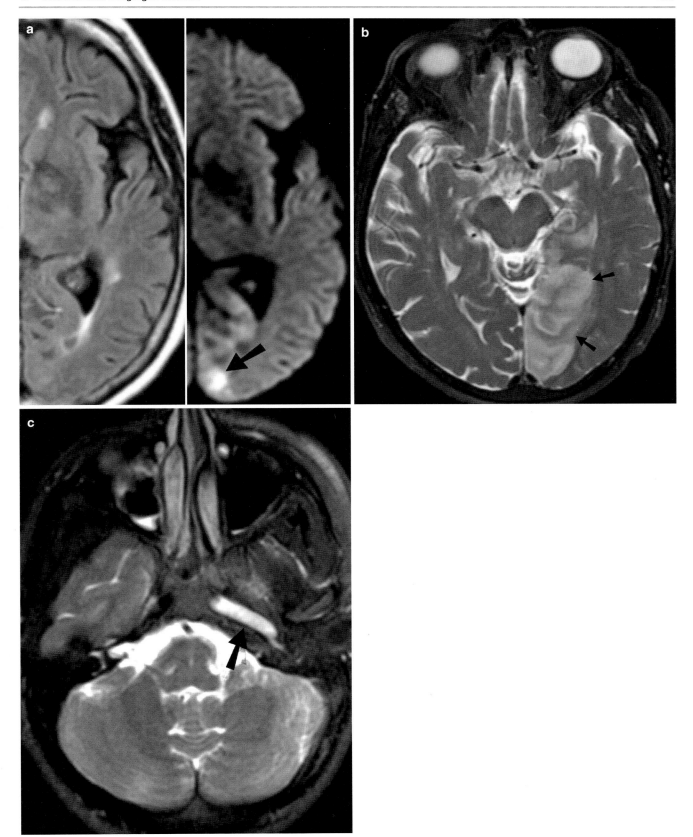

Fig. 18.5 Acute infraction on MRI. (**a**) Acute right PCA territory infarct which is not apparent on T2-weighted sequence, is clearly seen on DWI (*arrow*). (**b**) T2-weighted sequence shows acute left PCA terri-tory infarction (*arrows*). (**c**) Left ICA occlusion: T2-weighted sequence shows hyperintense signal within left ICA (*arrow*), indicating the pres-ence of thrombus in the arterial lumen

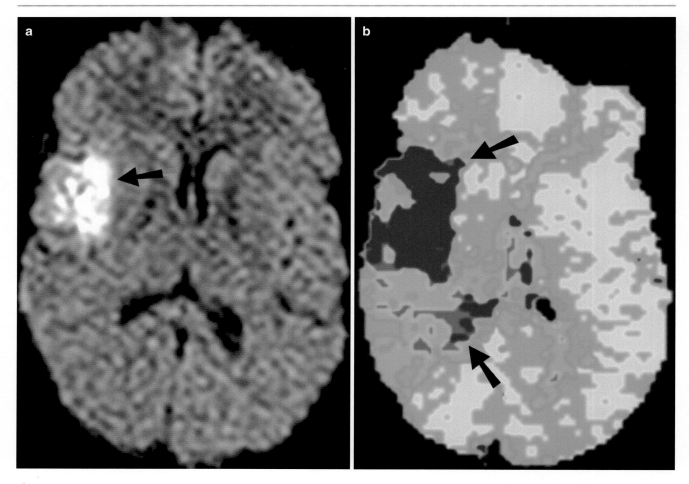

Fig. 18.6 Acute infarction on MR. (**a**) Diffusion-weighted sequence shows a hyperintense acute infarct in the right MCA territory. (**b**) MR perfusion image shows a large defect (*arrows*), suggesting the presence of a penumbra

The European Cooperative Acute Stroke Study (ECASS) classification of hemorrhagic transformation stratified the size of these hemorrhages with the clinical outcome [7].

HI (hemorrhagic infarct) (Fig. 18.7): petechial hemorrhages without space-occupying effect

HI1: small petechiae

HI2: more confluent petechiae

PH (parenchymal hematoma) (Fig. 18.8): hemorrhage (coagulum) with mass effect

PH1: <30 % of the infarcted area with mild space-occupying effect

PH2: >30 % of the infarcted area with significant space-occupying effect

Only PH2 independently modifies the risk of a worse clinical outcome both early and late after stroke onset. PH-1 has increased risk of early deterioration but not of a worse long-term outcome. HI is not associated with worse early or late outcome [8].

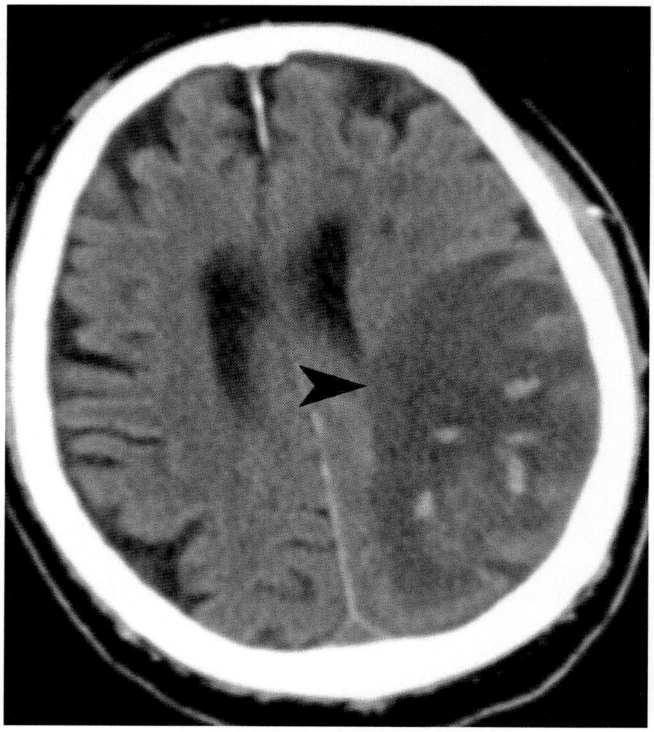

Fig. 18.7 Acute infarct with hemorrhage. Noncontrast CT shows petechial hemorrhages with left parietal infarct (*arrowhead*) (ECASS HI2)

Infarction from Septic Emboli

This is a subset of embolic infarctions, mostly seen with intravenous drug abuse, infective endocarditis, and cardiac

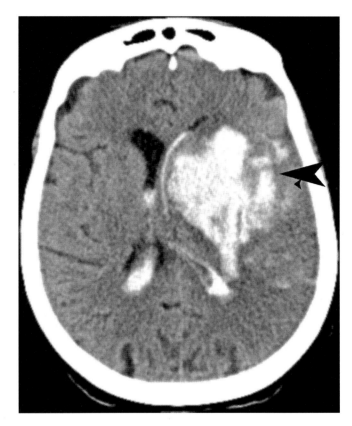

Fig. 18.8 Acute infarct with hemorrhage. Noncontrast CT shows intraparenchymal as well as intraventricular hemorrhage (*arrow*) within left MCA territory infarction (ECASS PH2), following IV tPA

valve abnormalities. The most common MRI finding in early stages of septic emboli is that of ordinary embolic infarction. Eventually changes related to infection show up, with disproportionate edema, enhancement, cerebritis, and finally frank abscess formation. Like other embolic infarctions, these show a higher tendency to bleed.

Watershed Infarction

Watershed or boundary zone infarctions occur from hypoperfusion at the junction between arterial territories and have two patterns (Fig. 18.9):

Superficial border zone: These are infarctions of the cortex and adjacent white matter located at the boundary zone between leptomeningeal collaterals from adjacent arterial territories (ACA/MCA, MCA/PCA, and ACA/PCA).

Internal border zone: They occur in the corona radiata and centrum semiovale, between lenticulostriate perforators and the deep-penetrating cortical branches of the MCA and between deep white matter branches of the MCA and the ACA.

Infarct Evolution

Subacute stage approximately extends from 2 to 14 days following the initial ischemic event. In this stage the infarcts become better circumscribed. Mass effect peaks by 3–5 days and then diminishes. When there is hemorrhagic transformation, MR signal characteristics of blood change with age. Contrast enhancement seen typically in this stage can be gyral or patchy (Fig. 18.10). It typically begins toward the

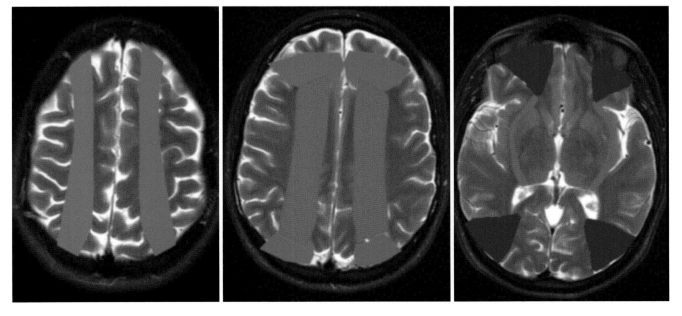

Fig. 18.9 Schematic representation of the superficial (*colored red*) and internal (*colored blue*) watershed zones in the cerebral hemispheres

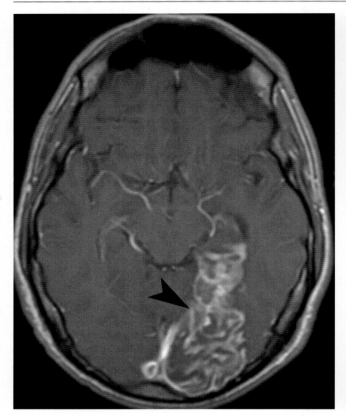

Fig. 18.10 Subacute infarction on MR. Contrast-enhanced T1-weighted image showing enhancing subacute infarct in left PCA territory (*arrowhead*)

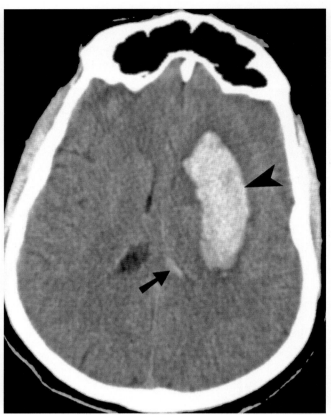

Fig. 18.11 Hypertensive hemorrhage. Noncontrast CT of the head demonstrates intraparenchymal hypertensive hemorrhage (*arrowhead*) in the left basal ganglia region with small intraventricular extension (*arrow*)

end of the first week, when mass effect has resolved, and persists for approximately 6–8 weeks. This discordance between enhancement and mass effect is a useful radiologic observation, because enhancing lesions with significant mass effect is unlikely to represent cerebral infarction [9].

The chronic stage of cerebral infarction begins weeks to months after the initial ischemic event, when the integrity of the blood–brain barrier is restored and edema has resolved. The infarcts are smaller and better defined than seen in earlier stages and no longer enhance. Gliosis or encephalomalacia and volume loss are the hallmarks of this stage.

Posttreatment Imaging

After treatment, CT is generally used to evaluate infarct progression or look for posttreatment hemorrhagic conversion. Special attention is paid to history and timing of any previous angiographic intervention, as dense contrast from this procedure can mimic blood.

Nontraumatic Intracranial Hemorrhage

Nontraumatic intracranial hemorrhage (ICH) accounts for about 15 % of strokes in the USA. The hemorrhages are typically parenchymal or subarachnoid but may be subdural, intraventricular, or rarely epidural. Further discussion in this section is limited to parenchymal hemorrhage.

Etiology

The causes of nontraumatic and noninfarct-related parenchymal ICH include hypertension, vascular malformations, amyloid angiopathy, neoplasm, coagulopathies, drug abuse, anticoagulants, thrombolytics, and venous thrombosis. Rarer causes like vasculitis and reversible cerebral vasoconstrictive syndrome can also be considered.

Hypertension is the most prevalent and modifiable risk factor for spontaneous ICH. The most frequent anatomic locations for hypertensive ICH are the putamen (Fig. 18.11), globus pallidus, external capsule, subcortical white matter, thalamus, internal capsule, and in the cerebellum and brain stem.

Cerebral amyloid angiopathy refers to the deposition of β-amyloid in small- and midsized arteries (and less frequently veins) of the cerebral cortex and the leptomeninges. Its prevalence is approximately 5–8 % in people in the seventh decade and 55–60 % of people who are 90 years or older [10]. It has been reported to account for 5–20 % of nontraumatic cerebral hemorrhages in elderly patients [11]. The hemorrhages are typically lobar (parietooccipital predominance) of different ages and affect elderly normotensive patients.

In a population-based study, 12 % of all cases of ICH were on anticoagulation medications at the time of their hemorrhage, compared with only 4 % of age-, race-, and gender-matched control [12].

Vascular malformations are the leading cause of spontaneous ICH in young adults. Arteriovenous malformations (AVM) and cavernous malformations (CM) account for most of the clinically evident hemorrhages. Brain tumors may have associated ICH, in up to 15 % of patients, but rarely is hemorrhage the presenting symptom of a previously undiagnosed brain mass [13]. Hemorrhagic primary brain tumors are generally high-grade tumors like glioblastoma multiforme and anaplastic astrocytoma. The intracerebral metastases that are most likely to hemorrhage are those caused by choriocarcinoma, melanoma, thyroid carcinoma, and renal cell carcinoma. However, most hemorrhagic metastases are caused by breast and lung carcinomas, as they are more common causes of brain metastases in the general population.

Illicit drugs associated with ICH include cocaine, amphetamines, phenylpropanolamine, phencyclidine, ephedrine, and pseudoephedrine. The predominant underlying mechanism is abrupt hypertension or in some cases vasculitis.

Hemorrhage from cerebral venous thrombosis is typically cortical in location, with subcortical extension [14]. Flame-shaped irregular zones of lobar hemorrhage in the parasagittal frontal and parietal lobes are typical findings in superior sagittal sinus thrombosis, whereas hemorrhage in the temporal or occipital lobes is more typical of transverse sinus thrombosis.

Imaging Evaluation

Noncontrast CT of the head is generally the initial investigation given the wide availability and high sensitivity for acute hemorrhage. Acute hematoma is hyperdense on CT with density between 50 and 70 Hounsfield units. After the third day, the blood density gradually decreases from periphery to the

Table 18.1 MR findings of hemorrhagic products

Stage of hematoma	Time	Signal on T1WI	Signal on T2WI
Hyperacute	First 6 h	Low	High
Acute	Up to 3 days	Iso to low	Low
Early subacute	4–7 days	High	Low
Late subacute	1 week to several months	High	High
Chronic	Months to years	Low	Low

central region. CT also provides information on the location, size, intraventricular extension, mass affect, hydrocephalus, or midline shift.

Contrast-enhanced MR imaging is the next imaging step in the subset of patients to evaluate for an underlying lesion. MR imaging of hemorrhage is more complex than CT, and the signal characteristics of the hematoma vary with its age (Table 18.1). Gradient-recalled echo or susceptibility-weighted sequences are sensitive for the detection of hemorrhage. Five stages of hemorrhage can be identified by MRI.

An important role of imaging is to evaluate for an underlying lesion. Heterogeneity of the hematoma (Fig. 18.12), enhancing component, hypodense filling defect on CT (Fig. 18.13), disproportionate surrounding edema, unusual or lobar location, unusual age, known primary tumor, additional enhancing lesions, abnormal calcification, and incomplete peripheral hypointense rim on T2 images suggest an underlying mass lesion. Contrast-enhanced MRI is more sensitive in detection of enhancing tumor component in or adjacent to the hematoma. Follow-up imaging may show delayed evolution of blood breakdown products, persistent edema, mass effect, or serpiginous flow voids. The underlying lesion may become more apparent as the hematoma resolves.

Underlying vascular malformation may be suggested by younger age of the patient and prominent vessels or linear calcification adjacent to the hematoma (Fig. 18.14). Catheter angiography is used to diagnose small AVMs that may be occult on both CT and MR, to fully characterize an AVM, and to perform therapeutic intervention. Repeat angiography after resorption of the hematoma is appropriate in selected patients with a high index of suspicion and a negative initial cerebral angiogram [11]. Cavernomas show characteristic "popcorn ball" morphology on MRI with complete T2 hypointense rim.

The direct signs of cerebral venous thrombosis can be seen on noncontrast CT (sensitivity of about 33 %) and include visualization of hyperattenuating thrombus in dural sinus (dense clot sign) (Fig. 18.15) [15]. The "cord sign" represents direct visualization of a hyperattenuating thrombosed cortical vein. Given this limited sensitivity of noncontrast CT, if the location of hematoma or the clinical features raise the possibility of venous thrombosis, further evaluation

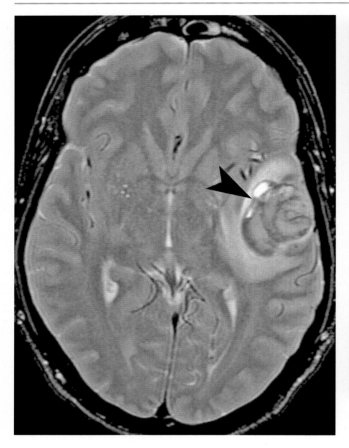

Fig. 18.12 Hemorrhagic primary intracranial tumor. T2-weighted image shows marked heterogeneity (*arrowhead*) of the hematoma in a patient with hemorrhagic glioblastoma multiforme

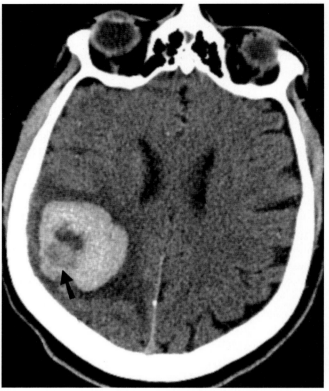

Fig. 18.13 Hemorrhagic metastatic melanoma. Noncontrast CT shows eccentric mass within the hematoma (*arrow*) in a patient with known melanoma

should be done by MRI and MRV or CTV. Contrast-enhanced CT can show "the empty delta sign," which represents the filling defect (non-enhancing thrombus) surrounded by the enhancing dural sinus wall. On MRI, thrombosed veins bloom on gradient-recalled images. There may also be intraluminal abnormal signal in the vein depending on the stage of the thrombus. Venographic techniques better demonstrate the thrombus and also show venous collaterals and resultant adjacent dural enhancement. Catheter angiogram can be done for confirmation and intervention.

Subarachnoid Hemorrhage

Subarachnoid hemorrhage (SAH) is most commonly of non-traumatic etiology, occurring secondary to ruptured aneurysm. Less common causes include AVM, vasculitis, venous

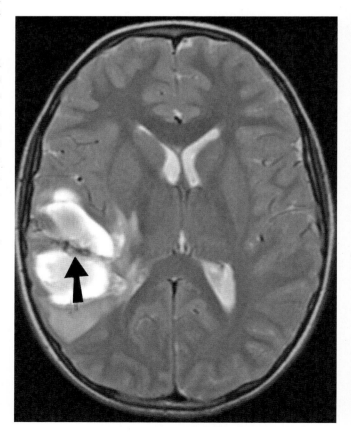

Fig. 18.14 Hemorrhagic AVM. T2-weighted sequence shows hyperintense subacute hematoma. Flow voids from vessels (*arrow*) is seen within the hematoma, suggests the presence of an underlying vascular abnormality

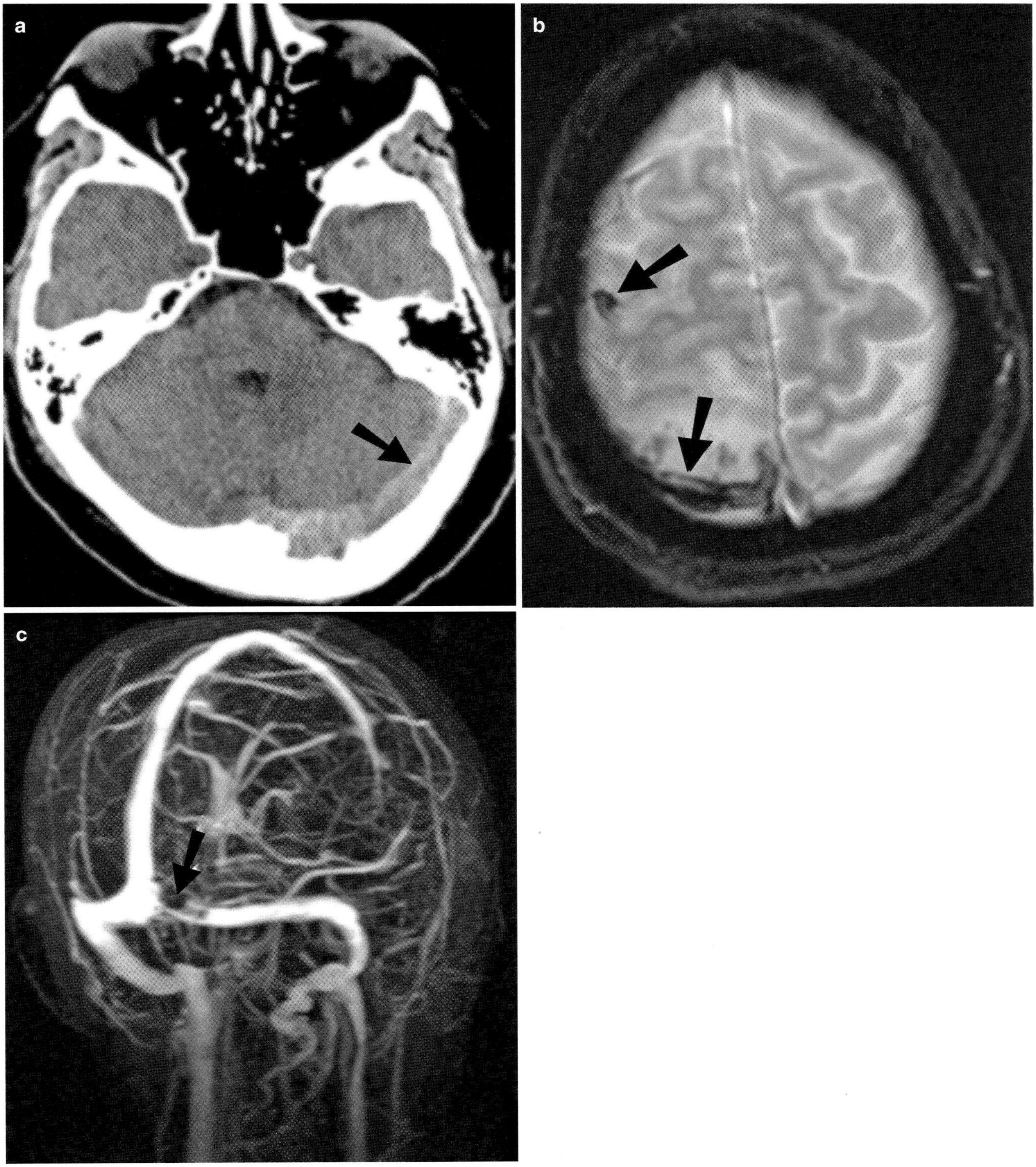

Fig. 18.15 Venous thrombosis, different patients. (**a**) Noncontrast CT shows hyperdense left transverse sinus, (*arrow*), secondary to thrombosis. (**b**) Gradient echo T2-weighted MR sequence shows blooming of thrombosed cortical veins (*arrows*). (**c**) MR venogram shows a focal filling defect within proximal left transverse sinus, from intraluminal thrombus

thrombosis, reversible cerebral vasoconstriction syndrome, and extension of parenchymal/intraventricular hemorrhage into subarachnoid space [16]. Saccular aneurysm is the most common type of cerebral aneurysm. Fusiform aneurysms are less common and are most often the result of atherosclerosis and dissection or found in association with congenital conditions. Septic emboli may result in mycotic aneurysms which are typically small and located in distal arterial branches. Aneurysms can be seen in feeding arteries, nidus, or draining veins of AVM.

Aneurysms are considered to be acquired lesions, occurring most frequently at the vascular bifurcations. The common locations of aneurysms are anterior communicating artery, clinoid/supraclinoid ICA, middle cerebral artery bifurcation or trifurcation, basilar artery (tip and the origin of superior cerebellar arteries), and vertebral artery (at the origin of the posterior inferior cerebellar arteries). Incidence of unruptured aneurysm is about 5 % [17]. When the aneurysms are multiple, the distribution of SAH and irregular/lobulated contour of the aneurysm is helpful in determining the ruptured aneurysm.

Approximately 10–15% of patients with SAH secondary to aneurysm rupture die before reaching the medical care and 25 % of the rest die over the succeeding 2 weeks [18]. The risk of rebleeding in untreated aneurysm is about 4 % within the first 24 h, 20 % within 2 weeks, and 50 % within 1 month [19].

Imaging Evaluation

The cornerstone of the diagnosis is a noncontrast head CT which has a diagnostic yield of approximately 90 %. SAH is seen as diffuse hyperdensity in subarachnoid space (Fig. 18.16). If hemorrhage is brisk, focal hematoma may form in the subarachnoid space. Careful attention should be paid to areas where a small amount of blood can be easily overlooked, such as posterior aspects of the sylvian fissures, interpeduncular cistern, deep cerebral sulci, occipital horns of the lateral ventricles, and the foramen magnum.

Exuberant inflammatory exudates in the subarachnoid space and recent iodinated contrast administration can result in subarachnoid hyperdensity and mimic SAH. Diseases causing diffuse cerebral edema as well as intracranial mass lesions and severe obstructive hydrocephalus can result in an appearance similar to SAH due to apposition of pial surfaces and resultant engorgement of pial veins [20].

Distribution of SAH, focal clot in subarachnoid space, and parenchyma hematoma may help in localization of ruptured aneurysm on NCT. The aneurysm may be seen as a

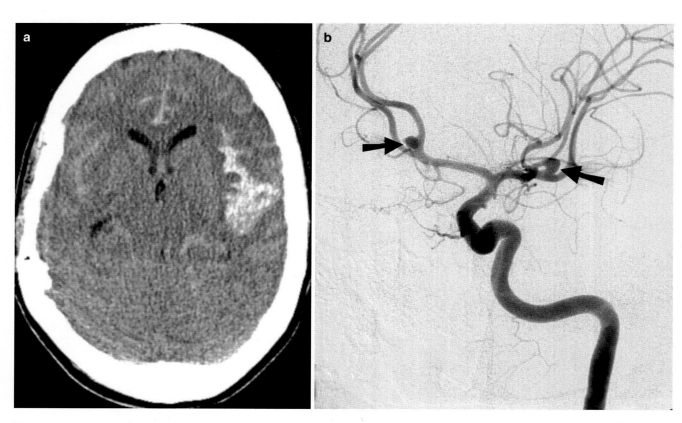

Fig. 18.16 Subarachnoid hemorrhage from ruptured circle of Willis aneurysm. (**a**) Noncontrast shows bilateral subarachnoid hemorrhage, most prominently involving the left sylvian fissure. (**b**) Subsequent digital subtraction angiogram shows left MCA and anterior communicating artery aneurysms (*arrows*). Given the focal hematoma in left sylvian fissure and lobulated contour, left MCA aneurysm is likely the source of bleeding

relatively hypodense area within the dense SAH. On CT, SAH generally resolves by 5–7 days. Smaller bleeds may resolve earlier. Focal clot, if present, may persist for a longer time.

Generally a lumbar puncture is performed to evaluate for xanthochromia in patients who have suspected SAH and a negative CT scan. Xanthochromia is representative of the presence of bilirubin in the CSF and requires at least 12 h to develop [18].

Computed Tomography Angiography (CTA)

CTA is generally the next investigation in SAH evaluation. The sensitivity of multidetector CTA is reported to be 94.8 % and the specificity 95.2 % for the detection on a per aneurysm basis and 99.0 and 95.2 % on a per patient basis, respectively [21]. In this study, a cutoff size of 2 mm was found as the inflection point at which CTA became less able to detect aneurysms. CTA demonstrates the location of aneurysm and evaluates for the presence of thrombus and wall calcification.

MRI

SAH has different MR imaging features than other intracranial hemorrhages. This is due to mixing of blood with CSF and resultant dilution, antifibrogenic elements in CSF and relatively high oxygen saturation of CSF (which limits amount of paramagnetic deoxyhemoglobin) [17]. Due to relative lack of magnetic inhomogeneity of SAH, gradient-recalled images are less sensitive for the detection SAH. T2-weighted fluid-attenuated inversion recovery (FLAIR) is the most sensitive sequence for SAH and shows subarachnoid hyperintensity. Larger amount of blood can demonstrate blooming on gradient-recalled images. Also, T1 images may show slight inhomogeneity of CSF with mild hyperintensity. FLAIR is comparable in its sensitivity to CT in detection of acute SAH. In our experience it is better than CT in subacute stage (Fig. 18.17). However, FLAIR is prone to artifacts, especially in the posterior fossa and adjacent to metallic hardware. Also other leptomeningeal inflammatory and neoplastic processes can result in subarachnoid hyperintensity in FLAIR images. SAH also causes reactive contrast enhancement in the meninges.

Magnetic Resonance Angiography (MRA)

The reported sensitivity of MRA in the detection of aneurysms 3 mm or larger is 90 %, but this number falls precipitously for smaller aneurysms with reported sensitivity of less than 40 %. MRA may be impractical in acute settings as most of the patients are ill and may not be able to lay still. This is a good modality to follow up unruptured aneurysms.

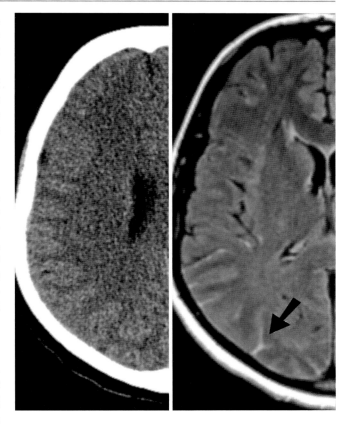

Fig. 18.17 Subacute SAH. Noncontrast CT fails to show sulcal hyperdensity, but FLAIR image clearly shows sulcal hyperintensity from subarachnoid hemorrhage (*arrow*)

Catheter Angiogram

This is the gold standard for aneurysm evaluation. If there is high suspicion for SAH and the noninvasive imaging fails to show an aneurysm, DSA should be done for further evaluation.

Angiogram can be negative in up to 10 % SAH, possibly due to vasospasm or clot filling up the aneurysm. A repeat catheter angiogram is usually performed at about the 7th day to look for aneurysms missed on the first study.

Vasospasm

After initial treatment and diagnosis of SAH, clinical deterioration can occur due to recurrent hemorrhage, hydrocephalus, vasospasm, and stroke. Vasospasm represents the leading cause of mortality and usually begins approximately 3 days after the initial bleed [17]. The proposed causes of SAH include reactive vasoconstriction, decreased vascular autoregulation, reversible vasculopathy, and relative hypovolemia [22].

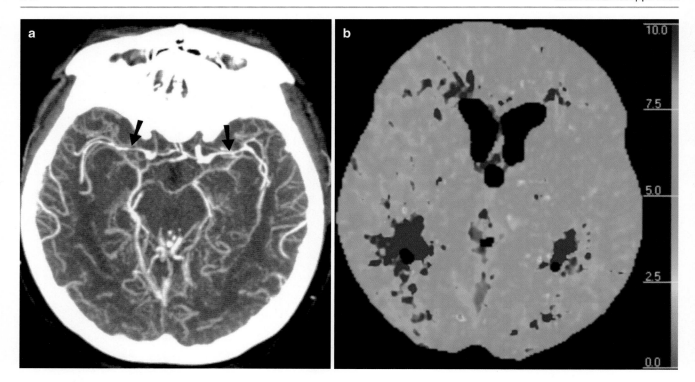

Fig. 18.18 Intracranial vasospasm. (**a**) CT angiogram shows vasospasm in bilateral middle cerebral arteries (*arrows*) and bilateral proximal posterior cerebral arteries. (**b**) Mean transit time (MTT) map from CT perfusion study shows prolonged MTT, more so on the left

The radiologic findings often precede such clinical deficits and thus offer the opportunity to potentially intervene to prevent neurologic injury.

The methods for diagnosing vasospasm include transcranial Doppler (TCD) ultrasonography, CTA, CTP, and DSA (gold standard). The validity of TCD as a monitor for VS has been controversial and is best, an adjunct to other tests. CTA has relatively good sensitivity and specificity in discovering severe VS of proximal arteries (Fig. 18.18a). It also has a high negative predictive value. MTT is reported to be the most accurate perfusion CT parameter for the diagnosis of vasospasm (Fig. 18.18b) [21]. DSA is the gold standard for diagnosis of vasospasm. Endovascular treatment options for vasospasm include intra-arterial vasodilator and angioplasty.

Stroke imaging has made significant progress in the last several years and is evolving. With technologic advances, together with better anatomic depiction, increased emphasis will be on functional imaging to determine tissue viability and the appropriateness of therapy.

References

1. Lloyd-Jones D, Adams RJ, Brown TM, Carnethon M, Dai S, De Simone G, et al. Executive summary: heart disease and stroke statistics–2010 update: a report from the American Heart Association. Circulation. 2010;121(7):948–54.

2. Rowley HA. The four ps of acute stroke imaging: parenchyma, pipes, perfusion, and penumbra. AJNR Am J Neuroradiol. 2001; 22(4):599–601.

3. Srinivasan A, Goyal M, Al Azri F, Lum C. State-of-the-art imaging of acute stroke. Radiographics. 2006;26 Suppl 1:S75–95.

4. Burdette JH, Ricci PE, Petitti N, Elster AD. Cerebral infarction: time course of signal intensity changes on diffusion-weighted MR images. AJR Am J Roentgenol. 1998;171(3):791–5.

5. Huang IJ, Chen CY, Chung HW, Chang DC, Lee CC, Chin SC, et al. Time course of cerebral infarction in the middle cerebral arterial territory: deep watershed versus territorial subtypes on diffusion-weighted MR images. Radiology. 2001;221(1):35–42.

6. Eastwood JD, Engelter ST, MacFall JF, Delong DM, Provenzale JM. Quantitative assessment of the time course of infarct signal intensity on diffusion-weighted images. AJNR Am J Neuroradiol. 2003;24(4):680–7.

7. Hacke W, Kaste M, Fieschi C, Toni D, Lesaffre E, von Kummer R, et al. Intravenous thrombolysis with recombinant tissue plasminogen activator for acute hemispheric stroke. The European Cooperative Acute Stroke Study (ECASS). JAMA. 1995;274(13):1017–25.

8. Berger C, Fiorelli M, Steiner T, Schabitz WR, Bozzao L, Bluhmki E, et al. Hemorrhagic transformation of ischemic brain tissue: asymptomatic or symptomatic? Stroke. 2001;32(6):1330–5.

9. Atlas SW. Magnetic resonance imaging of the brain and spine. Philadelphia: Lippincott Williams & Wilkins; 2008.

10. Masuda J, Tanaka K, Ueda K, Omae T. Autopsy study of incidence and distribution of cerebral amyloid angiopathy in hisayama, Japan. Stroke. 1988;19(2):205–10.

11. Fischbein NJ, Wijman CA. Nontraumatic intracranial hemorrhage. Neuroimaging Clin N Am. 2010;20(4):469–92.

12. Woo D, Sauerbeck LR, Kissela BM, Khoury JC, Szaflarski JP, Gebel J, et al. Genetic and environmental risk factors for intracerebral hemorrhage: preliminary results of a population-based study. Stroke. 2002;33(5):1190–5.

13. Salmaggi A, Erbetta A, Silvani A, Maderna E, Pollo B. Intracerebral haemorrhage in primary and metastatic brain tumours. Neurol Sci. 2008;29 Suppl 2:S264–5.
14. Leach JL, Fortuna RB, Jones BV, Gaskill-Shipley MF. Imaging of cerebral venous thrombosis: current techniques, spectrum of findings, and diagnostic pitfalls. Radiographics. 2006;26 Suppl 1:S19–41; discussion S42–3.
15. Poon CS, Chang JK, Swarnkar A, Johnson MH, Wasenko J. Radiologic diagnosis of cerebral venous thrombosis: pictorial review. AJR Am J Roentgenol. 2007;189(6 Suppl): S64–75.
16. Linn FH, Rinkel GJ, Algra A, van Gijn J. Incidence of subarachnoid hemorrhage: role of region, year, and rate of computed tomography: a meta-analysis. Stroke. 1996;27(4):625–9.
17. Yousem DM, Grossman RI. Neuroradiology: the requisites. 3rd ed. Philadelphia: Mosby; 2010.
18. Manno EM. Subarachnoid hemorrhage. Neurol Clin. 2004;22(2): 347–66.
19. Kassell NF, Torner JC, Haley Jr EC, Jane JA, Adams HP, Kongable GL. The international cooperative study on the timing of aneurysm surgery. Part 1: overall management results. J Neurosurg. 1990;73(1):18–36.
20. Provenzale JM, Hacein-Bey L. CT evaluation of subarachnoid hemorrhage: a practical review for the radiologist interpreting emergency room studies. Emerg Radiol. 2009;16(6):441–51.
21. Wintermark M, Ko NU, Smith WS, Liu S, Higashida RT, Dillon WP. Vasospasm after subarachnoid hemorrhage: utility of perfusion CT and CT angiography on diagnosis and management. AJNR Am J Neuroradiol. 2006;27(1):26–34.
22. Marshall SA, Kathuria S, Nyquist P, Gandhi D. Noninvasive imaging techniques in the diagnosis and management of aneurysmal subarachnoid hemorrhage. Neurosurg Clin N Am. 2010;21(2):305–23.

Imaging of Acute Orbital Pathologies

19

Ajay Singh

Introduction

There are 30,000 hospital admissions per year secondary to traumatic eye injuries, which occur commonly in patients with blunt or penetrating facial trauma. Majority of the traumas are secondary to motor vehicle collision or sports-related injury. Ocular trauma accounts for 7.5 % for eye admissions in the hospital [1]. Ocular trauma is the leading cause of noncongenital unilateral blindness in <20-year-olds and overall the second leading cause of blindness. Open-globe injury risk is highest for young adults and lowest for seniors [2].

Patients with significant eye injuries may have grossly normal eyes on physical exam and may subsequently become apparent. Prompt diagnosis is important in preserving visual acuity and preventing complications.

Traumatic injuries range from simple ecchymosis of the eyelid and subconjunctival hemorrhage to more serious lesions, including hyphema, choroidal or retinal rupture, optic nerve contusion, and rupture of the globe. Most common ocular injuries are superficial corneal ulcerations and foreign bodies. The more serious injuries include globe rupture, anterior chamber hemorrhage possibly complicated by glaucoma, intraocular foreign body, corneal perforation, posttraumatic cataract, and RD.

Classification and Mechanism

The visual pathway traumatic injuries by location can be divided into:
1. Intraocular
2. Intraorbital
3. Intracanalicular
4. Intracranial

Normal Anatomy (Fig. 19.1)

Orbit is a pyramid-shaped structure, constituted by seven bones. The medial wall is the thinnest and has four bones, namely, frontal process of maxilla, lacrimal bone, sphenoid, and lamina papyracea of the ethmoid. The lateral wall is constituted by the sphenoid wings and zygoma. The orbital roof is constituted by the orbital process of the frontal bone and lesser wing of the sphenoid. The floor is the weakest wall, constituted by maxilla, zygoma, and palatine bones.

Anterior chamber (AC) is crescent shaped between the lens and the cornea, measuring 2.5–3.5 mm in depth (Fig. 19.1). It is isointense to the vitreous on T1- and T2-weighted sequences. The posterior chamber lies between the posterior surface of the iris and anterior surface of the vitreous.

The vitreous constitutes 2/3rd volume of the eye (4 cc) and serves as the shock absorber. Because of 98 % water content, it has longer relaxation times than most tissues but shorter than that of water.

The intraocular lens measures 9 mm diameter and 4 mm in thickness. Anterior to the lens is the aqueous humor and posterior to the lens is the vitreous humor. It is the least hydrated organ (67 %) in the body and is therefore darker on MRI than surrounding tissues.

The walls of the globe include sclera (outer layer), uvea (middle layer), and retina (inner layer). It is not possible to distinguish between these three layers on CT or MRI in normal eye. Tenon's capsule surrounds the eyeball from optic nerve to the ciliary muscle.

Imaging

Radiographic assessment of the orbits can detect two-thirds of the orbital fractures but has very limited sensitivity for

A. Singh, MD
Department of Radiology,
Massachusetts General Hospital, Harvard Medical School,
10 Museum Way, # 524, Boston, MA 02141, USA
e-mail: asingh1@partners.org

A. Singh (ed.), *Emergency Radiology*,
DOI 10.1007/978-1-4419-9592-6_19, © Springer Science+Business Media New York 2013

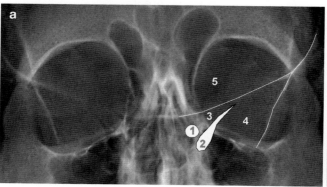

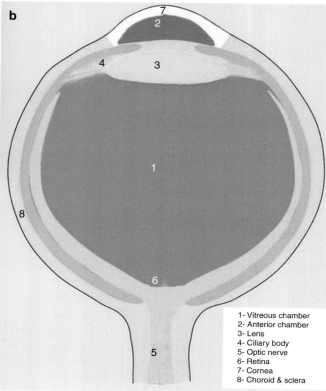

1- Vitreous chamber
2- Anterior chamber
3- Lens
4- Ciliary body
5- Optic nerve
6- Retina
7- Cornea
8- Choroid & sclera

Fig. 19.1 Normal orbital and ocular anatomy. (**a**) Plain radiograph (Water's view) demonstrates osseous anatomy. The superior orbital fissure (*2*) separates the roof from the lateral wall of the orbit. The lateral wall of the orbit is constituted by the greater wing of the sphenoid (*4*). The roof is constituted by the orbital plate of the frontal bone (*5*) and lesser wing of the sphenoid (*3*). The optic canal (*1*) is located in the roof, with in the lesser wing of the sphenoid. The floor is separated from the lateral wall by the inferior orbital fissure. (**b**) Drawing illustrates the axial anatomy of the globe. On imaging, it is not possible to distinguish sclera, choroids, and retina, unless retinal or choroidal detachment is present. The lens separates the aqueous humor from vitreous humor

soft tissue injuries. Ultrasound is contraindicated in patients where there is suspicion of globe rupture. MRI is not the primary modality in the evaluation of intraocular foreign body due to risk of damage by motion of a ferromagnetic foreign body and artifact produced by ferromagnetic foreign bodies. MRI is contraindicated if there is suspicion of metallic foreign body in the orbit.

CT is the modality of choice for traumatized eye and suspected ferromagnetic foreign body due to its wide availability in emergency departments, rapid scan time, no/minimal motion artifact, and high sensitivity in detection of foreign bodies [3].

Imaging Protocol

CT: Orbital protocol (0.625–1.25 mm slice thickness)
- Noncontrast CT
- Performed as part of the facial CT in axial plane
- Sagittal and coronal reformations performed at 1 mm interval
- Soft tissue and bone algorithm reconstructions
  MRI: Orbital protocol (3 mm slice thickness)
1. Axial and coronal T1 through orbits without fat sat
2. Coronal FSE T2 through orbits with fat sat

3. Post-gadolinium axial T1 with fat sat through orbits
4. Coronal T1 chiasm through globes with fat sat
5. Sagittal T1, axial FLAIR, axial T2, axial DWI through whole brain
6. Optional T1 axial through whole brain

Anterior Segment Injury and Lens Dislocation

Trauma accounts for more than half of the lens subluxation-dislocation. It is caused by disruption of the zonular attachments, which hold the lens in place. The lens is most commonly dislocated posteriorly, often lying in dependent vitreous humor. Spontaneous atraumatic dislocation, which is often bilateral, is associated with Marfan syndrome, homocystinuria, sulfite oxidase deficiency, hyperlysinemia, ED syndrome, aniridia, and congenital glaucoma. Most patients with lens dislocation will have a pars plana vitrectomy/lensectomy with an intraocular lens implantation.

The patients with traumatic hyphema have hemorrhage in anterior chamber, usually from tear of ciliary body and iris. Posttraumatic cataract is most often localized and not associated with significant loss of vision [4].

Imaging: Anterior chamber injuries are characterized by decrease in the depth of the anterior chamber, when compared with the normal eye. A dislocated lens is seen as high attenuation lenticular structure in the vitreous on CT, where it is generally free floating (Figs. 19.2 and 19.3). A ruptured lens capsule often results in decreased attenuation and subtle increase in the size of the lens.

Open-Globe Injury

Traumatic rupture of the globe results in loss of vitreous and posterior displacement of lens, causing deepening of the anterior chamber. Vitreal prolapse is associated with retinal detachment (RD), iridodialysis or ciliary body cleft, and contusion cataract (41 %) [5]. Globe ruptures (5 % of blunt injuries) are associated with grades III and IV hyphema.

Superior nasal limbus is the most common site of globe rupture because lower temporal quadrant is the most exposed site to trauma. The risk of trauma-induced globe ruptures is highest in eyes after cataract surgery and in females. The rupture of the globe most often occurs at the site of insertion of intraocular muscles because the sclera is thinnest at this site.

Imaging: The CT findings of globe rupture include vitreous hemorrhage, globe contour deformity, obvious loss of globe volume, absence of lens, intraocular air/foreign body, scleral discontinuity, increased depth of anterior chamber, and RD/CD (Figs. 19.4, 19.5, 19.6, 19.7, and 19.8). Flat tire sign is characterized by flattening of the posterior contour of the globe due to posterior collapse of the sclera and volume loss in the vitreous chamber.

Because of the decompression of the vitreous chamber, the lens may move back without disruption of the zonular attachments. This finding is seen as asymmetrically deep anterior chamber on CT. Discrepancy in depth of AC of 2 mm or more is abnormal. Absolute depth of AC measuring >5 mm is

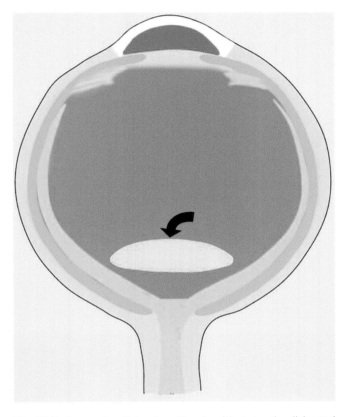

Fig. 19.2 Intraocular dislocation. Drawing illustrates the dislocated lens located posteriorly in the vitreous chamber

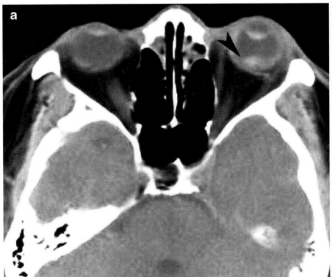

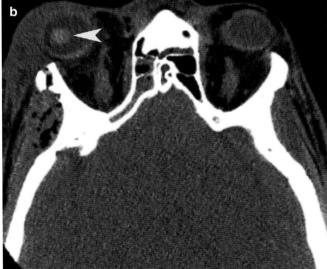

Fig. 19.3 Lens dislocation from penetrating trauma. (**a**) Axial CT shows posterior subluxation of the lens, increase in the depth of the anterior chamber, and vitreous hemorrhage (*arrowhead*). (**b**) Superior dislocation of the right lens (*arrowhead*) seen in a patient with right lateral orbital wall fracture and overlying soft tissue contusion from blunt trauma

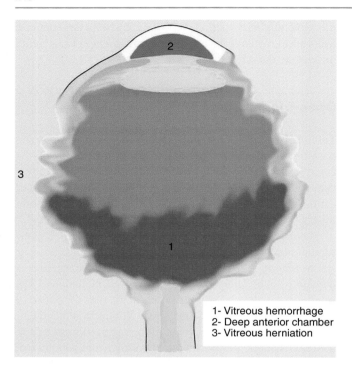

1- Vitreous hemorrhage
2- Deep anterior chamber
3- Vitreous herniation

Fig. 19.4 Ruptured globe. Drawing illustrates the imaging findings of distorted outline of the globe, increase in the depth of the anterior chamber with posterior location of the lens, and vitreous hemorrhage

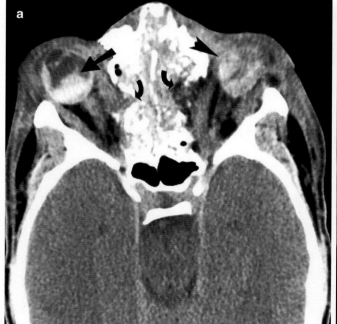

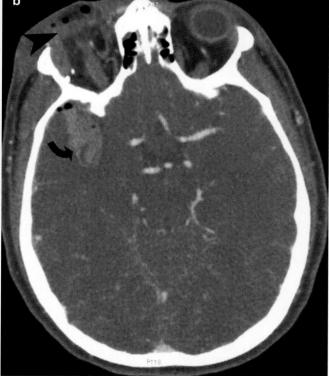

Fig. 19.5 Traumatic globe rupture. (**a**) Bilateral ruptured globes and orbital blowout fractures from wrench chain trauma. Axial CT shows bilateral open-globe injuries with vitreous hemorrhage. There is obvious distortion of the outline of the left globe (*arrowhead*). The right intraocular lens (*arrow*) is dislocated in to the vitreous chamber. There are bilateral blowout fractures involving the medial orbital walls (*curved arrows*). (**b**) Axial CT demonstrates globe rupture caused by shrapnel from a pipe bomb explosion. There is gross contour deformity and deflation of the globe (*arrowhead*). There is intracranial hemorrhage (*curved arrow*) caused by the shrapnel

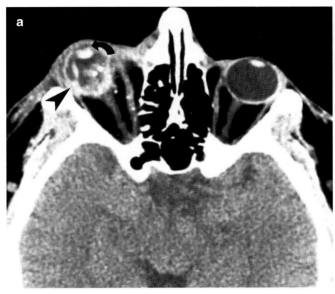

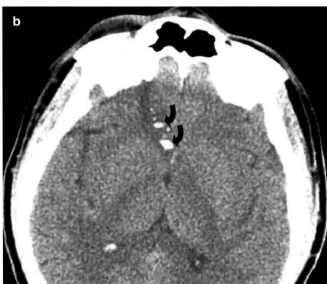

Fig. 19.6 Right globe rupture from bullet injury. (**a**) Axial CT shows increase in the depth of the anterior chamber (*curved arrow*), extensive vitreous compartment hemorrhage, and distortion in the shape of the globe (*straight arrow*). (**b**) Axial CT of the cerebral hemisphere shows the track of the bullet illustrated by bone fragments (*curved arrows*)

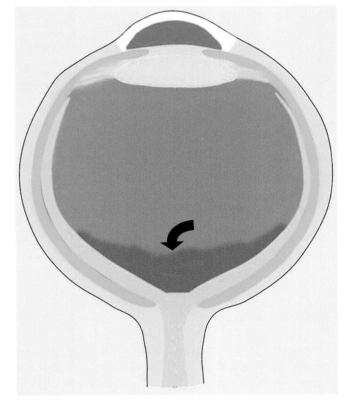

Fig. 19.7 Vitreous chamber hemorrhage. Drawing illustrates vitreous chamber hemorrhage (*curved arrow*), which can be an isolated finding or associated with globe rupture, lens dislocation, or orbital fractures

abnormal (normal AC depth = 2.5–3.5 mm). In the study by Arey et al., the sensitivity of CT to diagnose open-globe injury was 56–68 %, and the positive predictive value was 86–100 % [6].

Intraocular Foreign Body

Intraocular foreign body is often clinically overlooked, if not clinically suspected. While small nonreactive foreign bodies (gold, platinum, aluminum, and glass) can be left in the orbit, other foreign bodies made up of iron and copper must be removed due to risk of siderosis from iron and chalcosis from copper. Organic materials, such as wood, can cause abscess/chronic inflammation and therefore need to be removed.

Enucleation is usually necessary when a large foreign body enters the eye with resulting hemorrhage, lens dislocation, and vitreous loss. Intracranial injury should be excluded with imaging before performing enucleation.

Imaging: The high density of metallic foreign body is best diagnosed on CT (Figs. 19.9 and 19.10). The density of wood is highly variable, thereby resulting in lower sensitivity of CT and MRI in detection of organic foreign body (42 % vs 57 %) [7]. Wooden foreign bodies are most often of lower density and therefore can be mistaken for air. Geometric shape of air density should raise the suspicion of wooden foreign body. The sensitivity of helical CT and T1-weighted MRI sequence for the detection of intraocular glass is 57 and 11 %, respectively [8]. The sensitivity of CT for detection of more than 1.5 mm diameter glass fragment is much higher than a 0.5 mm fragment. MRI is contraindicated when a metallic foreign body is suspected.

Retinal Detachment

The retina is firmly attached anteriorly at the ora serrata and posteriorly at the optic disk. RD refers to the separation of the sensory retina from retinal pigmented epithelium. It can

Fig. 19.8 Vitreous chamber hemorrhage from blunt trauma in a 28-year-old male. Noncontrast axial CT and contrast-enhanced CT demonstrate left vitreous hemorrhage (*curved arrows*), left subdural hemorrhage (*arrowheads*)

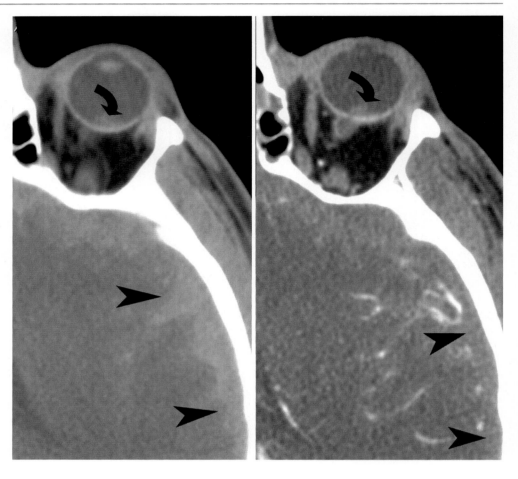

be caused by mass, vitreoretinopathy, toxocara endophthalmitis, Coat's disease, senile macular degeneration, and trauma.

Imaging: Exudative RD results in subretinal fluid rich in protein, resulting in high-density fluid on CT than seen with a rhegmatogenous RD. RD is seen on CT and MRI as a characteristic V-shaped configuration with apex at the optic disk and anterior end at the ora serrata (Figs. 19.11 and 19.12). On coronal MRI, it is seen as characteristic folding membranes converging at the optic disk.

Choroidal Detachment

CD is caused by accumulation of serous fluid or blood in potential subchoroidal space. The causes include intraocular surgery, trauma, or inflammatory disorders. Unlike RD, it does not extend to the optic disk and is restricted by anchoring effect of short posterior ciliary arteries and nerves.

Imaging: CT is the imaging modality of choice and shows focal, biconvex, lenticular mass in the ocular wall which is

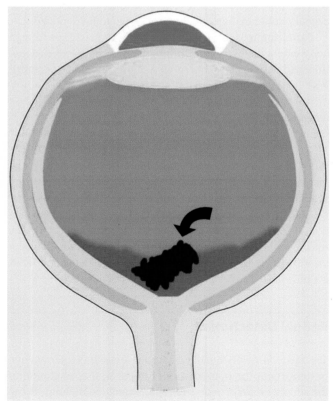

Fig. 19.9 Intraocular foreign body. Diagram illustrates an intraocular foreign body and hemorrhage in the vitreous chamber

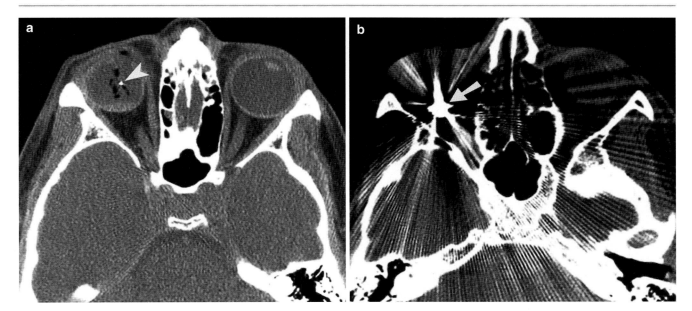

Fig. 19.10 Metallic intraocular foreign body. (**a**) Axial CT shows intraocular-dependent vitreous hemorrhage, intraocular and bullet fragment (*arrowhead*) from gunshot injury. (**b**) Axial CT at a more caudal level shows an intraconal metallic foreign body (*arrow*), producing streak artifacts at the posterior ocular wall

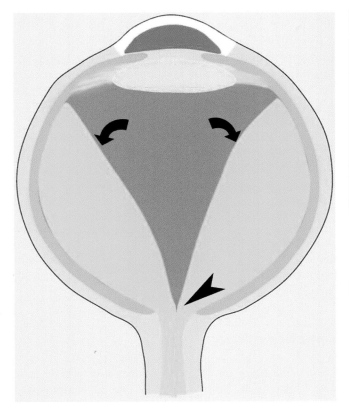

Fig. 19.11 Retinal detachment. Diagram illustrates V-shaped retinal detachment (*curved arrow*) arising posteriorly from the optic disk (*arrowhead*)

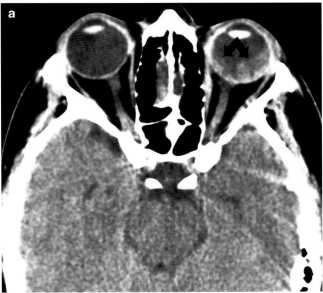

Fig. 19.12 Acute retinal detachment in a 39-year-old male. Axial CT (**a**) and axial FLAIR (**b**) sequence show retinal detachment with subretinal hemorrhage (*bifid arrow*) which is of high density on CT and hyperintense on FLAIR sequence

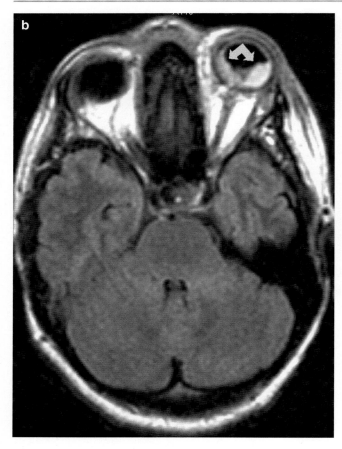

Fig. 19.12 (continued)

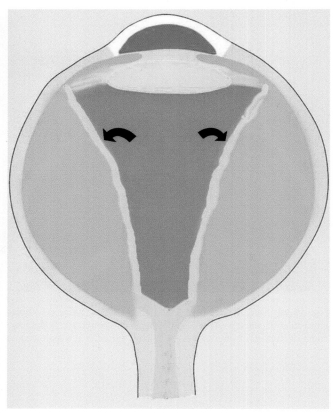

Fig. 19.13 Choroidal detachment. Diagram illustrates fluid accumulation of fluid which is confined by choroid (*curved arrows*) on the inside and sclera on the outside

posteriorly restricted by short posterior ciliary arteries and nerves (Figs. 19.13 and 19.14a).

MRI shows choroidal hematoma as a focal, well-demarcated lenticular mass in the wall of the eyeball (Fig. 19.14b). Within the first 48 h, the hematoma is isointense to slightly hypointense to the vitreous body on T1-weighted images. After 5 days choroidal hematoma appears hyperintense on T1-weighted images. Choroidal hematoma usually increases in signal intensity on T1- as well as T2-weighted images and becomes hyperintense by the second week on all MRI sequences.

Associated Injuries

The injuries associated with ocular trauma include retrobulbar hemorrhage, optic nerve injury, orbital wall fractures, herniation of intraorbital contents through the orbital fracture, muscle entrapment/contusion, intraorbital emphysema, intracranial injuries, and maxillofacial fractures (Figs. 19.15, 19.16, 19.17, and 19.18). Orbital floor is the most common and orbital roof is the least common site for orbital wall fracture. Type 2 and 3 Le Fort fractures involve the orbital walls.

Le Fort 2 fracture is a pyramidal-shaped fracture of the maxilla with superior extension to the inferior orbital rim and medial orbital wall. Le Fort 3 fracture is called craniofacial dissociation and involves the orbital floor, medial wall, as well as the lateral wall.

Optic Nerve Injury

Optic nerve injury can be due to compression from an optic canal fracture or more commonly due to compromised vascular supply to the optic nerve. Injury to the optic nerve can be seen as hyperintensity of the optic nerve on T2-weighted images (Fig. 19.19).

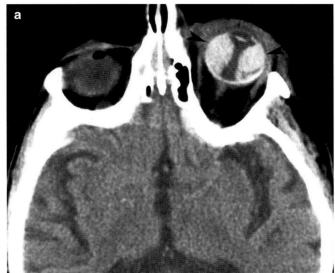

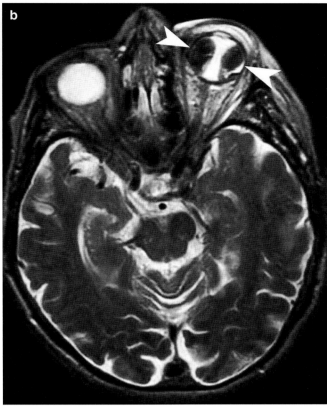

Fig. 19.14 Choroidal detachment from blunt trauma in a 92-year-old female. (**a**) Axial CT shows choroidal detachment (*arrow heads*) with high-density blood in the subchoroidal space. There is preseptal soft tissue contusion extending lateral to the left lateral orbital wall. (**b**) T2-weighted MRI sequence demonstrates acute choroidal detachment with hypointense subchoroidal fluid (*arrowheads*), indicating the presence of acute blood products

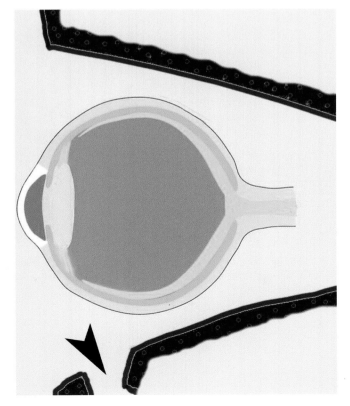

Fig. 19.15 Orbital blowout fracture. Diagram illustrates orbital floor fracture (*curved arrowhead*) which is the most common orbital wall to fracture from blunt force causing increase in the intraorbital pressure

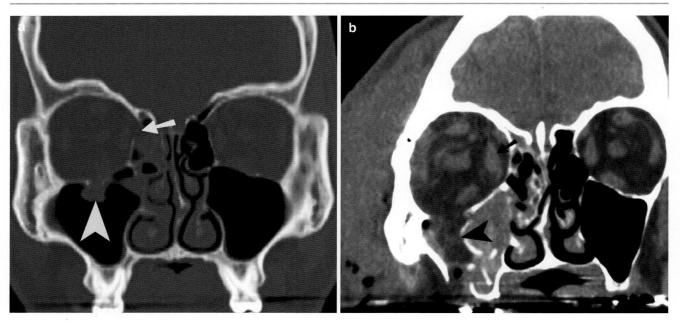

Fig. 19.16 Orbital blowout fracture. (**a**) Coronal CT reconstruction shows fracture of the medial (*arrow*) and inferior orbital wall. There is herniation (*arrowhead*) of intraorbital fat into the right maxillary sinus. (**b**) Coronal CT reconstruction in a different patient demonstrates the asymmetric right medial rectus muscle thickening (*arrow*). There is herniation of intraorbital fat (*arrowhead*) through the inferior orbital wall fracture

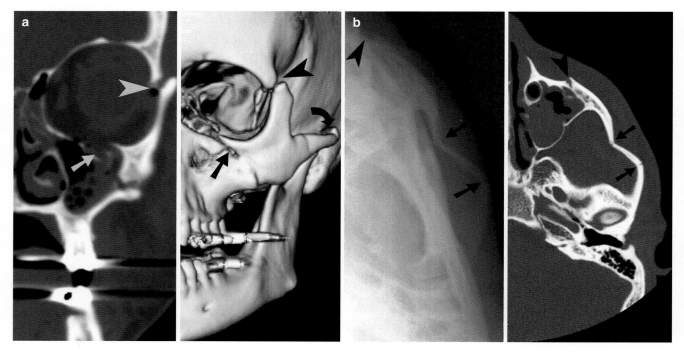

Fig. 19.17 Orbital wall fractures. (**a**) Coronal CT reformation and 3D reconstruction in a patient show zygomaticomaxillary fracture involving the lateral orbital rim (*arrowhead*), zygomatic arch (*curved arrow*), and inferior orbital rim (*straight arrow*). (**b**) Base of skull radiograph and axial CT demonstrates zygomaticomaxillary fracture involving the zygomatic arch (*straight arrows*) and orbital floor (*arrowhead*)

Fig. 19.18 Intraconal and extraconal hemorrhage after blunt trauma. (**a**) Axial and coronal CT shows right proptosis secondary to intraconal hemorrhage (*arrowheads*). There is scleral thickening at the optic disk, secondary to scleral contusion. (**b**) Axial CT in a patient who was punched in the left eye shows left retrobulbar hemorrhage leading to proptosis. (**c**) Coronal CT reconstruction in a patient who fell down an elevator shaft demonstrates extraconal hemorrhage (*arrowhead*) along the superior orbital wall. There is also inferior orbital wall fracture (*arrow*) with hemorrhage in the right maxillary sinus

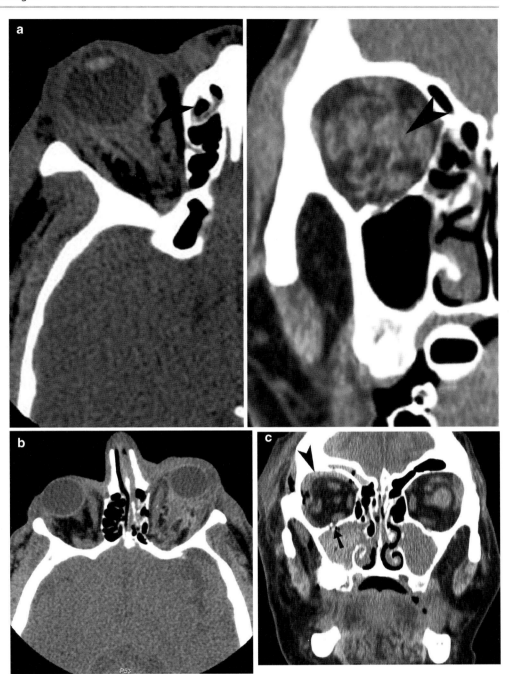

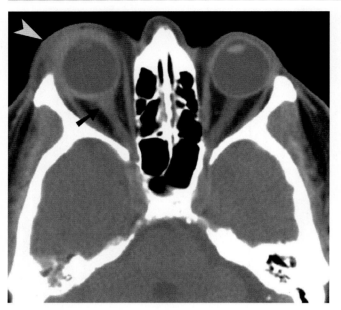

Fig. 19.19 Optic nerve contusion. Axial CT shows thickening and increased density (*arrow*) of the right optic nerve with adjacent scleral thickening. There is also right preseptal contusion (*arrowhead*) caused by blunt trauma

Carotid Cavernous Fistula

It is most commonly caused by posttraumatic tear in the internal carotid artery with communication with the cavernous sinus. Because of the reversal of flow in the venous tributaries of the cavernous sinus, there is prominence of the superior ophthalmic vein on CT imaging. The diagnosis can be confirmed on CT angiogram or conventional angiogram (Fig. 19.20).

Orbital Infections

Orbital infections are classified as preseptal (periorbital) or postseptal (orbital), depending on their location in relation to orbital septum. The orbital septum is a periosteal reflection off the bony margin of the orbit. Based on CT, it is not possible to distinguish preseptal edema from periorbital cellulitis. Periorbital cellulitis is treated less aggressively, compared to postseptal infection, with antibiotics therapy.

The postseptal infections can be intraconic, extraconic (between periosteum and recti muscles), and subperiosteal (between orbital wall and periosteum). The postseptal infections are more serious as they may lead to cavernous sinus thrombosis, brain abscess, and meningitis.

Orbital Subperiosteal Abscess

Orbital subperiosteal abscess is most often caused by maxillary, ethmoidal, or frontal sinusitis due to close anatomic relationship with the orbit. Spread of the infection can cause loss of vision, endophthalmitis, cavernous sinus thrombosis, brain abscess, and meningitis.

The CT findings include opacification of the ethmoidal and maxillary sinuses with rim-enhancing, lenticular-shaped subperiosteal abscess, most commonly along the medial orbital wall (Fig. 19.21). Occasionally, air is present within the subperiosteal abscess. Unlike ethmoidal sinusitis, which causes subperiosteal abscess along the medial orbital wall, frontal sinusitis most often causes the subperiosteal abscess to be along the orbital roof.

Optic Neuritis

Optic neuritis refers to acute inflammatory or demyelinating disorder of the optic nerve. Although majority of the cases are idiopathic, some cases are due to multiple sclerosis. Majority of the patients are in the 15–50-year age group and have rapid progression of visual loss within 2 weeks. Although the diagnosis is typically made on clinical examination, MRI imaging is used when there are atypical clinical features.

The MRI features include T2 hyperintensity with enlarged optic nerve. It frequently enhances on postcontrast T1-weighted imaging (Fig. 19.22). There may be associated white matter abnormalities on T2-weighted sequence which can predict the subsequent development of multiple sclerosis. The 5-year risk of developing subsequent multiple sclerosis is 51 % in patients with three or more lesions and 16 % in patients without white matter abnormalities [9].

Teaching Points

1. CT is the imaging modality of choice in the detection of intraocular foreign bodies, globe rupture, lens dislocation, intra/extraconal injury, and associated orbital/facial injuries.
2. The role of MRI is more limited in the evaluation of acute ocular trauma; however, it can be utilized when a ferromagnetic foreign body is excluded by radiography or CT imaging.
3. Ultrasound is contraindicated when globe rupture is suspected.

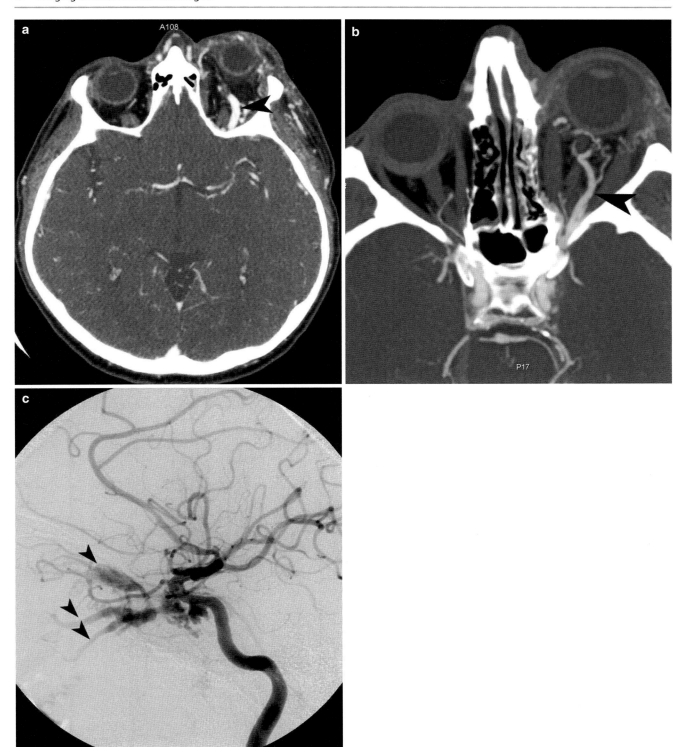

Fig. 19.20 Posttraumatic carotid cavernous fistula. (**a, b**) Contrast-enhanced CT demonstrates prominence of the left superior ophthalmic vein (*arrowhead*) secondary to carotid cavernous fistula. (**c**) Left internal carotid angiogram demonstrates communication with the cavernous sinus as well as its venous tributaries

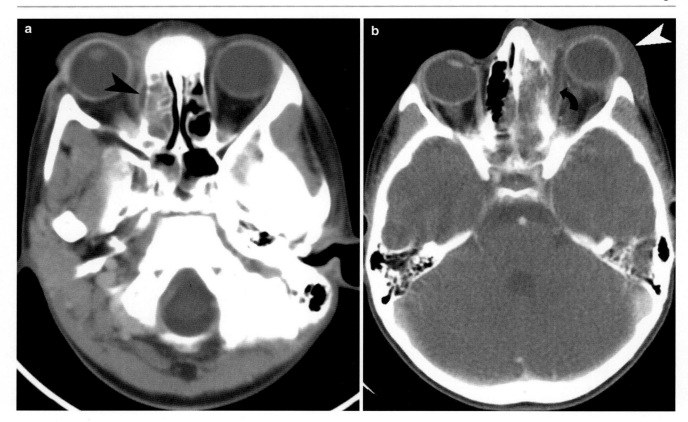

Fig. 19.21 Orbital abscess. (**a**) Contrast-enhanced CT demonstrates orbital subperiosteal abscess (*arrowhead*) along the right medial orbital wall, secondary to ethmoidal sinusitis. (**b**) Contrast-enhanced CT shows left ethmoidal sinusitis with abscess (*curved arrow*) formation along left medial orbital wall, leading to proptosis. The abscess has extended beyond the subperiosteal confines to involve extraconic compartment medial to the medial rectus. There is also extension of inflammation anteriorly to cause periorbital cellulitis (*arrowhead*)

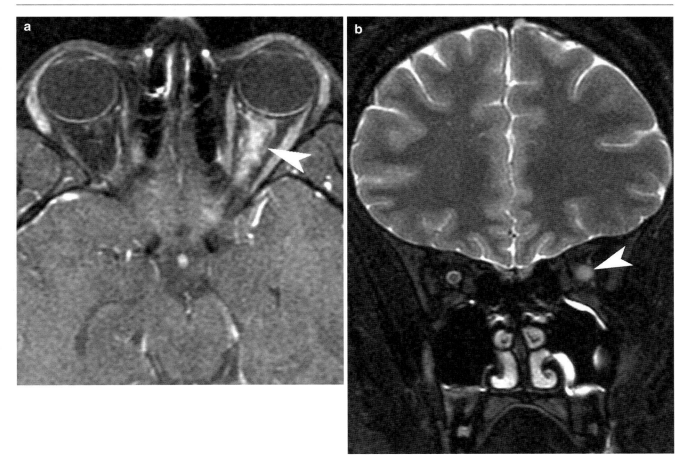

Fig. 19.22 Optic neuritis. Axial post-gadolinium T1-weighted (**a**) and coronal T2-weighted (**b**) sequence demonstrate thickening and enhancement of the left optic nerve (*arrowhead*)

References

1. Maltzman BA, Pruzon H, Mund ML. A survey of ocular trauma. Surv Ophthalmol. 1976;21(3):285–90.
2. Schrader WF. Epidemiology of open globe eye injuries: analysis of 1026 cases in 18 years. Klin Monbl Augenheilkd. 2004;221(8): 629–35.
3. Lakits A, Prokesch R, Scholda C, Bankier A. Orbital helically computed tomography in the diagnosis and management of eye trauma. Ophthalmology. 1999;106(12):2330–5.
4. Canavan YM, Archer DB. Anterior segment consequences of blunt ocular injury. Br J Ophthalmol. 1982;66(9):549–55.
5. Viestenz A, Kuchle M. Blunt ocular trauma. Part II. Blunt posterior segment trauma. Ophthalmology. 2005;102(1):89–99; quiz 100–1.
6. Arey ML, Mootha VV, Whittemore AR, Chason DP, Blomquist PH. Computed tomography in the diagnosis of occult open-globe injuries. Ophthalmology. 2007;114:1448–52.
7. Nasr AM, Haik BG, Fleming JC, Al-Hussain HM, Karcioglu ZA. Penetrating orbital injury with organic foreign bodies. Ophthalmology. 1999;106(3):523–32.
8. Gor DM, Kirsch CF, Leen J, Turbin R, Von Hagen S. Radiologic differentiation of intraocular glass: evaluation of imaging techniques, glass types, size, and effect of intraocular hemorrhage. AJR Am J Roentgenol. 2001;177(5):1199–203.
9. Optic Neuritis Study Group. Visual function 5 years after optic neuritis: experience of the Optic Neuritis Treatment Trial. The Optic Neuritis Study Group. Arch Ophthalmol. 1997;115(12): 1545–52.

Joshua Leeman, Jonathan E. Leeman,
and Ajay Singh

Introduction

A vast number of traumatic injuries can involve the upper extremity. In this chapter, the specific injuries seen most commonly in a busy emergency department will be described, with emphasis on the mechanism of injury, radiographic appearance, and complications. Radiographic appearances of injuries will be emphasized as the radiograph is typically the initial imaging tool utilized in the emergency setting, and frequently the diagnosis can be made using radiography alone.

Scapulothoracic Dissociation

Scapulothoracic dissociation is a rare but devastating and potentially life-threatening injury. It most commonly results from severe traction of the shoulder girdle in the case of a motorcyclist who holds on to the handlebars while being thrown from the vehicle. It is usually accompanied by avulsion of the brachial plexus and rupture of the subclavian or axillary artery.

Imaging

On frontal radiograph there is lateral displacement of the scapula, as indicated by wide separation between the medial edge of the scapula and the spinous processes. The injury is often accompanied by other osseous injuries including

J. Leeman, MD • J.E. Leeman, MD
Department of Radiology, Shady Side Hospital,
Pittsburgh, PA, USA

A. Singh, MD(✉)
Department of Radiology, Massachusetts General Hospital,
Harvard Medical School,
10 Museum Way, # 524, Boston, MA 02141, USA
e-mail: asingh1@partners.org

acromioclavicular separation, sternoclavicular dislocation, and distracted fracture of the clavicle. Adjacent soft tissue masses representing hematomas suggest severe injury to vascular structures [1].

As it is the result of severe trauma, scapulothoracic dissociation is often overlooked initially because of concomitant hemodynamic shock or head injuries. Brachial plexus avulsion can result in flail arm which usually requires above-the-elbow amputation.

Clavicle Fracture

Clavicle fractures represent 50 % of fractures involving the shoulder girdle [2]. They are usually the result of a direct fall on the shoulder during athletic activity or falling on an outstretched hand. Fractures of the clavicle are common in the pediatric population and can also result from anterior pressure on the shoulder during childbirth.

Imaging

The majority of fractures occur in the middle third of the clavicle and are easily detectable on radiography. Because of the unopposed action of the sternocleidomastoid muscle, there is often superomedial displacement of the medial segment of the clavicle. The inferior displacement of the lateral clavicle fragment results from the weight of the upper extremity (Fig. 20.1).

Complications

Clavicle fracture can be associated with injury to the subclavian artery, subclavian vein, or brachial plexus. There may be associated sternoclavicular or acromioclavicular subluxation, as well as pneumothorax. Malunion and nonunion can lead to shortening of the shoulder girdle and chronic pain [3].

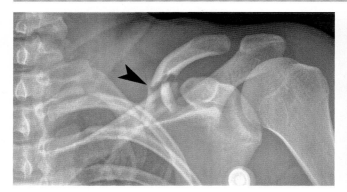

Fig. 20.1 Clavicle fracture. AP view of the clavicle shows a comminuted fracture at the distal third of the clavicle (*arrowhead*)

Sternoclavicular Dislocation

Sternoclavicular dislocation accounts for only 2–3 % of shoulder girdle dislocations and can occur after indirect blunt trauma to the shoulder [4]. The dislocation allows for free rotation of the head of the clavicle with the intact costoclavicular ligament serving as a fulcrum. Anterior dislocation from an anterolateral blow is significantly more common than posterior dislocation from a posterolateral blow.

Imaging

Sternoclavicular dislocation can result in asymmetry of the clavicular heads. Compared to plain radiography, CT can better distinguish anterior from posterior dislocation. It is also able to detect associated injury to mediastinal structures such as great vessels, recurrent laryngeal nerve, trachea, and esophagus, in patients with posterior dislocation (Fig. 20.2).

Acromioclavicular Dislocation

Acromioclavicular dislocation is a common injury usually resulting from direct trauma in contact sports, such as football or hockey. Dislocation can also result from a fall on an outstretched hand.

AP radiographs with a 10–15° cephalic tilt (Zanca view) are recommended for assessment of the acromioclavicular region. Dislocations are classified into the following types:

Type 1: Isolated sprain of the acromioclavicular ligament (AC). Plain films are normal aside from soft tissue swelling.

Type 2: Subluxation with rupture of the AC ligament and sprain of the coracoclavicular ligament (CC). The distal clavicle will typically be situated less than 5 mm superiorly to the acromion.

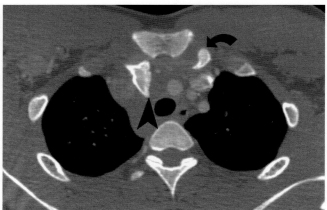

Fig. 20.2 Posterior dislocation of clavicle. Axial CT image depicts posterior dislocation of the right clavicle head (*arrowhead*) which is now situated within the superior mediastinum. The left sternoclavicular articulation (*curved arrow*) is normal

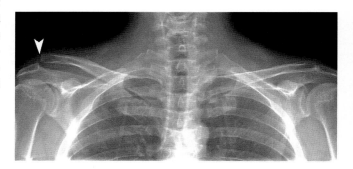

Fig. 20.3 Acromioclavicular dislocation. AP view shows a type III acromioclavicular injury with elevation of the acromion more 5 mm from its normal position (*arrowhead*). This degree of displacement indicates rupture of both CC and AC ligaments

Type 3: Complete rupture of AC and CC ligaments with superior migration of the clavicle greater than 5 mm above the acromion (Fig. 20.3). Coracoid fracture and injuries to the insertion of the trapezius or deltoid muscles can occur as a result of type 3 dislocations.

Glenohumeral Joint Dislocation

Because of its inherent instability, the glenohumeral joint is the most commonly dislocated joint in the body. Anterior dislocation is far more common than posterior and often results from an anterior blow to an abducted arm and less frequently from a direct injury to the shoulder. Posterior dislocation may be a consequence of electric shock or seizure and can therefore be bilateral. Inferior glenohumeral dislocation, known as luxatio erecta, results from hyperabduction of the arm and is suspected in a patient with an abducted arm, with the wrist resting on the head. Superior dislocation from an upward blow on an adducted arm represents the rarest type and is almost always associated with rotator cuff tear.

Imaging

In the setting of anterior glenohumeral dislocation, the AP radiograph will show the humeral head situated medial and inferior with respect to the glenoid, such that it lies directly inferior to the coracoid process (Fig. 20.4a). If posteriorly dislocated, the AP view will depict an increased distance between the humeral head and the glenoid and loss of the normal overlap of the humeral head and glenoid. However, it should be noted that a large effusion may have an identical appearance. The axillary projection (45° posterior oblique with 45° of inferior angulation) and scapular Y projection (60° anterior oblique) afford an excellent appraisal of the congruence of the glenohumeral joint (Fig. 20.4b). These latter

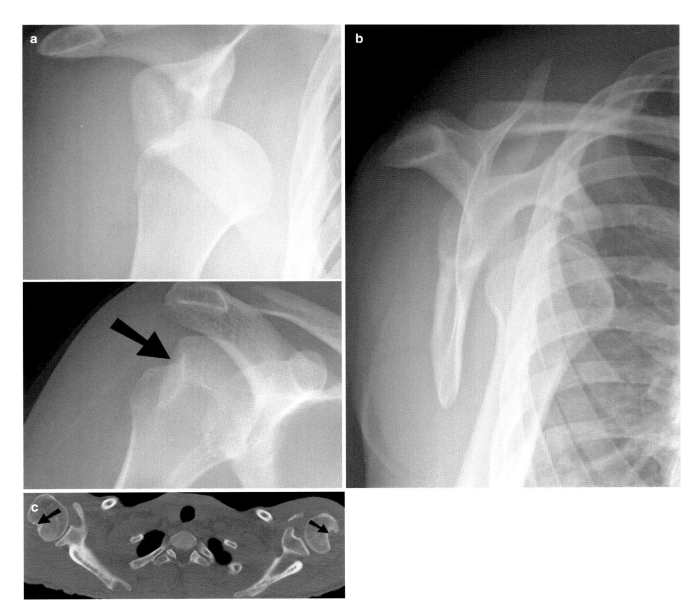

Fig. 20.4 A. Glenohumeral dislocation. (**a**) AP view of the shoulder illustrates the typical appearance of anterior glenohumeral dislocation with the humeral head situated in a subcoracoid position (*top*). A postreduction AP view shows a wedge-shaped defect at the posterolateral aspect of the humeral head typical of a Hill-Sachs lesion (*arrow*). (**b**) Scapular Y view clearly demonstrates anterior dislocation of the humeral head which now lies under the coracoid process. (**c**) Axial CT shows wedge-shaped Hill-Sachs deformities on the posterolateral aspects of both humeral heads (*arrows*) after bilateral anterior dislocations. (**d**) MIP reconstruction of contrast-enhanced CT shows abrupt occlusion of the axillary artery (*arrowhead*) caused by anterior glenohumeral dislocation

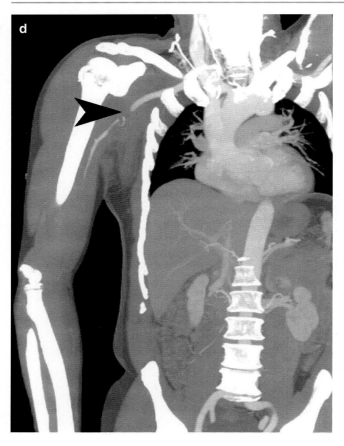

Fig. 20.4 (continued)

views are often best for distinguishing between an anterior and posterior dislocation when the AP view is confusing.

Anteroinferior dislocation, or subcoracoid dislocation, can result in fracture of the posterolateral aspect of the humeral head (Hill-Sachs lesion), best seen as a linear or wedge-shaped defect that is evident on radiography (Fig. 20.4c). As the humeral head impacts against the glenoid rim, fracture of the anteroinferior glenoid (Bankart lesion) with avulsion of the labroligamentous complex can also occur. With nonoperative treatment, anterior dislocations will recur in approximately 50 % of cases [5].

Conversely, a reverse Bankart lesion, or posteroinferior fracture of the glenoid rim, can result from posterior dislocation. In evaluation of glenohumeral dislocation, CT is most appropriate for identifying bony fragments or associated vascular injury, while MRI can more clearly identify soft tissue damage (Fig. 20.4d).

Scapular Fracture

An isolated fracture of the scapula is uncommon and is usually the consequence of direct blunt trauma. It is usually accompanied by tenderness, fracture crepitus, and an adducted upper extremity.

Imaging

Fractures of the scapular body can be horizontal, vertical, or comminuted. CT is optimal for delineation of these fractures and identification of associated fractures.

Since scapular fractures are often accompanied by other injuries, they are frequently missed on AP chest radiographs as the associated injuries are either more clinically urgent (lung contusion, pneumothorax, widened mediastinum) or more obvious (clavicle and rib fractures).

Proximal Humerus Fractures

A fracture of the proximal humerus represents a common injury in the elderly population, most often occurring after a fall on an outstretched hand. Alternatively, a direct blow to the lateral shoulder can cause a head-splitting fracture by forcing the humeral head directly into the glenoid fossa. Most commonly, proximal humeral fractures occur at the surgical neck.

Imaging

The Neer classification system describes the severity of proximal humerus fractures according to the displacement of the four bone segments (greater tuberosity, lesser tuberosity, head, and surgical neck) [6]. Displacement is defined as greater than 1 cm or greater than 45° of separation from the anatomic position of the bone fragment. The majority of fractures are one-part fractures that are not associated with significant displacement of any segments.

Since the anterior circumflex humeral artery is closely associated with the surgical neck of the humerus, fractures may compromise the blood supply to the humeral head and result in avascular necrosis. Other complications of displaced fractures include rotator cuff tear and nonunion.

Supracondylar Fractures

Pediatric supracondylar fractures of the humerus are most frequently caused by axial loading on the elbow from a fall on an outstretched hand. Low impact falls can also result in supracondylar fractures in osteoporotic elderly patients.

Imaging

The radiographic findings include an elevated anterior or posterior fat pad, caused by hemarthrosis. A posterior fat pad sign may represent the sole finding in a patient with radiographically occult fracture [7]. Anterior displacement

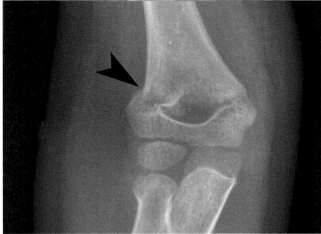

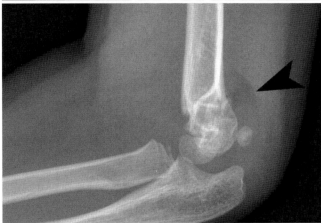

Fig. 20.5 Supracondylar fracture. AP projection of the elbow depicts a focal cortical step-off of the supracondylar humerus (*arrowhead*), indicative of supracondylar fracture (*top*). A lateral projection of the elbow shows the elevated posterior fat pad (*arrowhead*) which normally should not be seen and indicates an effusion. Also, the anterior humeral line passes through the anterior margin of the capitellum

of the anterior humeral line which ordinarily transects the middle third of the capitellum is also a common finding (Fig. 20.5).

Supracondylar fractures are traditionally classified by the Gartland system: class I is a non-displaced fracture; class II fractures have anterior cortical disruption; and class III fractures have both anterior and posterior disruption [8].

Radial Head Fractures

Radial head fractures are usually the result of axial loading from a fall on an outstretched hand where the radial head is forced into the capitellum. Less commonly, it occurs secondary to posterior elbow dislocation. Fractures are classified into four types: type I is non-displaced, type II is a displaced marginal fracture, type III fracture is comminuted, and type IV fracture is associated with elbow dislocation.

Imaging

On radiography, the fracture line may be subtle or radiographically occult. AP, lateral, and radiocapitellar views (angled 45° cephalad) may be obtained. Lateral radiographs may reveal or can reveal anterior and posterior fat pad signs which indicate hemarthrosis and are suggestive of an underlying radial head fracture. The radial head should be aligned with the capitellum in all views and any disruption of the radiocapitellar line indicates radial head dislocation.

Radial head fractures can be associated with elbow dislocation and fractures of the capitellum or coronoid process. Avulsion of the medial epicondyle may also result from excessive, valgus stress.

Medial and Lateral Condyle Fractures

Fractures of the humeral condyles represent a small fraction of elbow injuries with lateral fractures being more common than medial. Fractures of the condyles in the pediatric population are often Salter-Harris type IV fractures with involvement of epiphysis, physis, and metaphysis. Either condyle may be fractured as a result of a direct force applied to the elbow at an angle during flexion.

Radiographic findings may be subtle in the immature elbow, particularly distinguishing between condylar fractures and epicondylar fractures, which are extra-articular. Comparison with the contralateral extremity anatomy may be valuable. Stress views may be helpful with the application of valgus or varus forces under anesthesia. MRI, arthrography, or oblique radiographic views may also reveal slight displacement [9].

Associated injuries include elbow dislocation or associated fracture of the radial head. Additionally, fracture nonunion, valgus deformity, or ulnar neuritis can complicate recovery [10].

Medial Epicondyle Avulsion

Avulsion of the medial epicondyle of the humerus is a common sports-related injury in adolescents. It is the result of extreme valgus force on the apophysis secondary to contraction of the forearm flexors during pitching or arm wrestling.

If avulsion involves a bony fragment, it may be apparent on AP radiography. If bone is not fractured, then MRI or ultrasound is essential to assess for soft tissue injury.

Because of its close association with the medial epicondyle, damage to the ulnar nerve may occur.

Elbow Dislocation

Elbow dislocation is almost always caused by a fall on an outstretched hand triggering a posterior dislocation. Injury

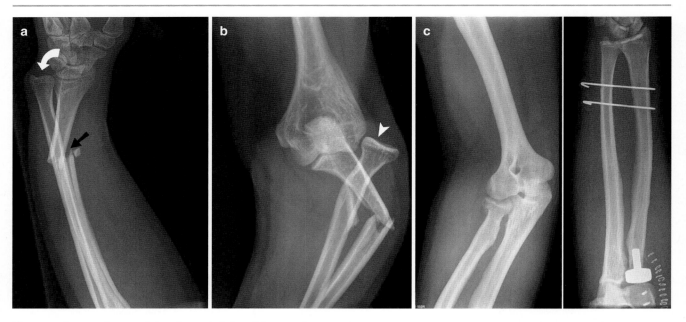

Fig. 20.6 Forearm fracture dislocations. (**a**) Galeazzi fracture dislocation: Lateral view of the forearm depicts a fracture of the shaft of the radius (*straight arrow*) with associated disruption at the distal radioulnar joint (*curved arrow*). (**b**) Montaggia fracture dislocation: Radiograph demonstrates fracture of the proximal ulnar shaft with dislocation of the radial head (*arrowhead*). (**c**) AP view of the elbow (*left*) shows a subtle non-displaced radial head fracture as a component of the Essex-Lopresti complex. After surgical repair, a radial head prosthesis is in place and there is normal alignment at the distal radioulnar joint with K-wire fixation (*right*)

progresses in three stages: Stage 1 is associated with posterolateral ulnar subluxation with disruption of the lateral ulnar collateral ligament. A stage 2 injury is characterized by perching of the coronoid process inferior to the trochlea. When the coronoid rests posterior to the trochlea, the injury is classified as stage 3.

Ligamentous disruption can be best visualized on T2-weighted MR imaging and reveals complete tear of the lateral ulnar collateral ligament. The other findings may include disruption of the radial collateral ligament as well as injury to the brachialis muscle or tendon.

Complex dislocations may be associated with fractures (radial head, radial neck, coronoid process, or capitellum) or neurovascular injury (brachial artery or ulnar nerve). Late complications include myositis ossificans, leading to limitation of range of motion of the elbow.

Forearm Fracture Dislocations

Galeazzi fracture dislocation involves fracture through the midshaft of the radius with associated subluxation or dislocation of the distal radioulnar joint (Fig. 20.6a). In an adult, a radial fracture is almost always accompanied by injury to the distal radioulnar joint. The Galeazzi fracture dislocation is uncommon in children, with only approximately 5 % of pediatric radial shaft fractures accompanied by disruption at the distal radioulnar joint [9].

Monteggia fracture dislocation is defined as fracture of the ulnar diaphysis with dislocation of the radial head (Fig. 20.6b). It most commonly involves a proximal ulnar fracture with anterior apex angulation and anterior radial head dislocation. As a rule, an angulated fracture of the radius or ulna is seen with fracture or dislocation of the other bone in the forearm. The combination of a fracture of the radial head and dislocation at the distal radioulnar joint is known as the Essex-Lopresti complex (Fig. 20.6c). A nightstick fracture is defined as an isolated fracture of the ulna, often in the distal shaft.

Distal Radius Fractures

The majority of forearm fractures are at the distal radius and typically occur from a fall on an outstretched hand in pronation and dorsiflexion (Figs. 20.7 and 20.8). The radial fracture is most commonly extra-articular and transversely oriented.

The quadrator pronatus sign suggests a distal radius fracture that may be otherwise radioccult. This sign is identified on lateral radiographs as anterior displacement, bowing, or obliteration of the quadrator pronatus fat stripe which parallels the quadrator pronatus muscle and represents accumulation of fluid, usually blood, within the pronator quadratus muscle (Fig. 20.7a).

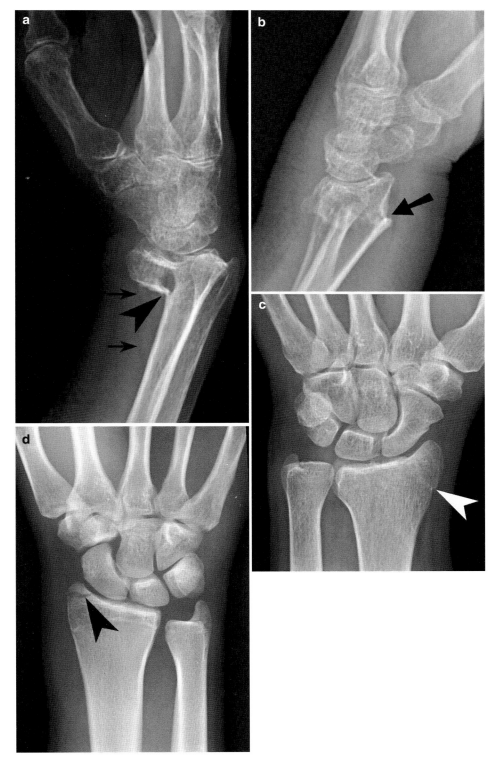

Fig. 20.7 Distal radius fractures. (**a**) Pronator quadratus sign: The radiolucent stripe of fat (*arrows*) along the anterior border of the pronator quadratus is bowed anteriorly because of edema/hemorrhage in the pronator quadratus muscle, secondary to the distal radial fracture (*arrowhead*). (**b**) Colles' fracture: Lateral view of the distal radius demonstrates a transversely oriented fracture (*arrow*) of the distal radius with dorsal displacement of the distal fragment. (**c, d**) Chauffeur's fracture: AP view of the wrist joint in two different patients demonstrates acute fractures of the radial styloid process (*arrowheads*). (**e**) Reverse Bartons fracture: There is intra-articular fracture of the distal radius (*arrowhead*) through the volar aspect of the articular surface. Compared to Barton's fracture which is intra-articular fracture through the dorsal rim of the distal radius

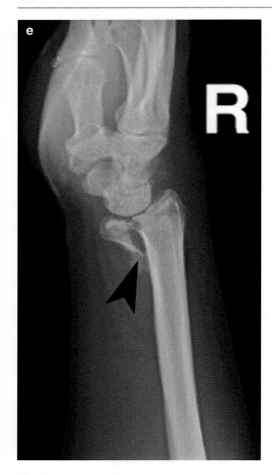

Fig. 20.7 (continued)

Colles' Fracture

It involves dorsal impaction and angulation of the distal radius fracture fragment, leading to the "dinner fork" deformity (Fig. 20.7b). Smith fracture or reverse Colles' fracture is characterized by volar impaction, displacement, and angulation of the distal radial fracture fragment.

Chauffeur's Fracture

It is an intra-articular fracture of the radial styloid due to avulsion of radiocarpal ligament and is also known as "Hutchinson" fracture (Fig. 20.7c, d).

Barton's Fracture

It refers to an intra-articular fracture involving the dorsal aspect of the distal radius and may be accompanied by fracture of the radial styloid (Fig. 20.7e).

Torus (buckle) fracture (Fig. 20.8a) of the distal radius is the most common fracture of distal forearm in children. It is a greenstick fracture where the cortex buckles on the compressed side and is intact on the opposite side.

Salter-Harris type 1 fracture (Fig. 20.8b) of distal radius occurs due to fall on outstretched hand and occurs in first decade of life. The hyperextension and supination cause dorsal displacement of the distal epiphyseal center. It is often associated with fracture of distal radius (50 %). After healing, abnormalities in the growth of the radius are uncommon.

Treatment is based on reestablishing normal radius length, with appropriate radial volar tilt and congruence at the radiocarpal and distal radioulnar joint. Acute carpal tunnel syndrome with median nerve palsy is a known complication of Colles' fracture, and carpal tunnel syndrome has been reported to develop even many years after the initial injury [10].

Carpal Fractures

Scaphoid fracture is the most common isolated carpal bone fracture, representing approximately 75 % of carpal bone fractures [11–13]. Fall onto a dorsiflexed wrist is the usual mechanism and results in impingement of the scaphoid by the radial styloid with tensile loading of the scaphoid waist. Thus, 70 % of fractures occur through the scaphoid waist [11].

Triquetral fractures make up the second most common carpal fracture and result from severe dorsiflexion with ulnar deviation of the wrist. The mechanism of injury involves impaction of the triquetrum against the ulnar styloid with avulsion of a bone fragment from the dorsal triquetral surface.

Hamate bone fractures are less common and result from a direct blow to the ulnar aspect of the wrist when an individual is holding an object such as a golf club or baseball bat. Fractures can occur through the base of the hamate hook or through the body of the hamate.

Fractures of the remaining carpal bones including the capitate, lunate, and pisiform are less common and may be seen following a direct forceful blow to the wrist in the setting of other fracture dislocations.

Imaging

In the setting of acute scaphoid fracture, initial radiographs may be normal. A dedicated scaphoid view may be helpful and involves positioning the wrist in maximal ulnar deviation with the x-ray beam directed in an anteroposterior direction with approximately 15° of craniocaudal angulation. Alternatively, a repeat radiograph can be obtained 7–10 days later and may show bone resorption at the fracture site (Fig. 20.9a, b). CT or MRI may be more sensitive for depiction of the acute fracture.

Fig. 20.8 Distal radial fractures. (a) Buckle fracture: AP view of the wrist demonstrates a greenstick buckle fracture (*arrowhead*) of the distal radial mataphyses. (b) Salter-Harris type 1 fracture: Radiograph of the wrist demonstrates dorsal displacement of the distal radial epiphyseal center due to Salter-Harris type 1 injury through the physis (*arrowhead*)

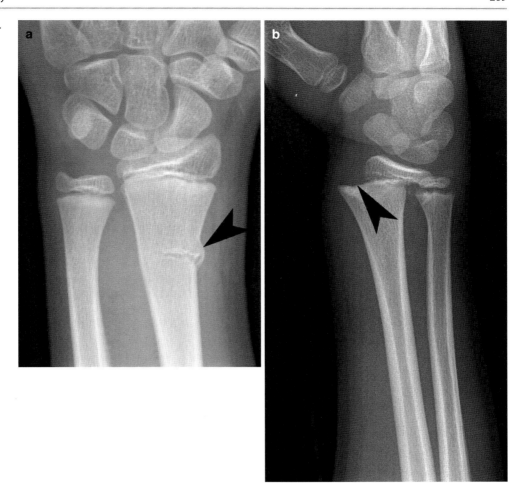

Triquetral fractures are typically occult on frontal radiographs, but a lateral projection may show a bone chip dorsal to the proximal carpal row with associated soft tissue swelling (Fig. 20.9c, d). A hamate hook fracture may be suggested on a frontal radiograph by indistinctness or lack of the normally seen "eye" of the hamate hook. Alternatively, a carpal tunnel view or CT with axial reconstruction may show this fracture to better advantage.

Since the blood supply of the scaphoid is via a single artery passing from the distal pole to feed the proximal pole, a fracture through the scaphoid waist predisposes to avascular necrosis (AVN). Although the initial radiograph may be normal, later they show changes of AVN, such as cystic change, sclerosis, cortical collapse, and fragmentation. MRI may initially show heterogeneous areas of low signal on T1- and T2-weighted sequences, indicative of areas of sclerosis (Fig. 20.9b). Homogenous gadolinium enhancement indicates an intact blood supply, whereas lack of enhancement confirms irreversible necrosis.

Nonunion of a scaphoid fracture may result from a delay in diagnosis or fixation. Ultimately, a fibrous union may form

between the two scaphoid poles with low signal material filling the fracture gap on T1- and T2-weighted imaging. Scaphoid nonunion with advanced collapse (SNAC wrist) represents end-stage nonunion and involves carpal collapse with proximal migration of the capitate between the two scaphoid poles with dorsal angulation of the lunate.

Hamate fractures are often not visualized on plain radiography. Carpal tunnel view, 20° supine oblique view, and reverse oblique views can be used to increase sensitivity of plain radiography in demonstrating hamate fractures. Statistically, the most common fracture of hamate involves the hook and can be best seen on carpal tunnel view (Fig. 20.10). CT or MRI can be performed if the plain radiography findings are nondiagnostic for hamate fracture.

Perilunate Instability Injuries

The mechanism of perilunate instability injuries typically involves falling on an outstretched hand or extreme loading applied to a hyperflexed or extended wrist. Mayfield et al.

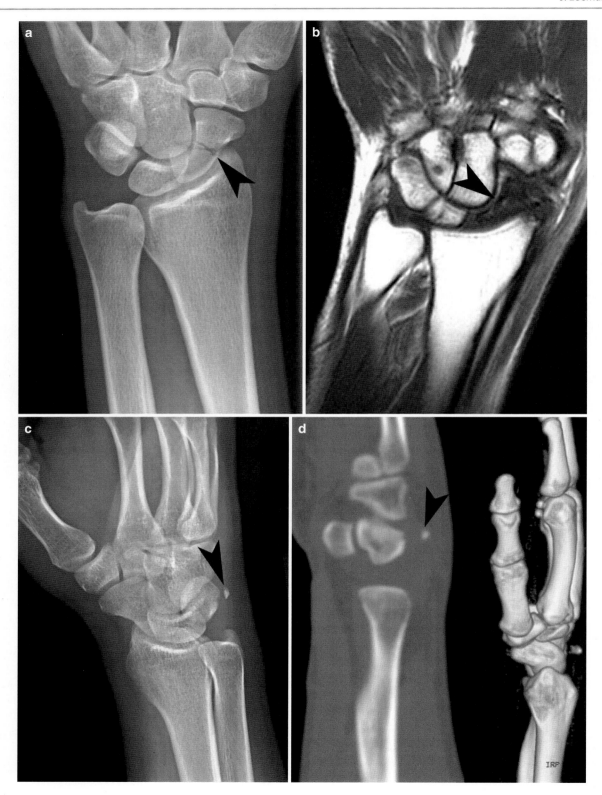

Fig. 20.9 Carpal bone fractures. (**a**) Scaphoid fracture: AP view of the wrist demonstrates a fracture lucency extending through the scaphoid waist (*arrowhead*), the most commonly fractured site in the scaphoid bone. (**b**) Avascular necrosis of scaphoid: Coronal T1-weighted sequence demonstrates diffuse low signal within a collapsed scaphoid bone (*arrowhead*) secondary to avascular necrosis. (**c**) Triquetrum fracture: Oblique view of the wrist shows a small fracture fragment (*arrowhead*) dorsal to the triquetrum. (**d**) Triquetrum fracture: Sagittal reformation and 3D volume-rendered reconstruction demonstrate a small fracture fragment (*arrowhead*) dorsal to the triquetrum

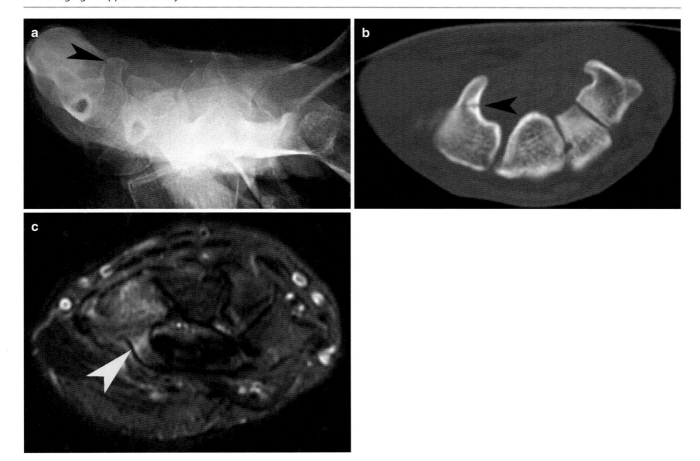

Fig. 20.10 Hamate fracture. (**a**) Carpal tunnel view of the wrist showing a fracture through the hook of hamate (*arrowhead*). (**b**) Axial CT through the wrist shows a fracture through the hook of hamate (*arrowhead*). (**c**) Axial T2-weighted sequence with fat suppression shows linear high signal (*arrowhead*) intensity bone marrow edema due to the fracture of the hook of hamate

identified four stages of perilunate instability based on the severity of injury (Fig. 20.11a, b). These include (1) scapholunate dissociation, (2) capitolunate dislocation, (3) lunotriquetral dissociation, and (4) lunate dislocation [12].

Scapholunate dissociation is the least severe injury and involves disruption of the scapholunate and radioscaphoid ligaments, leading to the dorsal intercalatated segmental instability (DISI) injury pattern. Normally, on the lateral projection, the scapholunate angle measures 30–60°. The DISI pattern represents volar tilt of the scaphoid with dorsal tilt of the lunate, which increases the scapholunate angle above 60°. On the posteroanterior radiograph, widening of the scapholunate interval greater than 3 mm gives rise to the "Terry Thomas" sign. Associated volar rotation of the scaphoid leads to the distal scaphoid pole viewed en face giving rise to the "signet ring" sign on the AP projection. Scapholunate dissociation eventually leads to further widening of the scapholunate interval with loss of cartilage at the radioscaphoid joint and proximal migration of capitate (scapholunate advanced collapse or SLAC wrist).

Capitolunate dislocation, also known as perilunate dislocation, is defined as dorsal dislocation of the capitate while the longitudinal alignment of the lunate and radius is preserved (Fig. 20.11a).

Lunotriquetral dissociation results from rupture of lunotriquetral ligaments and may include perilunate dislocation but is considered more severe. On the AP view, the scaphoid is volar flexed and so the "signet ring" sign may be identified. On the lateral radiograph, the lunate is volar flexed, leading to a scapholunate angle less than 30° or volar intercalated segmental instability (VISI deformity).

Lunate dislocation, the most severe injury in the perilunate instability spectrum, involves volar dislocation of the lunate, while the capitate remains in normal alignment with the radius. On the lateral projection, the lunate appears as a "spilled teacup" and is oriented approximately 90° with respect to the radius. On the frontal projection, the lunate takes on a triangular or "pie" shape, in contrast to its normal trapezoidal appearance (Fig. 20.11c, d).

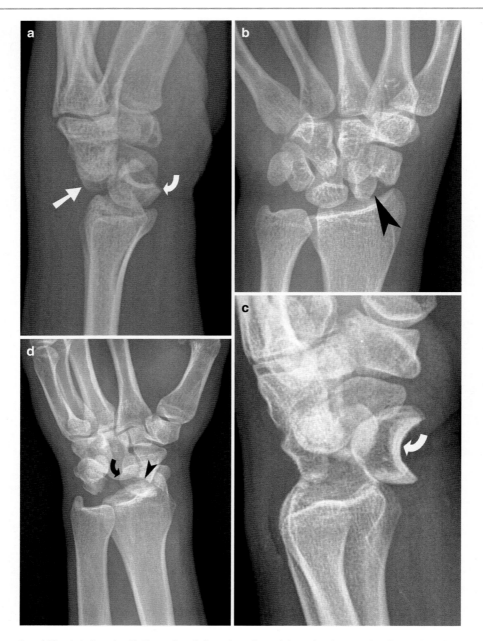

Fig. 20.11 Perilunate instability injuries. (**a**, **b**) Lateral and frontal view of the wrist shows the classic appearance of perilunate dislocation with dorsal dislocation of the capitate (*straight arrow*). Note that the lunate (*curved arrow*) maintains a normal alignment with the radius. There is fracture seen through the waist of the scaphoid with displacement of the proximal fragment (*arrowhead*). (**c**, **d**) Lateral and frontal view of the wrist shows volar dislocation of lunate (*curved arrow*) in a "spilled teacup" configuration. The capitate remains well aligned with the radius. The AP view in the same patient depicts an abnormal pie-shaped appearance of the lunate secondary to volar flexion. There is fracture seen involving the scaphoid (*arrowhead*)

Metacarpal Injuries

A transverse fracture of the neck of the fifth metacarpal, and less frequently the fourth metacarpal, with volar angulation is the most common metacarpal fracture and is called boxer's fracture. It typically results from axial loading of the metacarpal when the closed fist strikes a wall or jaw. Often, a butterfly fragment that is impacted volarly can be identified. A posteroanterior view of the hand will demonstrate shortening at the metacarpal neck (Fig. 20.12). A lateral view will demonstrate volar angulation at the fracture site.

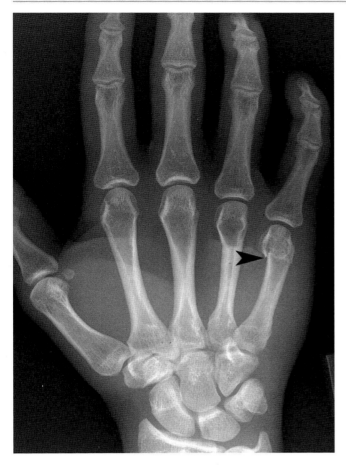

Fig. 20.12 Boxer fracture. AP view of the hand depicts an impacted fracture through the neck of the fifth metacarpal (*arrowhead*) with shortening of the overall length of the metacarpal

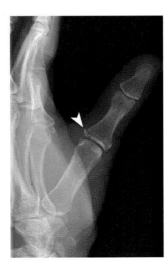

Fig. 20.13 Gamekeeper's thumb. AP view of the thumb shows an avulsed fragment (*arrowhead*) at the base of the proximal phalanx, at the attachment site of the ulnar collateral ligament

Gamekeeper's Thumb

A complete or partial tear of the ulnar collateral ligament of the thumb ("Gamekeeper's thumb") classically occurs when a falling skier improperly plants his pole resulting in sudden abduction and valgus stress at the first metacarpophalangeal (MCP) joint. Disruption most commonly occurs at the distal attachment of the ulnar collateral ligament (UCL), at the base of the proximal phalanx. Radial collateral ligament injury is significantly less common than UCL injury and results from forceful adduction at the MCP joint irrespective of thumb position.

Initial radiographic evaluation may reveal an avulsed bone fragment from the proximal phalanx at the distal attachment site of the UCL (Fig. 20.13). Abduction stress radiographs can demonstrate greater than 30° of radial deviation at the MCP joint or greater than 20° difference compared to the contralateral side, findings indicative of complete disruption of the ulnar collateral ligament. MRI may reveal abnormal signal within the ligament in the case of a partial tear. In the setting of a complete tear, discontinuity with proximal retraction of the ligament may be seen, referred to as the "yo-yo on a string" appearance.

A complete tear with proximal retraction of the ulnar collateral ligament may lead to abnormal interposition of the adductor aponeurosis between the retracted proximal UCL and its distal attachment, a complication known as the Stener lesion which complicates approximately 29 % of cases [13]. This lesion mandates surgical repair to avoid chronic instability of the joint.

Injury at the Carpometacarpal Joint of the Thumb

An intra-articular fracture at the base of the first metacarpal, known as a Bennett fracture, is often accompanied by displacement or distraction of the metacarpal shaft due to continued traction by the adductor pollicis and abductor pollicis longus muscles, while the small ulnar fracture fragment is held in place by ligamentous attachments (Fig. 20.14). A Bennett fracture is treated with open reduction and fixation.

A Rolando fracture is a comminuted fracture of the metacarpal base. Soft tissue swelling in isolation may be indicative of injury to the anterior longitudinal ligament, which is the most important stabilizer at the base of the thumb. MRI may depict a partial or complete thickness tear of the ligament. Surgical repair of the comminuted Rolando fracture may be more challenging than Bennett fracture, with a higher likelihood of eventually developing posttraumatic osteoarthritis.

Phalangeal Injuries

Phalangeal tuft fractures are commonly associated with occupational injury and result from a direct loading mechanism such as having a heavy object drop on the finger. These fractures may be simple or comminuted. Formation of an epidermoid cyst secondary to dermal elements seeding the fracture site is a known complication [14].

Disruption of the extensor mechanism with an avulsion fracture at the dorsal base of the distal phalanx can occur when the finger is maximally extended and a sudden forceful flexion is caused, such as when the fingertip is struck by a baseball (Fig. 20.15a). This injury is known as mallet finger deformity due to the fixed flexion deformity at the distal interphalangeal (DIP) joint.

A similar injury occurs when the finger is in a flexed position and undergoes abrupt extension, classically occurring when an athlete grabs an opponent's jersey, leading to an avulsion fracture at the distal attachment of the volar plate at the DIP joint at the insertion of the flexor digitorum profundus tendon (Fig. 20.15b). This injury most commonly occurs at the ring finger and results in loss of ability to flex the DIP joint.

In descending order of frequency, phalangeal dislocations may occur dorsally ("Coach's finger"), laterally, or volarly. Phalangeal dislocations most commonly occur at the proximal interphalangeal (PIP) joint. Dorsal or volar dislocations are often associated with volar plate disruption with or without avulsion fracture at its distal attachment site at the base of the middle phalanx. Lateral dislocation secondary to valgus or varus stress leads to disruption of one of the collateral ligaments.

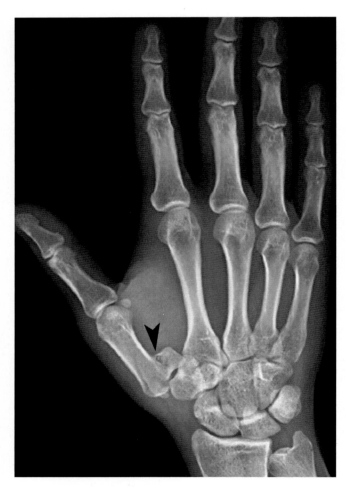

Fig. 20.14 Bennett fracture. AP view of the hand shows an intra-articular fracture at the base of the thumb (*arrowhead*). Note the metacarpal shaft is displaced in a radial direction, secondary to traction by abductor pollicis longus

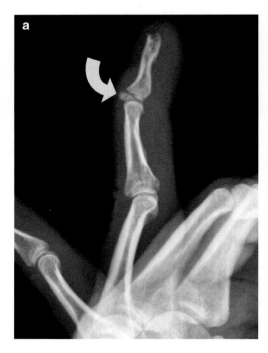

Fig. 20.15 Phalangeal fractures. (**a**) Baseball fracture: Lateral view of the index finger shows fixed flexion deformity at the distal interphalangeal joint due to an avulsion fracture (*arrow*) at the extensor tendon attachment site. (**b**) Lateral view depicts an avulsion fracture at the site of attachment of flexor digitorum profundus (*arrowhead*) with fixed extension at the distal interphalangeal joint

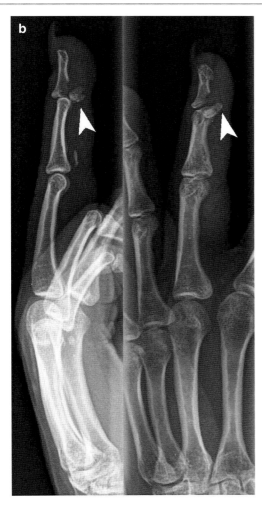

Fig. 20.15 (continued)

References

1. Lavelle WF, Uhl R. Scapulothoracic dissociation. Orthopedics. 2010;33(6):417–21.
2. Preston CF, Egol KA. Midshaft clavicle fractures in adults. Bull NYU Hosp Jt Dis. 2009;67(1):52–7.
3. Smekal V. Shaft fractures of the clavicle: current concepts. Arch Orthop Trauma Surg. 2009;129(6):807–15.
4. Restrepo CS, Martinez S, Lemos DF, Washington L, et al. Imaging appearances of the sternum and sternoclavicular joints. Radiographics. 2009;29(3):839–59.
5. Kuhn JE. Treating the initial anterior shoulder dislocation – an evidence-based medicine approach. Sports Med Arthrosc. 2006;14(4):192–8.
6. Neer CS. Displaced proximal humeral fractures. I. Classification and evaluation. J Bone Joint Surg Am. 1970;52(6):1077–89.
7. Mirzayan R, Skaggs DL. The posterior fat pad sign in association with occult fracture of the elbow in children. J Bone Joint Surg Am. 1999;81(10):1429–33.
8. Gartland JJ. Management of supracondylar fractures of the humerus in children. Surg Gynecol Obstet. 1959;109(2):145–54.
9. Walsh HP, McLaren CA, Owen R. Galeazzi fractures in children. J Bone Joint Surg Br. 1987;69(5):730–3.
10. Goyal V, Bhatia M, Behari M. Carpal tunnel syndrome after 22 years of Colle's fracture. Neurol India. 2003;51(1):113–4.
11. Hauger O, Bonnefoy O, Moinard M, Bersani D, Diard F. Occult fractures of the waist of the scaphoid: early diagnosis by high-spatial-resolution sonography. AJR Am J Roentgenol. 2002;178(5):1239–45.
12. Mayfield JK, Johnson RP, Kilcoyne RK. Carpal dislocations: pathomechanics and progressive perilunar instability. J Hand Surg Am. 1980;5(3):226–41.
13. Hinke DH, Erickson SJ, Chamoy L, Timins ME. Ulnar collateral ligament of the thumb: MR findings in cadavers, volunteers, and patients with ligamentous injury (gamekeeper's thumb). AJR Am J Roentgenol. 1994;163(6):1431–4.
14. Hamad AT, Kumar A, Anand KC. Intraosseous epidermoid cyst of the finger phalanx: a case report. J Orthop Surg (Hong Kong). 2006;14(3):340–2.

Lower Extremity Trauma

Rathachai Kaewlai and Ajay Singh

Imaging of extremity trauma usually starts with conventional radiography, which is a cornerstone of orthopedic trauma workup. Standard AP and lateral views are usually diagnostically adequate for assessment of lower extremity trauma. However, superimposed bony structures in complex areas such as ankle and foot can make image interpretation difficult. Extensive bone and joint injuries, though visible on radiography, may also be challenging for accurate treatment planning. In this regard, multidetector computed tomography (MDCT) with multiplanar reformations (MPR) will provide a more accurate detection of occult bone and joint injuries and better depiction of complex fractures and dislocations.

Magnetic resonance (MR) imaging has excellent soft tissue contrast and can provide valuable information on identification of occult fractures, stress fractures, cartilaginous/labral injuries, compartment syndromes, and tendon/ligamentous disruptions. However, the use of MR imaging has mainly been limited by cost and availability. In this chapter, the authors discuss common fractures, easily missed fractures, fracture classifications, and their imaging characteristics.

Pelvis

Standard views: AP, PA with 25° caudal angulation (Ferguson) of the pelvis

Frequent types of fractures:

    Isolated fractures of the pubic rami

    Pelvic ring disruption

R. Kaewlai, MD
Department of Radiology, Ramathibodi Hospital,
Mahidol University,
Ratchatewi, Bangkok, Thailand

A. Singh, MD (✉)
Department of Radiology, Massachusetts General Hospital,
Harvard Medical School,
10 Museum Way, # 524, Boston, MA, 02141, USA
e-mail: asingh1@partners.org

Fractures of the pelvis are usually caused by direct injury or by force transmitted longitudinally through the femur. There are two major groups of pelvic fractures: isolated fractures and pelvic ring disruption.

Any part of the pelvis may be affected by an isolated fracture. The commonest one is through the pubic ramus (superior, inferior, or both). Isolated fractures can also be seen involving the iliac wing (Duverney), sacrum, anterior inferior iliac spine (rectus femoris avulsion), anterior superior iliac spine (sartorius avulsion), and ischial tuberosity (hamstring avulsion) (Fig. 21.1).

Pelvic ring disruption refers to osseous or joint disruption at two points of the pelvic ring (sacrum and two innominate

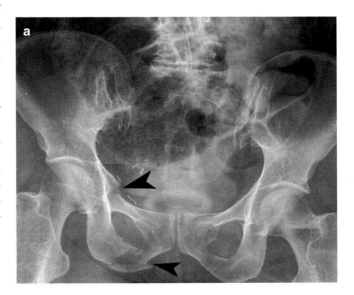

Fig. 21.1 Pelvic fracture. (**a**) An AP radiograph of the pelvis shows displaced vertically oriented fractures (*arrowheads*) of the right superior and inferior pubic rami and widening of the right sacroiliac joint, representing an anteroposterior compression (APC) type of pelvic ring disruption. (**b**) A focused AP radiographic view and corresponding CT image of the right iliac wing show an isolated fracture of the right iliac wing (*arrows*), which is considered a stable pelvic injury

A. Singh (ed.), *Emergency Radiology*,
DOI 10.1007/978-1-4419-9592-6_21, © Springer Science+Business Media New York 2013

Fig. 21.1 (continued)

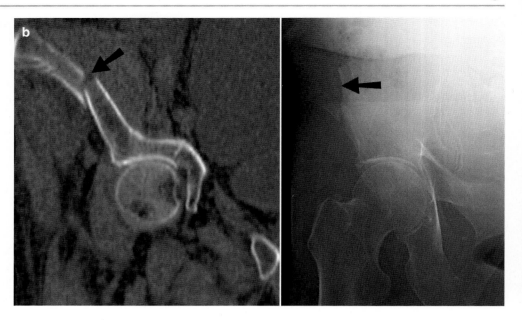

bones) approximately opposite to one another. The anterior injury often involves either a fracture through both pubic rami or pubic symphysis diastasis. The posterior injury is usually a subluxation of the sacroiliac joint or a fracture through the ilium or sacral ala. The most widely used classification of pelvic ring disruption is the Young-Burgess system and describes four patterns, according to the direction of forces to the pelvis [1]:

1. Anteroposterior compression: Vertically oriented fractures of the pubic rami, pubic symphysis diastasis, and disruption of the sacroiliac joints. They may be associated with urethral and urinary bladder rupture (Fig. 21.2).
2. Lateral compression: It produces coronal or horizontal fractures of the pubic rami, sacral compression fracture, iliac wing fracture, and central hip dislocation.
3. Vertical shear: It results in vertically oriented fractures of the pubic rami, sacrum, and iliac wings. There is extensive ligamentous disruption, often resulting in severe pelvic instability, sciatic nerve, and pelvic vascular injury.
4. Combined mechanism.

In general, a single break in the pelvic ring is considered stable, while two or more breaks of the pelvic ring are unstable. Most sacral fractures are vertically oriented and are associated with fractures of the pelvis or lumbosacral dislocation.

Denis classification: It divides sacrum into three zones [2]:

Zone I fractures: They are located lateral to the sacral foramina and rarely cause neurological deficit.

Zone II fractures: These fractures are usually vertically oriented (Figs. 21.3a, b). They pass through sacral foramina and are often associated with L5 nerve root injury.

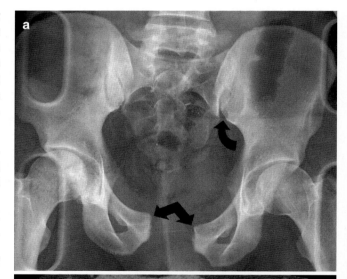

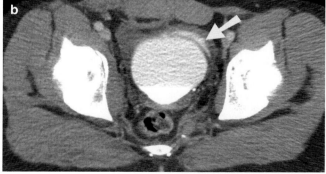

Fig. 21.2 Pelvic fracture. (**a**) An AP radiograph of the pelvis shows widening of the pubic symphysis (*double arrow*) and the left sacroiliac joint (*arrow*), indicative of an anteroposterior compression (APC) type of pelvic ring disruption. (**b**) An axial CT cystography image reveals an extraperitoneal bladder rupture (*arrow*)

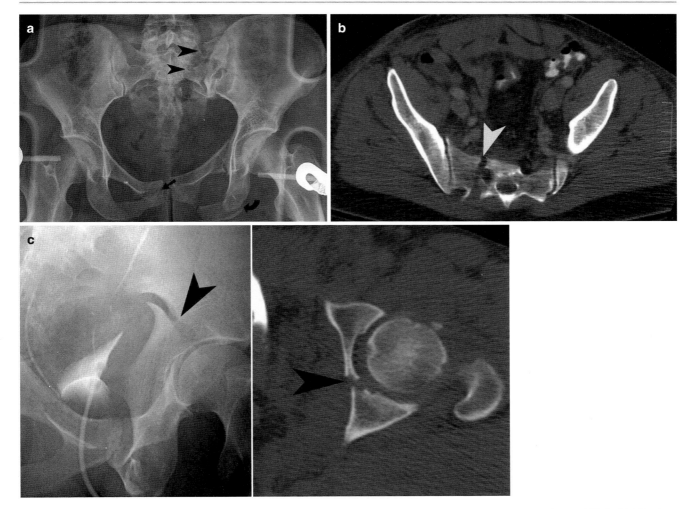

Fig. 21.3 Pelvic fractures. (**a**) An AP radiograph of the pelvis shows a vertical fracture through the left sacral ala (*arrowheads*), widening of the left sacroiliac joint, multiple bilateral pubic rami fractures (*straight* and *curved arrow*). (**b**) An axial CT image of another patient shows a zone II right sacral fracture (*arrowhead*). (**c**) An iliac oblique Judet view of the left hip demonstrates a disrupted ilioischial line by a displaced posterior column fracture (*arrowhead*). An accompanying axial CT image confirms the finding of a column fracture, which is seen as a coronally oriented fracture line (*arrowhead*) through the posterior half of the acetabulum

Zone III fractures: These fractures involve the central canal and have the highest frequency of neurological deficit.

Acetabulum

Standard views: AP and Judet views of the hip (two oblique views centered on the hip, tilted 45° medially or laterally from a true AP direction)

Frequent types of fractures:

Posterior wall

Transverse

Transverse plus posterior wall

T-shaped

Associated both column

Imaging performed in acetabular fracture is to evaluate for wall involvement, intra-articular entrapped bone fragment and associated femoral head fracture. On the AP view of the hip, six lines relating to the acetabulum and surrounding structures have been described: iliopubic or iliopectineal line, ilioischial line, radiographic teardrop, roof of the acetabulum, anterior rim of the acetabulum, and posterior rim of the acetabulum. Disruption of any of these normal lines indicates the possible presence of abnormality [3] (Fig. 21.3c).

1. Iliopectineal line: It extends from the sciatic notch to pubic tubercle and is discontinuous in anterior column fractures.
2. Ilioischial line: It is drawn from the sciatic notch to internal cortex of the ischium and is discontinuous with posterior column fracture. The breaks in the anterior and posterior rim of the acetabulum indicate either a column or wall fracture. The radiographic teardrop is a composite

U-shaped shadow at the anteroinferior portion of the acetabular fossa, without true structural correlate.

On lateral view, the pelvis is divided into anterior and posterior columns. The anterior column (iliopubic component) consists of pubis and ilium, whereas the posterior column (ischial component) consists of ischium, ischial spine, and ischial tuberosity. The posterior wall fractures are the most common acetabular fractures and are often associated with multiple fragments as well as posterior hip dislocation.

Hip

Standard views: AP and true lateral views of the hip
Frequent sites of fractures:
Femoral neck fractures
Posterior hip dislocations
Frequently missed injuries:
Nondisplaced femoral neck fractures
Fractures of the greater trochanter
Fractures of the femoral head

Hip Dislocations

Dislocations of the hip are infrequent injuries since strong force is required to produce such trauma. There are several types of hip dislocations, which are defined by the relationship of the femoral head relative to the acetabulum.

Posterior dislocation, which is the most common type of hip dislocation, is characterized by posterior displacement of femoral head in relation to the acetabulum (Fig. 21.4). It is classically the result of a head-on motor vehicle collision, in which the occupant's knees strike the dashboard, while the knees are in flexed position. It commonly occurs in association with fractures of the posterior acetabular rim. On radiography, there is a lack of congruency of the femoral head and the acetabular fossa with the femoral head located superolateral to the acetabulum. In approximately half of cases, there is associated fracture of the posterior acetabular rim. Common complications of posterior hip dislocation are injury to the sciatic nerve, femoral head fracture, avascular necrosis of the femoral head, posttraumatic ossification, and osteoarthritis.

Anterior hip dislocation is the second most common type of hip dislocation, accounting for 10–15 % of all hip dislocations. It is caused by forced abduction and lateral rotation of the limb, usually from motor vehicle collision. On radiography, the femoral head is often located inferomedial to the acetabulum. The dislocated femoral head appears slightly larger than on the contralateral side because of magnification (dislocated femoral head is located further away from the cassette) and the lesser trochanter is visualized in full profile. There is association with femoral head and acetabular fracture [4].

Central hip dislocation describes the medial displacement of the femoral head into the pelvis, causing comminuted fracture of the medial wall of the acetabulum. It is usually

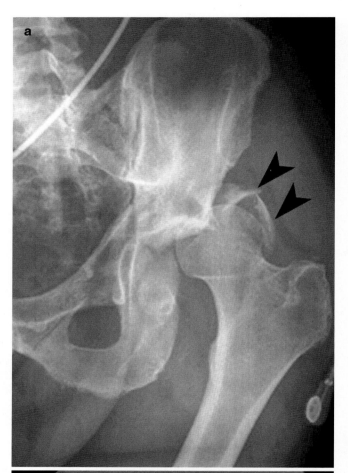

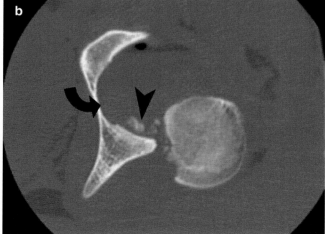

Fig. 21.4 Posterior dislocation at the hip joint. (**a**) An AP radiograph of the pelvis shows an apparent superolateral location of the left femoral head relative to the acetabulum, which is characteristic of posterior hip dislocation. *Arrowheads* point to associated acetabular fracture fragments. (**b**) An axial CT image shows an empty left acetabulum (*arrow*) with several bone fragments (*arrowhead*) in the hip joint from associated posterior wall acetabular fracture

caused by a heavy lateral blow upon the femur, for example, fall from height onto the side. Retroperitoneal bleeding, subsequent retroperitoneal infection, and residual joint incongruity frequently complicate this injury.

Postreduction radiograph is required to determine the adequacy of reduction and to identify potential intra-articular fragments. Asymmetry of hip joint space or unequal widths between the radiographic teardrop and femoral head should raise suspicion of large effusion, interposed soft tissue, or intra-articular fragments. CT is the imaging method of choice to evaluate for intra-articular loose body.

Fractures of the Proximal Femur

Fractures of the femoral head are relatively infrequent in isolation given the protection of the femoral head by the acetabulum (Figs. 21.4b and 21.5a). When they occur, they are usually associated with hip dislocation and are caused by impaction or shearing by the acetabulum. Pipkin classification is the standard mean to classify femoral head fractures, with a main criterion of whether the fracture is above or below the fovea [5].

Pipkin Classification:

Type 1 is a fracture below the fovea.

Type 2 is the fracture above the fovea.

Type 3 is a femoral head fracture associated with a neck fracture.

Type 4 is a femoral head fracture associated with an acetabular fracture.

Type 3 and 4 fractures often require operative intervention, while the need for operative fixation of type 1 and 2 fractures depends on several factors including intra-articular fragment, irreducible dislocation, and involvement of the weight-bearing portion. The fractures of the femoral head are at an increased risk of avascular necrosis or nonunion because main arterial supply (medial femoral circumflex artery) may be injured.

Femoral neck fractures may result from a significant injury such as a fall but can also be seen in minor trauma among osteoporotic individuals. Garden classification is most commonly used to describe these fractures [6].

Garden I is an incomplete or impacted fracture, in which the inferior aspect of the neck trabeculae is still intact. It commonly results in a slight valgus angulation of the femoral neck.

Garden II is a complete fracture without displacement (Fig. 21.5b).

Garden III is a complete fracture with partial displacement. Shortening and external rotation of the affected limb is commonly seen.

Garden IV is a complete fracture with total displacement (no continuity between the proximal and distal fragments).

While displaced fractures are readily visualized on radiography, imaging features of nondisplaced fractures are often subtle. These features include:

1. Disruption of a normal S or reversed S curve of the outline of the femoral head joining the concave outline of the femoral neck.
2. Sclerotic line of impacted fracture.

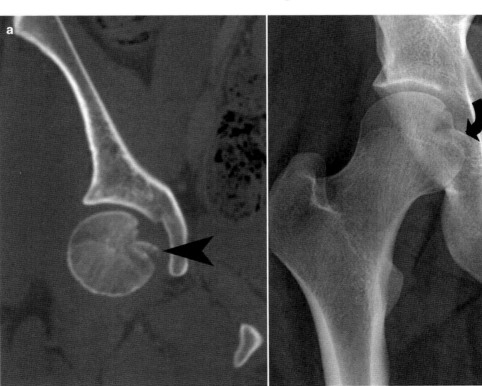

Fig. 21.5 Proximal femoral fractures. (**a**) An AP radiograph of the right hip reveals a depression at the femoral head (*arrow*), later confirmed by a corresponding CT scan as a depressed fracture (*arrowhead*) involving the fovea capitis. (**b**) A coronal STIR MR image of the pelvis in another patient demonstrates bone marrow edema of the left femoral neck with a linear hypointense line (*arrowhead*) in the medial aspect of the femoral neck, perpendicular to the bony cortex, representing a stress fracture. (**c**) An AP radiograph of the right hip of another patient shows an intertrochanteric fracture with a displaced lesser trochanter fragment

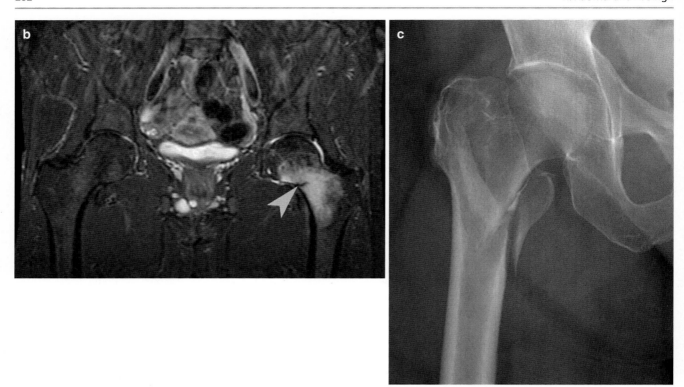

Fig. 21.5 (continued)

3. Abnormal angulation of the major trabeculae groups. On a lateral radiograph, one should look for posterior comminution of the fracture, since its presence indicates a higher chance of nonunion.

The blood supply to the femoral head is through three routes, including the vessels in the ligamentum teres, capsular vessels, and branches of the nutrient vessels. There is an increased risk of avascular necrosis following femoral neck fractures because of nutrient and capsular vessel disruption. The frequency of avascular necrosis in displaced and nondisplaced fractures is 30–40 and 10 %, respectively [7]. If radiography is negative but there is still a high clinical suspicion, CT with multiplanar reconstruction or MRI should be considered.

Intertrochanteric fractures occur along the line between greater and lesser trochanter (Fig. 21.5c). Since the joint capsule attaches anteriorly to the intertrochanteric line and posteriorly to the medial half of the femoral neck, trochanteric fracture is theoretically extracapsular and heals well relative to the femoral neck fractures. It is important to distinguish stable from unstable trochanteric fractures. This can be determined by assessing the medial cortex and comminution of the posterior cortex (on lateral view). Comminuted fracture line at the medial cortex, displaced lesser trochanter fracture, and lesser trochanter fragment containing calcar femorale are generally considered unstable. Presence of a fracture gap medially and posteriorly will allow fracture displacement into varus or retroversion, causing instability. Unlike fractures of the femoral neck, trochanteric fractures are almost free from serious complications.

Subtrochanteric fractures are fractures located between the lesser trochanter and 5 cm below. It is usually a result of direct trauma and may occur in isolation or with intertrochanteric fractures. The fractures are usually displaced by muscle pulls, resulting in shortening and varus deformity.

Fractures of the Femoral Shaft, Supracondyle, and Condyle

Fractures of the distal femur usually occur with high-velocity trauma in young adults and low-energy trauma in osteoporotic bone of elderly persons. Therefore, it is commonly associated with several other injuries such as fractures of the patella, hip and tibial shaft, and ligamentous disruptions of the knee. Femoral shaft fractures occur at any age and are equally common in the uppermost, middle, and lower thirds of the shaft. Their pattern may be transverse, oblique, spiral, comminuted, or greenstick. Radiographic evaluation must include the hip and knee joints since joint dislocations may coexist.

The fractures of the supracondylar and condylar regions are divided into three types: extra-articular (transverse), partial articular, and complete articular. The key components

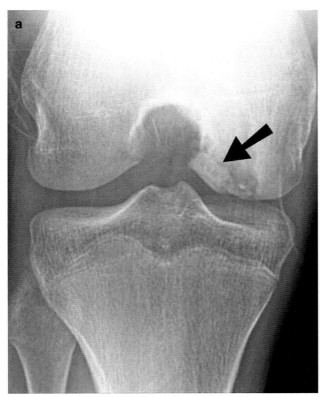
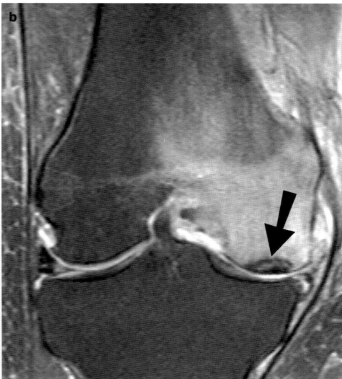

Fig. 21.6 Osteochondral injury. (**a**) A tunnel radiographic view of the right knee shows an osteochondral fracture (*arrow*) of the lateral aspect of the medial femoral condyle. (**b**) A coronal fat-suppressed T2W MR image of the right knee in a different patient reveals bone marrow edema of the medial femoral condyle with an osteochondral fragment in the subarticular portion (*arrow*). There is soft tissue edema in the medial aspect of the knee. The medial collateral ligament is intact

in dividing distal femoral fractures are presence of (1) a fracture line extending into the intercondylar notch (intercondylar split), (2) osteochondral fragments in the area of or between the intercondylar split, and (3) coronal-plane (Hoffa) fracture. Partial articular fractures are an intra-articular fracture that involves either the medial, lateral condyle, or in a coronal plane (best seen on a lateral radiograph). Complete articular fractures produce separate articular and metaphyseal segments, in which each can be simple or multifragmentary.

Osteochondritis dissecans (OCD) of the knee (Fig. 21.6) may present in a similar fashion to acute traumatic osteochondral fractures, although they differ. The condition is characterized by sequential degeneration or aseptic necrosis and recalcification. It can occur in persons of any age group but is most frequent between 10 and 20 years old, with male predominance. Most of the cases (85 %) involve the medial femoral condyle in the posterolateral aspect [8]. Radiography shows OCD as a well-circumscribed crescent-shaped area of radiolucency above the subchondral bone, separated from femoral condyle. MRI is helpful to help determining the vascularity of the lesion, bilaterality, occult lesions, and degree of loosening of the lesion.

Knee

Standard views: AP, lateral, both obliques (optional patellar sunrise if suspicious for patellar injuries)

Frequent sites of fractures:

    Patellar fractures

    Tibial plateau fractures

Frequently missed injuries:

    Tibial plateau fractures

    Segond fractures

    Maisonneuve fractures

Knee Dislocations

Knee dislocations may occur as a result of either high- or low-velocity trauma, in which the mechanism of injury will reflect the incidence of associated neurovascular injuries. Five types of knee dislocations are described with tibia in relation to the femur, which include anterior (most common), posterior (2nd most common), lateral, medial, and rotary.

On an initial radiographic assessment, the findings are usually obvious (Fig. 21.7a). One should look for associated

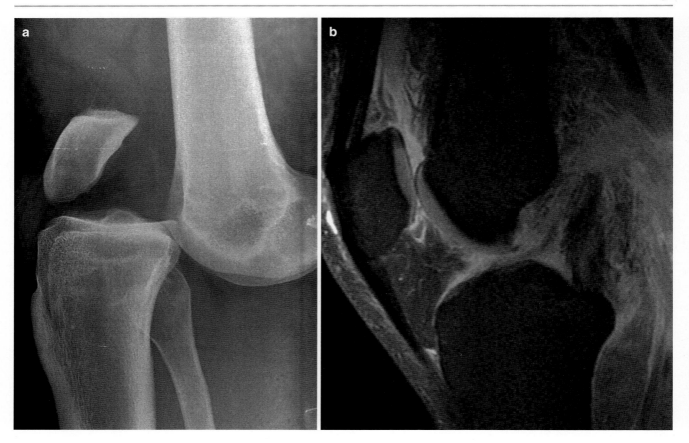

Fig. 21.7 Knee dislocation. (**a**) A lateral radiographs of the left knee demonstrate an apparent anterior knee dislocation with the tibia and fibula displacing anteriorly relative to the distal femur. The patella moves with the distal fragments. (**b**) A sagittal T2W MR image with fat suppression shows extensive ligamentous disruptions and soft tissue injuries of the knee joint

injuries such as fractures of the tibial plateau, proximal fibula, Gerdy's tubercle, intercondylar eminence, and fibular head. Tears of the ACL and PCL often occur along with at least one collateral ligament, which can be confirmed on MR imaging (Fig. 21.7b). Popliteal artery is at risk of intimal injury and subsequent occlusion [9]. Conventional or CT angiography is usually indicated in high-velocity knee dislocations to exclude intimal injury even if the distal pulse returns following the reduction.

Fractures of the Tibia Plateau

Tibial plateau fractures are the most common fractures of the proximal tibia. Since the lateral tibial plateau is weaker than the medial counterpart, it is more frequently fractured. This classically is a result of a direct trauma to the lateral side of the knee such as in pedestrian versus car collision (bumper fracture).

Schatzker [10] classifies the tibial plateau into six types according to the location and pattern of injury:

Type I is a split fracture of the lateral plateau.
Type II is a split-compression fracture.

Type III is an isolated compression lateral plateau fracture (Fig. 21.8a, b).
Type IV is a depressed fracture of the medial plateau.
Type V is a bicondylar fracture and type VI is a diaphyseal-metaphyseal separation.

The radiographic appearance of depressed-type fracture can be difficult to discern because the x-ray beam of a routine anteroposterior view of the knee is not tangential to the tibial joint surface. The secondary signs of tibial plateau fractures include the presence of a fat-blood level or fat-blood interface sign within the suprapatellar bursa, seen on the lateral crosstable radiographic view of the knee. CT with multiplanar reconstruction is helpful for detecting occult fractures, fracture staging, and treatment planning.

Avulsion Fractures Around the Knee

Segond fracture is an avulsion of the lateral aspect of the proximal tibia due to a pull of lateral capsular ligament from the proximal tibia posterior to the Gerdy's tubercle. On AP radiography, it appears as a small elliptical bone fragment lying immediately distal to the lateral tibial plateau and

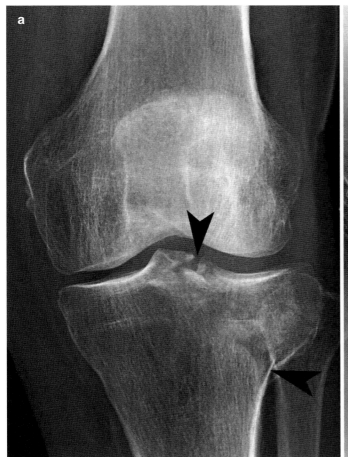
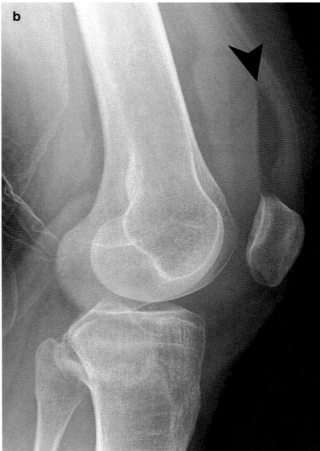

Fig. 21.8 Tibial plateau fracture. (**a**) An AP radiographic view of the left knee shows abnormal increased medullary sclerosis on the lateral plateau with cortical disruptions (*arrowheads*) at the plateau near the tibial spine and laterally at the metadiaphysis. (**b**) A lateral crosstable radiograph reveals a fat-blood interface (*arrowhead*) in the suprapatellar bursa, indicating lipohemarthrosis and implying an intra-articular fracture

parallel to the long axis of the tibia (Fig. 21.9a, b). It is often associated with more serious injuries such as anterior cruciate ligament or meniscal tear. The other similar entity that occurs on the medial side of the tibia, called medial Segond-type fracture, describes a cortical avulsion of the medial tibial plateau in association with posterior cruciate ligament tear.

Injury to the Gerdy's tubercle is an avulsion of the iliotibial tract at its attachment to the lateral proximal tibia. The detached fragment is usually much larger than and lies more anterior and distal to that of Segond fracture fragment. It is best seen on the oblique external rotation radiographic view and is associated with lateral capsular, lateral collateral, and ACL injuries.

Avulsion of the tibial eminence may involve anterior, posterior, or both tibial spines. The most common site is at the anterior aspect from a pull of ACL (Fig. 21.9c). The fragment may be displaced or nondisplaced, in which the degree of displacement dictates a different type of tibial eminence avulsion. The injury is commonly seen in children between ages of 8 and 14 but can also be seen in adults. Radiographic findings may be difficult to recognize and include a presence of small bone fragment in the intercondylar notch and hemarthrosis, best seen on lateral radiography. Avulsion of the fibular styloid process is the fracture at the attachment site of the biceps tendon and fibular collateral ligament, which is commonly associated with disruption of the ACL, popliteus tendon, and arcuate ligament.

Patellar Fractures

Patellar fractures may be a result of two types of injury: (1) a sudden violent contraction of the quadriceps (i.e., abnormal flexion of the knee against contracted quadriceps) and (2) a fall or direct blow to the patella. The former tends to cause a clean fracture line with separation of the fragments, whereas the latter causes a comminuted fracture (Fig. 21.10a). Displacement of the fracture fragments indicates disruption

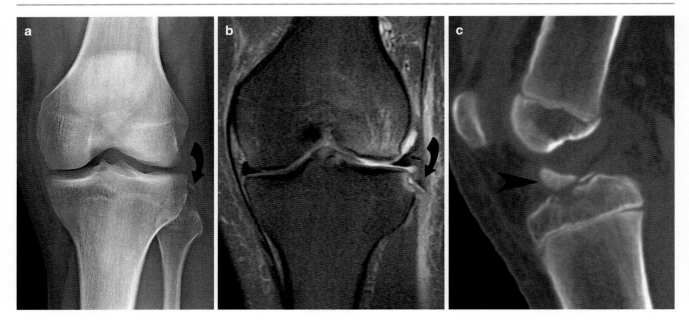

Fig. 21.9 Proximal tibial fractures. (**a**) An AP radiograph of the left knee shows a small flake of bone (*arrow*) just lateral to the edge of the lateral tibial plateau. (**b**) A coronal T2W MR image with fat suppression shows an avulsion of the lateral collateral ligament, joint effusion, and opposing bone contusions associated with a Segond fracture (*arrow*). (**c**) A sagittal CT image of the knee of a different patient shows an avulsion fracture (*arrow head*) of the tibial spine due to a pull of the anterior cruciate ligament

of the patellar retinaculum. Nondisplaced fracture can be difficult to visualize on AP radiographic view but usually can be discerned on the lateral projection. Small peripheral fractures may be confused with bipartite patella, which tends to have a sclerotic rim and is located in a characteristic superolateral aspect of the patella (Fig. 21.10b). If in doubt, a contralateral knee radiograph is usually helpful because bipartite patella often occurs bilaterally.

Soft tissue injuries to the extensor mechanism may occur to the quadriceps tendon, or patellar tendon (Fig. 21.11a, b). The findings on radiograph include high- or low-lying patella, joint effusion, and thickening or distortion of the affected tendon. Chronic repetitive traction injury of the immature osteochondral junction at the inferior pole of the patella represents a Sinding-Larsen-Johansson disease [11] (Fig. 21.10c, d), in which it presents with point tenderness at the inferior pole of the patella associated with soft tissue swelling after strenuous sporting activity. This condition is seen in active adolescents typically between ages of 10 and 14. On radiography, there may be focal thickening of the proximal patellar tendon with hazy adjacent Hoffa's fat pad and osteolysis at the distal pole of the patella. Ultrasound and MRI may show thickening of the tendon with abnormal echogenicity and signal intensity representing tears of posterior fibers of the patellar tendon. The indirect force to the patellar tendon may cause acute bony avulsion at the inferior pole of the patella or tibial tubercle. Patellar sleeve avulsions are seen as thin, curvilinear bone fragment off the parent bone.

Patellar Dislocations

The two major mechanisms that result in patellar dislocation are sudden forceful contraction of the quadriceps with sudden flexion and external rotation of the tibia on the femur and direct trauma to the patella with the knee in flexion. Majority of patellar dislocations are in lateral direction (Fig. 21.12a). The predisposing factors include patella alta, ligamentous insufficiency, and genu valgum.

When the patella is spontaneously relocated, the radiologic diagnosis is more difficult and the role of imaging is to search for associated injuries such as osteochondral or patellar fractures. On lateral radiographic view, there may be patella alta, osteochondral fragment, or joint effusion. Axial patellar (or sunrise) radiographic view may show patellar tilt or osteochondral fragment. The osteochondral fracture fragment often arises from the medial patellar facet or lateral femoral condyle and can be anywhere in the joint space, including in the suprapatellar pouch, posterior to the patella, intercondylar notch, beside the femoral condyles.

Since the loose body may contain only cartilage, making it invisible on plain radiography, MR imaging is the most appropriate imaging method for detection and grading of this injury. The MR imaging appearance includes bone marrow edema in the inferomedial patella and anterolateral aspect of the lateral femoral condyle, rupture of the medial patellar retinacula, and abnormal patellofemoral cartilage (softening, fissuring, or focal defect) (Fig. 21.12b, c).

Fig. 21.10 Patellar fracture. (**a**) A lateral radiograph of the knee reveals a transverse nondistracting fracture of the patella (*arrowhead*) with a moderate-sized joint effusion. (**b**) An AP radiograph of the knee of another patient demonstrates a bipartite patella (*arrow*), which is a well-corticated bone fragment in a characteristic superolateral aspect of the patella. (**c**, **d**) Lateral knee radiograph and sagittal fat-suppressed T2W MR image of a patient with Sinding-Larsen-Johansson disease shows a corticated fragment (*arrow*) at the inferior aspect of the patella with associated bone marrow edema (*arrowhead*) and thickened, T2 hyperintense patellar tendon at its deep portion of the patellar attachment

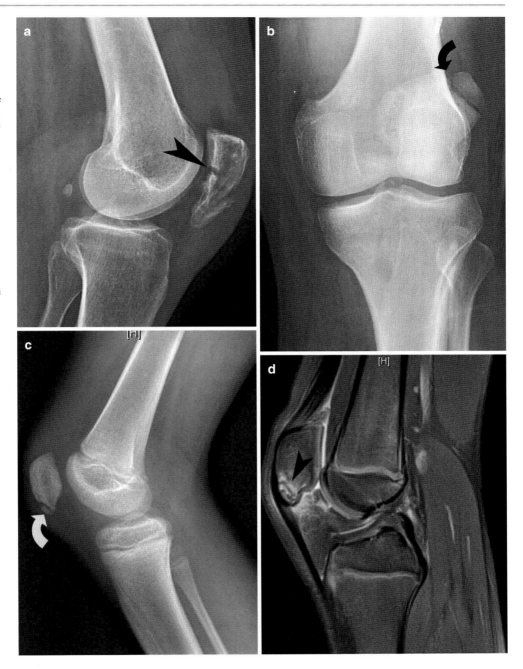

Fractures of the Shafts of the Tibia/Fibula

Most fractures of the shafts of the tibia and fibula occur either from angulatory force or rotational force. The former tends to cause transverse or short oblique fractures, while the latter often produces spiral fractures. They are usually displaced. The tibial fractures are usually open because the tibia is close to the skin and is poorly protected by muscles.

The fractures of the fibula alone often occur in association with injury to the lateral collateral ligament, peroneal nerve, and anterior tibial artery. It can also be the result of rotational

injury of the ankle where there is significant ankle injury with transmission of force superiorly through the interosseous membrane, exiting through a proximal fibular fracture (Maisonneuve fracture) [12]. The ankle should always be imaged if an isolated fibular fracture is seen regardless of the level of the fibular fracture.

Tibia is among the most common site of stress fracture, caused by nonviolent, repetitive stress to tibia that does not allow sufficient recovery between stress applications. Tibial stress fractures are common in athletes in endurance and jumping sports because of their weight-bearing activities. Most early

Fig. 21.11 Soft tissue injuries of the extensor mechanism. (**a**) A lateral radiograph of the right knee shows an abnormally high position of the patella with thickening of the patellar tendon, indicating a patellar tendon rupture in an acute setting. (**b**) A lateral radiograph shows low position of the patella with a soft tissue defect at the quadriceps attachment to the patella, representing a quadriceps tendon tear

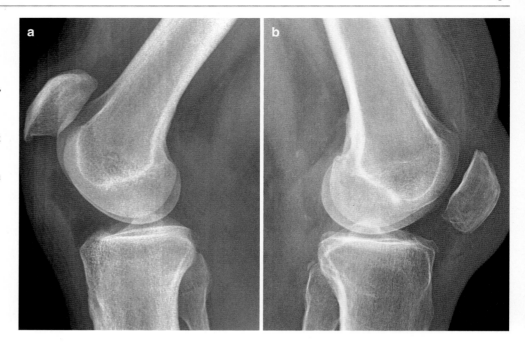

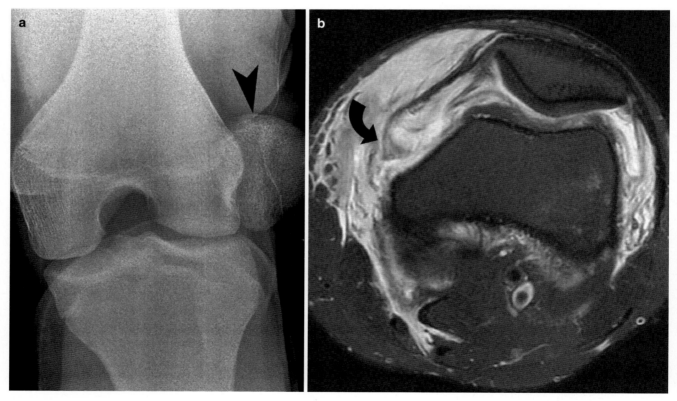

Fig. 21.12 Patellar dislocation. (**a**) An AP radiograph of the left knee shows an obvious lateral dislocation of the patella (*arrow*). (**b, c**) Axial fat-suppressed T2W MR images of other different patients demonstrate a tear of the medial patellar retinaculum (*arrow*), extensive soft tissue edema, and irregular cartilage of the femoral condyle (**b**) and characteristic pattern of bone marrow edema in the inferomedial aspect of the patella (*arrowhead*) and anterior aspect of the lateral femoral condyle (*arrow*) (**c**)

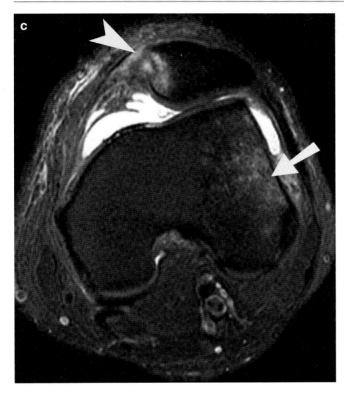

Fig. 21.12 (continued)

radiography shows no abnormality, especially when fractures are immature. Bone scan may help in diagnosing it by showing focal increased periosteal activity but this is a nonspecific finding. Currently, MRI is the imaging method of choice because of its high sensitivity and specificity (Fig. 21.13).

Ankle and Foot

Standard views:

Ankle: AP, lateral, mortise views of the ankle

Calcaneus: Lateral and axial views of the calcaneus

Foot: PA, lateral, and oblique of the foot

Phalanx: PA, lateral, and oblique of the phalanx

Ankle Fractures

Ankle fractures resulting from an axial-loading force are called pilon or tibial plafond fractures (Fig. 21.14a). The fractures are a combination of ankle fracture (medial malleolus, anterior tibial margin, posterior tibial surface) with distal tibial metaphyseal fracture and intra-articular comminution. In most cases, there is an associated fibular fracture signifying the valgus shearing force that causes injuries to the lateral aspect of the ankle joint.

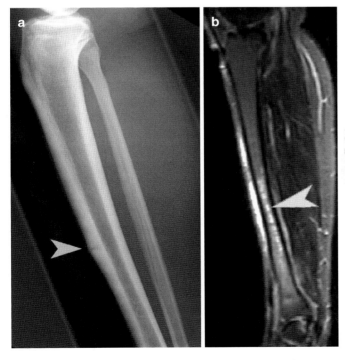

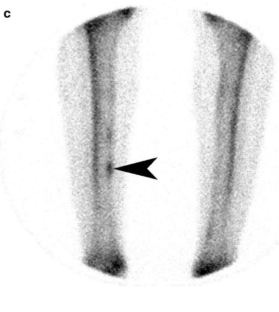

Fig. 21.13 Stress fracture of tibia. (**a–c**) A lateral radiograph of the tibia/fibula (**a**), sagittal fat-suppressed STIR MR image (**b**), and bone scan (**c**) show characteristic imaging features of a tibial stress fracture. There is a linear lucent line perpendicular to the cortex at the anterior aspect of the mid-tibia with surrounding sclerosis, evidence of bone marrow edema on MRI, and localized increased uptake on bone scan (*arrowheads*)

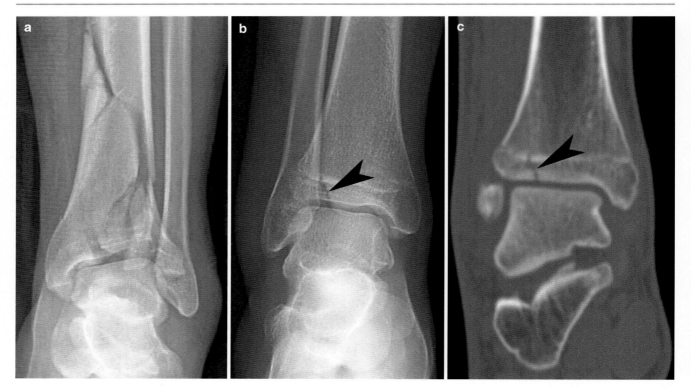

Fig. 21.14 Pilon and Tillaux fracture. (**a**) An AP ankle radiograph shows a comminuted fracture of the tibial plafond with disruption of the articular surface, or a pilon fracture. (**b**) An AP radiograph of the right ankle of another patient shows a vertical fracture line (*arrowhead*) involving the lateral aspect of the distal tibial epiphysis, which extends transversely and laterally along the physeal plate. (**c**) The coronal-reformatted CT image confirms the nature of the Tillaux fracture (*arrowhead*), which is a Salter Harris type III epiphyseal plate injury

Tillaux fracture describes an avulsion of the lateral distal tibial margin seen as a vertical fracture line extending from the distal articular surface of the tibia superiorly to the lateral tibial cortex (Fig. 21.14b). In children, this is considered a Salter Harris epiphyseal plate injury type III. The medial aspect of the distal tibial growth plate fuses earlier than the lateral counterpart; therefore, the lateral side is weaker and prone to trauma. In adults, this is usually a ligamentous injury without bony fractures, so-called Tillaux lesion.

Ankle fractures often results from a combination of forces to the ankle joint, either rotational (less severe) or axial-loading types. The latter often results in comminuted intra-articular fracture of the distal tibia.

Rotational ankle fractures are divided into three types based on Weber classification into type A, B, and C injuries [13, 14]. It utilizes the level of the fibular fracture to determine the extent of injury to the tibiofibular ligamentous complex. In general, the higher the fibular fracture, the more extensive the damage to the tibiofibular ligament complex and greater the risk of ankle joint instability. An oblique fracture line is typically seen with impaction injuries, while a horizontal/transverse fracture line is characteristic of avulsive trauma.

Weber classification:

1. Weber type A: Inversion injury (supination-adduction), in which there is a horizontal fracture of the lateral malleolus, is below the level of the tibiofibular syndesmosis or rupture of the lateral collateral ligament (LCL). The syndesmotic ligaments are intact; therefore, the ankle mortise is stable. If the force is progressive, there may be an oblique fracture of the medial malleolus or posteromedial aspect of the medial malleolus (Fig. 21.15a).

2. Weber type B: Eversion injury (supination-external rotation), in which there is an oblique fracture of the lateral malleolus at the level of the syndesmosis. In these injuries, there may be a horizontal fracture of the medial malleolus or deltoid ligament rupture, fracture of the posterolateral tibia, and partial disruption of the tibiofibular ligament complex. Injury to the deltoid ligament is assumed if there is a greater than 5 mm widening of the medial clear space either on static or stress radiograph.

3. Weber type C: Fibular fracture occurs above the level of the ankle joint and is oblique in orientation. It is an eversion injury that results from pronation-external rotation.

Maisonneuve fracture [12] is a part of the spectrum of pronation-external rotation ankle injuries, in which the fibular fracture occurs proximally with a tear of the tibiofibular syndesmosis and distracting medial ankle injuries. The diagnosis of Maisonneuve fracture should be considered when one encounters an isolated fracture of the posterior lip of the distal tibia, isolated displaced fracture of the medial malleolus,

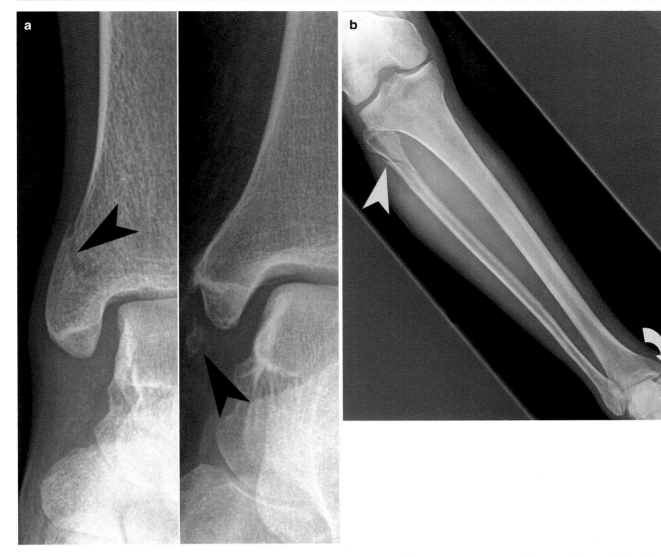

Fig. 21.15 Maleolar fracture. (**a**) Two focused radiographs of the right ankle demonstrate an oblique fracture of the medial malleolus (*arrowhead* in the first picture) compared with a well-corticated accessory ossicle (*arrowhead* in the second picture). (**b**) An AP radiograph of the right tibia/fibula shows a transverse fracture of the medial malleolus (*arrow*) and an oblique fracture of the fibular neck (*arrowhead*), representing a Maisonneuve fracture

and widening of the medial or lateral clear spaces without fracture of the lateral malleolus on ankle film (Fig. 21.15b). Full view of the tibia and fibula should be obtained to identify potential proximal fibular fractures.

Injuries of the Hindfoot

The calcaneus is the most frequently fractured tarsal bone, accounting for 60 % of all tarsal fractures. Calcaneal fractures most frequently occur in young individuals (20– 40 years), with axial-loading mechanism (most commonly falls from a height onto the heels). Both heels may be injured at the same time; bilateral calcaneal fractures are present in 5–10 % of cases. During trauma, the talus is driven down into the calcaneus causing a fracture.

There are two major forms of calcaneal fractures: an isolated fracture without displacement (usually in the tuberosity) or a compression injury (Fig. 21.16). Minor fracture without compression usually occurs in the tuberosity and can be overlooked if only a lateral projection of the calcaneus is taken. Avulsion fracture of the Achilles tendon may cause a tuberosity fracture particularly in diabetic patients.

Compression fracture of calcaneus is a serious injury that may cause significantly impaired function. On lateral radiograph, the upper surface of the calcaneus is flattened and Bohler's angle reduced. A Bohler's angle measures the angle between the line of the subtalar joint and the upper surface of

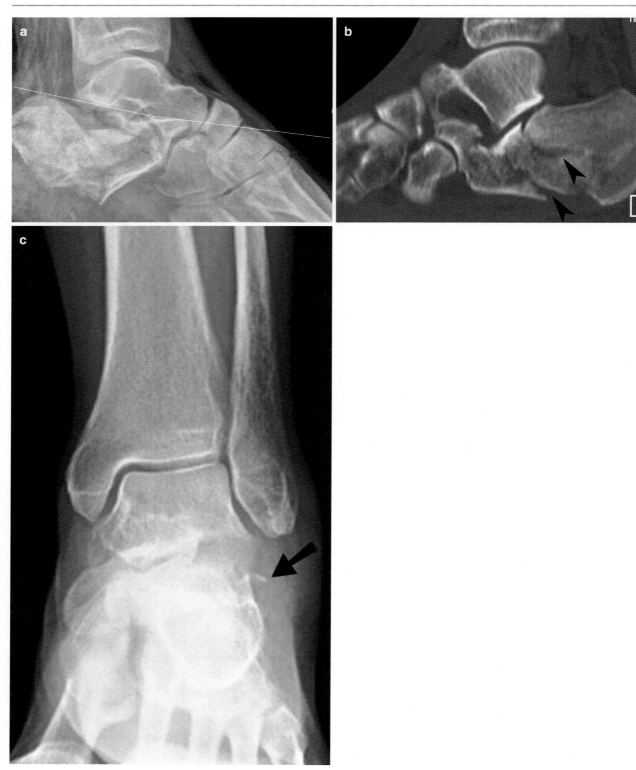

Fig. 21.16 Calcaneal fracture. (**a, b**) A lateral radiograph and sagittal-reformatted CT image of the calcaneus show a comminuted compression fracture of the calcaneus (*arrowheads*) with subtalar joint extension and reduced Bohler's angle. (**c**) An AP ankle radiograph of another patient demonstrates an avulsion fracture (*arrow*) of the dorsolateral aspect of the calcaneus at the origin of the extensor digitorum brevis muscle

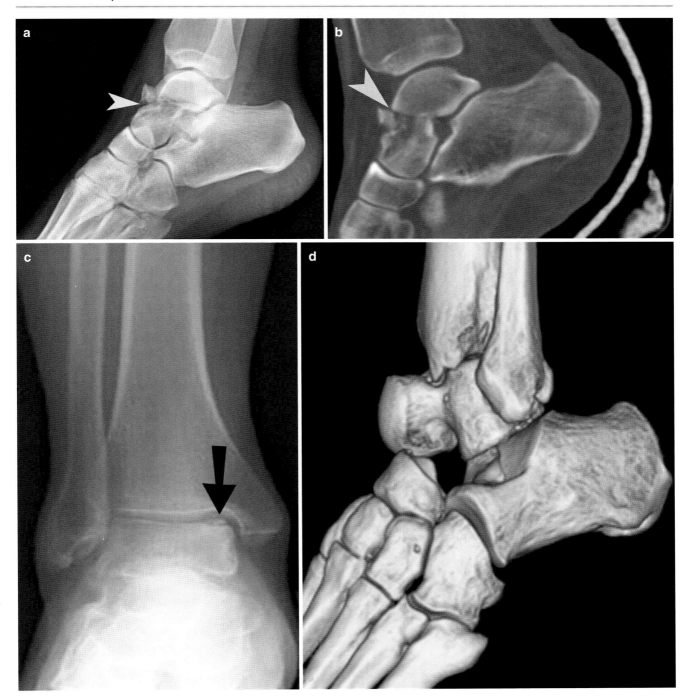

Fig. 21.17 Talar fracture. (**a**, **b**) A lateral radiograph and sagittal-reformatted CT image of the foot demonstrate a talar neck fracture (*arrowheads*) without subtalar or tibiotalar joint subluxation/dislocation. (**c**) An AP ankle radiograph of another patient shows a small bone fragment in the medial aspect of the talar dome (*arrow*), representing osteochondritis dissecans. (**d**) A 3D CT image of the ankle shows an obvious dislocation of the subtalar joint, in which there is disruption of the talonavicular and talocalcaneal articulations

the tuberosity to determine the severity of the compression and the status of the posterior facet of the calcaneus. The angle is normally between 20° and 40° [15].

Talar fractures are the second most common tarsal bone fractures. They are usually caused by forced dorsiflexion force, in which the force is transmitted to the head of the talus and the bone gives way in the neck. In severe injuries, the body of talus may be dislocated posteriorly out of the ankle mortise. The most common site of talar fracture is the neck (Fig. 21.17). The fracture line is located anterior to the lateral process of the talus and is often vertically oriented. Hawkins classification divides talar neck fracture into four types [16]:

Fig. 21.18 Lisfranc fracture dislocation. (**a**, **b**) A PA radiographic view and 3D CT image of the foot demonstrate a disrupted alignment of the Lisfranc joint (*arrowhead*), with lateral/dorsal dislocation of the 1st through 5th digits and fractures of the metatarsal bases (*arrows*). This is a homolateral Lisfranc fracture/dislocation

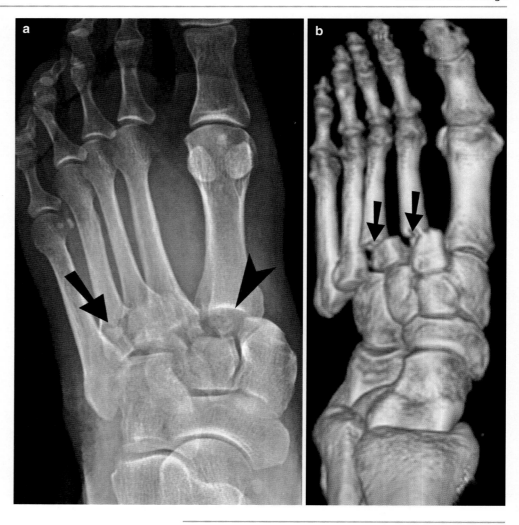

Type I is a fracture without dislocation or subluxation.

Type II is a fracture with subtalar subluxation or dislocation.

Type III is a fracture with subtalar and tibiotalar dislocation.

Type IV is a fracture with subtalar subluxation and talonavicular dislocation.

The risk of developing AVN increases with higher fracture type due to damage to the nutrient vessels at the time of the injury. Fractures extending into or posterior to the lateral process of talus are defined as fractures of the body (intra-articular). The fractures of the lateral process are easily overlooked and can be misdiagnosed clinically as severe sprain. These fractures are best visualized on the mortise view.

Subtalar or peritalar dislocations are rare and describe concomitant dislocations of the subtalar and talonavicular joints but normal tibiotalar relationship. Medial dislocation is the most frequent type but a lateral counterpart is more severe (Fig. 21.17d). Total talar dislocation is defined when there is concomitant dislocation of the subtalar, talonavicular, and tibiotalar joints, which is the most severe of all tarsal injuries.

Injuries of the Midfoot and Forefoot

The tarsal bones are responsible for maintaining the relationship between the forefoot and hindfoot. The navicular is the most frequently injured bone of the midfoot. These are commonly due to sports-related injuries, falls, or motor vehicle collisions. Uncommonly, navicular fractures occur from an avulsive force to the talonavicular or naviculocuneiform ligaments. An accessory navicular (os tibiale externum) can be mistaken as a fracture, although this is bilateral in 90 % of the time.

Lisfranc [17] (tarsometatarsal) injuries are a complex injury commonly resulting from plantar hyperflexion across the long axis of the foot. The key anatomic structure related to this injury is the Lisfranc ligament, which is a strong plantar ligament connecting the medial cuneiform and the second metatarsal base. Injuries may cause a tear of this ligament and/or fractures of the medial cuneiform or base of the second metatarsal. Two major types of Lisfranc injuries are homolateral and divergent (Fig. 21.18). When the four lateral metatarsals or all metatarsals dislocate laterally, this is called

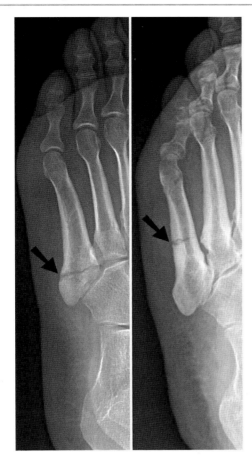

Fig. 21.19 Fifth metatarsal fracture. Two different cases demonstrate zone II (*left image*) and zone III (*right image*) fractures of the fifth metatarsal base (*arrows*)

Stress fractures (Fig. 21.20) are a result of repetitive trauma below the threshold for acute fracture but considerable enough to cause microtrabecular failure. Lower extremity stress fractures are common in athletes and military recruits. The diagnosis is based on history of repetitive overuse and the lack of acute traumatic event. Frequent locations are metatarsals, calcaneus, and lower leg. The most frequently affected metatarsal bone is the second metatarsal, which typically occurs in the diaphysis. In the calcaneus, the posterior aspect (heel) is the most common location. The fracture line is perpendicular to the trabecular cancellous

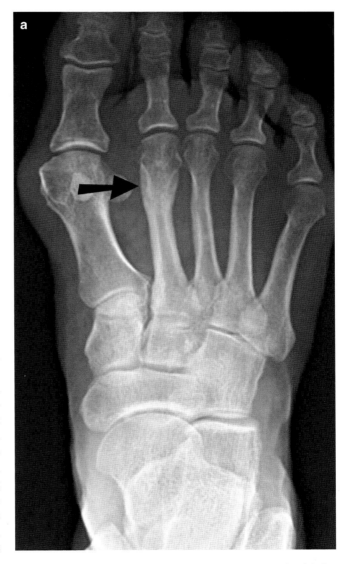

Fig. 21.20 Stress fracture. (**a, b**) A PA radiograph and axial fat-suppressed STIR MR image of the foot of two different patients show a stress fracture (*arrow*) of the 2nd metatarsal bone at the neck. On radiography, there is bony callus formation of a healed stress fracture. On MRI, bone marrow edema with surrounding callus formation and T2 hyperintensity is seen. (**c**) A lateral calcaneal radiograph shows a linear lucent line at the heel with surrounding sclerosis (*arrowhead*), representing a calcaneal stress fracture

homolateral. If the first metatarsal dislocates medially but the rest is dislocated laterally, it is a divergent type.

There are three distinct patterns of fractures of the fifth metatarsal, according to the location of the fracture line (Fig. 21.19). Zone 1 injuries describe an avulsion fracture at the base of the fifth metatarsal due to a pull of a lateral band of the plantar aponeurosis during sudden inversion of the hindfoot. Zone 2 injuries are true Jones fractures, which involve the metadiaphyseal junction of this bone, extending to the intermetatarsal and/or tarsometatarsal joints. Zone 3 injuries are fractures of the proximal fifth metatarsal. Mimics of fractures of the fifth metatarsal base include an apophysis, which is oriented longitudinally to the axis of the metatarsal.

Phalangeal fractures are the most common injury to the forefoot with the proximal phalanx being the most frequent site. They are often a result of crushing injuries, as from the fall of a heavy object onto the foot. The former often causes a comminution, while the latter produces a spiral or oblique fracture with greater deformity due to varus or valgus forces.

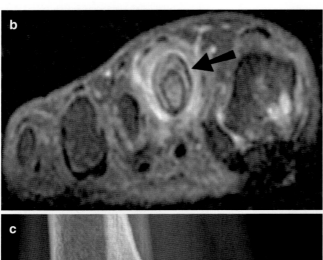

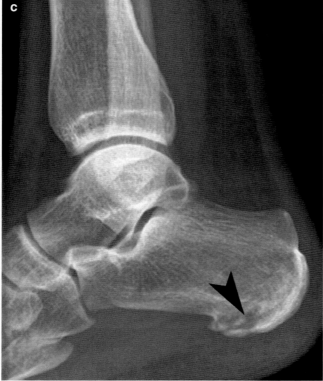

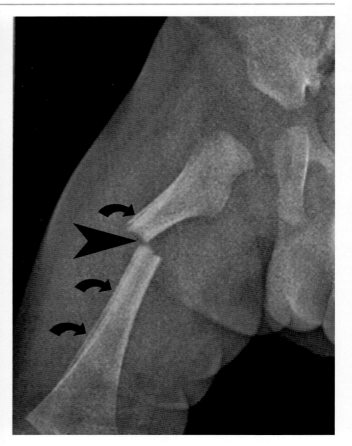

Fig. 21.21 Nonaccidental trauma. An AP radiograph of the right femur as a part of bone survey in a young child demonstrates a displaced transverse fracture (*arrowhead*) of the proximal third of the femur superimposed on an ongoing healing process as evident by solid periosteal reaction (*arrows*) along the femur

Fig. 21.20 (continued)

lines. Radiography has a poor sensitivity for detection in an early phase because of the lack of callus formation unless there is a superimposed acute fracture. MRI is very sensitive and specific for evaluation of these injuries. Linear region of T1 and T2 hypointensity (fracture line) with surrounding T2 hyperintensity (bone marrow edema) is characteristic.

Nonaccidental Trauma

Fractures are the second most common findings in nonaccidental trauma after dermatologic findings such as bruises, contusions, and burns. Skeletal survey is commonly performed in children under the age of 2 years suspected of nonaccidental trauma. This study helps showing fractures; in which up to half can be clinically occult. The role of radiologists is to detect and describe fractures with knowledge of the clinical history in cooperation with other specialists such as pediatricians. Several fractures are highly specific for inflicted injury including rib (especially posterior), classic metaphyseal lesion (CML, also known as corner fracture or bucket-handle fracture), spiral fracture of the femur, and fractures of the sternum, spine, and scapula (Figs. 21.21 and 21.22). Other fractures that should raise a suspicion of nonaccidental trauma are bilateral fractures, multiple fractures at various ages of healing, vertebral body fractures, epiphyseal separation, and digital fractures [18]. The CML is a fracture through the immature metaphysis of the long bone, resulting from twisting injury. It is frequently found in the femur, tibia, and humerus. Radiographic appearance differs when one views it from a different angle. A bucket-handle fracture fragment is seen en face, while a triangular "corner" fracture is depicted when viewed in profile [19].

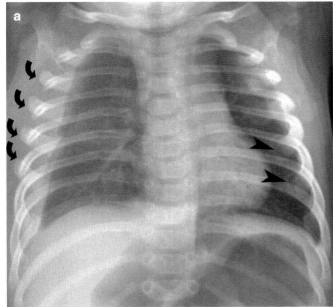

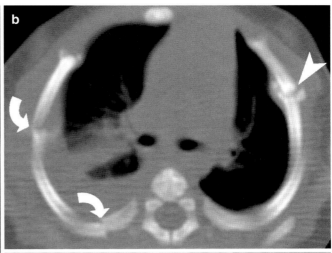

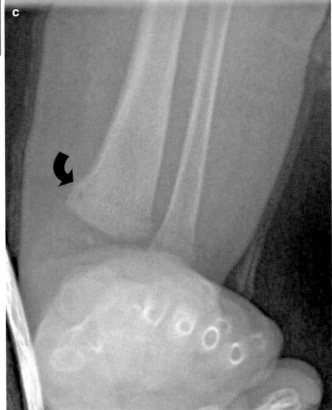

Fig. 21.22 Nonaccidental trauma. (**a**, **b**) Plain radiograph and CT of the chest demonstrates multiple right-sided acute rib fractures (*arrows*). There are multiple healing left-sided rib fractures (*arrowheads*). (**c**) Plain radiograph of the same patient demonstrates a healed distal tibial metaphyseal fracture (*arrow*)

References

1. Young JW, Burgess AR, Brumback RJ, Poka A. Pelvic fractures: value of plain radiography in early assessment and management. Radiology. 1986;160:445–51.
2. Denis F, Davis S, Comfort T. Sacral fractures: an important problem. Retrospective analysis of 236 cases. Clin Orthop Relat Res. 1988;227:67–81.
3. Saks BJ. Normal acetabular anatomy for acetabular fracture assessment: CT and plain film correlation. Radiology. 1986;159:139–45.
4. DeLee JC, Evans JA, Thomas J. Anterior dislocation of the hip and associated femoral-head fractures. J Bone Joint Surg Am. 1980; 62:960–4.
5. Pipkin G. Treatment of grade IV fracture-dislocation of the hip. J Bone Joint Surg Am. 1957;39-A:1027–42. Passim.
6. Garden RS. Low-angle fixation in fractures of the femoral neck. J Bone Joint Surg Br. 1961;43B:17.

7. Barnes R, Brown JT, Garden RS, Nicoll EA. Subcapital fractures of the femur. A prospective review. J Bone Joint Surg Br. 1976;58: 2–24.

8. Aichroth P. Osteochondritis dissecans of the knee. A clinical survey. J Bone Joint Surg Br. 1971;53:440–7.

9. Green NE, Allen BL. Vascular injuries associated with dislocation of the knee. J Bone Joint Surg Am. 1977;59:236–9.

10. Schatzker J, McBroom R, Bruce D. The tibial plateau fracture. The Toronto experience 1968--1975. Clin Orthop Relat Res. 1979; (138):94–104.

11. Medlar RC, Lyne ED. Sinding-Larsen-Johansson disease. Its etiology and natural history. J Bone Joint Surg Am. 1978;60:1113–6.

12. Pankovich AM. Maisonneuve fracture of the fibula. J Bone Joint Surg Am. 1976;58:337–42.

13. Danis R. Theorie et pratique de l' osteosynthese. Paris: Masson & Cie; 1949.

14. Weber BG. Die verletzungen des oberen sprunggelenkes. Bern: Huber; 1972.

15. Chen MY, Bohrer SP, Kelley TF. Boehler's angle: a reappraisal. Ann Emerg Med. 1991;20:122–4.

16. Hawkins LG. Fractures of the neck of the talus. J Bone Joint Surg Am. 1970;52:991–1002.

17. Lisfranc J. Nouvelle methode operatoire pour l'amputation partielle du pied dans son articulation tarso-metatarsienne: methode precedee des nombreuses modifications qu'a subies celle de Chopart. Paris: Gabon; 1815.

18. Kleinman PK, Marks Jr SC, Richmond JM, Blackbourne BD. Inflicted skeletal injury: a postmortem radiologic-histopathologic study in 31 infants. AJR Am J Roentgenol. 1995;165:647–50.

19. Kleinman PK, Marks SC, Blackbourne B. The metaphyseal lesion in abused infants: a radiologic-histopathologic study. AJR Am J Roentgenol. 1986;146:895–905.

Imaging of Spinal Trauma

Parul Penkar, Rathachai Kaewlai, Ajay Singh,
Laura Avery, and Robert A. Novelline

Introduction

Spine trauma accounts for significant mortality and morbidity. The annual incidence of spinal cord injury (SCI), excluding those who died at the scene of the accident, is approximately 40 cases per million population in the USA or approximately 12,000 new cases each year [1]. Spine trauma can result from blunt or penetrating trauma such as motor vehicle collisions, falls, diving injuries, industrial accidents, gunshot wounds, assault, and other miscellaneous causes. Pathological fractures usually occur from underlying osteoporosis, rheumatoid arthritis, malignancy, infection, and metabolic or endocrine conditions and usually cause compression fractures.

CT as Initial Cervical Spine Screening Modality

Most cervical spine fractures occur predominantly at two levels, at the level of C2 and at the level of C6 or C7. Unfortunately, 20–30 % of these fractures can be missed on plain radiographs. Current data and American College of Radiology Appropriateness Criteria recommend use of multidetector-row computed tomography (MDCT) as the initial screening examination in suspected cervical trauma instead of radiographs [2].

P. Penkar, MD • L. Avery, MD
Department of Radiology,
Massachusetts General Hospital, Boston, MA, USA

R. Kaewlai, MD
Department of Radiology,
Ramathibodi Hospital and Mahidol University,
Ratchatewi, Bangkok, Thailand

A. Singh, MD (✉) • R.A. Novelline, MD
Department of Radiology, Massachusetts General Hospital,
Harvard Medical School, 10 Museum Way, # 524,
Boston, MA 02141, USA
e-mail: asingh1@partners.org

The multicentric National Emergency X-Radiography Utilization Study (NEXUS) criteria which were based on clinical data and radiography of 34,069 patients found that their criteria had an overall sensitivity of 99.6 % in identifying patients at risk for cervical spine injury [3, 4]. Another clinical prediction prospective study on 8,924 patients, the Canadian C-spine Rule Study which was based on three main questions found that their clinical criteria had 100 % sensitivity and 42.5 % specificity for identifying clinically important cervical spine injuries [5]. It is debatable if radiography should be obtained in patients with low risk for cervical spine injury, but recent ACR Appropriateness Criteria recommends no imaging in patients who satisfy any of the "low-risk" criteria and CT imaging in patients who do not fall in the low-risk category [2, 4, 5].

NEXUS Criteria

Imaging is unnecessary if all of the five following criteria are met:
1. Absence of posterior midline cervical tenderness
2. No focal neurological deficits
3. Normal level alertness
4. No evidence of intoxication
5. No painful distracting injures

A retrospective study at our institution showed that in patients with low clinical suspicion for cervical spine trauma who had plain film radiography, the overall positivity rate for acute cervical spine fractures was 0.0 %. This data indicates that radiography for patient with low risk for cervical spine trauma may have too low a yield to justify its use and could be explained by the fact that the radiographs were done on patients who do not meet the validated NEXUS criteria or Canadian C-spine rule (Fig. 22.1a) [6, 7]. In a meta-analysis of seven studies with strict inclusion criteria, the pooled sensitivity of radiography for detecting patients with cervical spine injury was 52 %, while the combined sensitivity of CT was 98 % [2, 8–10].

A. Singh (ed.), *Emergency Radiology*,
DOI 10.1007/978-1-4419-9592-6_22, © Springer Science+Business Media New York 2013

In case if cervical plain radiographs are obtained for trauma due to unavailability of emergent CT, an adequate cervical spine series must include five views: a true lateral view, which must include all seven cervical vertebrae and the cervicothoracic junction; an anteroposterior view; an open-mouth odontoid view; and both the oblique views. A swimmer's view may be necessary to adequately show the lower cervical spine. Any film series that does not include these five views or which does not visualize all seven cervical vertebrae and the junction of C7–T1 is inadequate.

Flexion and extension views of the cervical spine are contraindicated in case of cervical spine fracture. They were used in the past for suspected ligamentous injuries; however, currently they have been replaced by MRI for suspected soft tissue trauma. In rare instances, they have been used for detecting new malalignment or exaggeration of the existing listhesis in patients with degenerative changes and in patients with equivocal MRI findings.

Cervical Spine Lines and Spaces

The cervical spine lines should be continuous curves through the bony elements regardless of the degree of flexion or extension, and any misalignment of these lines should be viewed as a sign of ligamentous injuries or occult fractures. The exception to this finding would be from anterior pseudosubluxation ligamentous laxity, which can occur at the C2–C3 level and less commonly at the C3–C4 level. Normal cervical spine

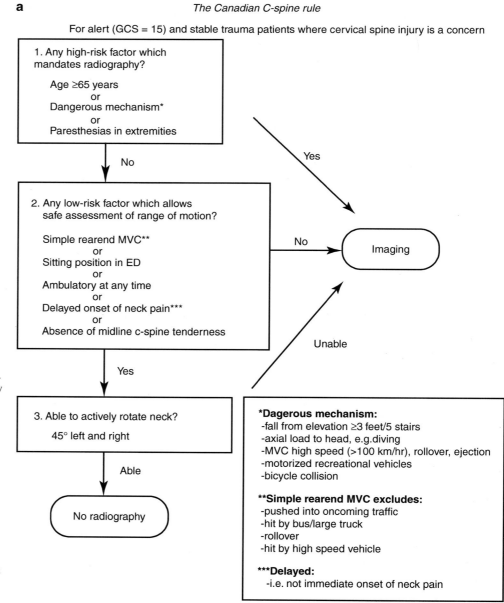

Fig. 22.1 (**a**) The Canadian C-spine rule (Adapted with permission from Stiell et al. [27]). (**b, c**) Normal lines on lateral view of the cervical spine. (**b**) On the lateral radiograph of the cervical spine, the anterior spinal line (*3*), posterior spinal line (*2*), and spinolaminar line (*1*) are located along the anterior cortex of vertebral bodies, posterior cortex of vertebral bodies, and spinolaminar junctions, respectively. (**c**) Discontinuous anterior spinal line (*3*), posterior spinal line (*2*), and spinolaminar line (*1*) are seen on lateral radiograph of the cervical spine in a patient with type 2 dens fracture (*arrowhead*)

a   *The Canadian C-spine rule*

For alert (GCS = 15) and stable trauma patients where cervical spine injury is a concern

1. Any high-risk factor which mandates radiography?

Age ≥65 years
or
Dangerous mechanism*
or
Paresthesias in extremities

No

2. Any low-risk factor which allows safe assessment of range of motion?

Simple rearend MVC**
or
Sitting position in ED
or
Ambulatory at any time
or
Delayed onset of neck pain***
or
Absence of midline c-spine tenderness

Yes

3. Able to actively rotate neck?

45° left and right

Able

No radiography

Yes

No

Unable

Imaging

*Dagerous mechanism:
-fall from elevation ≥3 feet/5 stairs
-axial load to head, e.g.diving
-MVC high speed (>100 km/hr), rollover, ejection
-motorized recreational vehicles
-bicycle collision

**Simple rearend MVC excludes:
-pushed into oncoming traffic
-hit by bus/large truck
-rollover
-hit by high speed vehicle

***Delayed:
-i.e. not immediate onset of neck pain

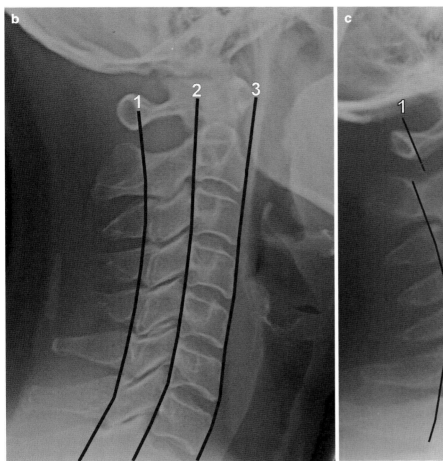
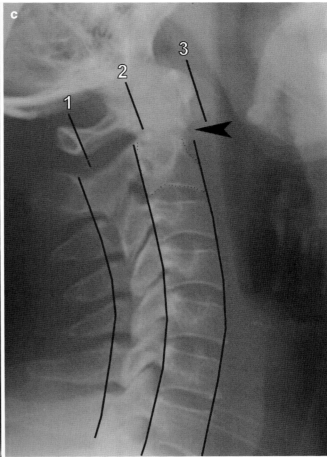

Fig. 22.1 (continued)

lordosis can sometimes be reversed due to the presence of cervical collar, patient positioning, or muscle spasm.

There are four basic lines to evaluate alignment on lateral view of the cervical spine (Fig. 22.1b, c). These lines include anterior spinal line, posterior spinal line, spinolaminar line, and posterior spinous process line.

Predental Space or Atlanto-Dens Interval Space

The space between the odontoid process and the anterior portion of the ring of C1 should be less than 3.5 mm in adults and less than 5 mm in children. An increase in this space is presumptive evidence of a fracture of C1 or of the odontoid process, although it may also represent ligamentous injury at this level.

Prevertebral Space

Prevertebral soft tissue swelling (more than 6 mm at C2, more than 22 mm at C6) is highly specific for a fracture but not very

sensitive. Soft tissue swelling in symptomatic patients should be considered an indication for further radiographic evaluation.

Interspinous and Intervertebral Distance

The spinous processes are examined to evaluate for abnormal widening or fanning of the spinous processes. If abnormal widening of the intervertebral or interspinous distance or angulation of more than 10° is present, a ligamentous injury or fracture should be considered.

Basion-axial interval (BAI) is the distance from the basion (inferior tip of the clivus) to a line drawn along the posterior body of C2, which should measure less than 12 mm.

Vertical basion-dens distance should measure less than 12 mm.

Indication for CT or MR Angiogram

Concomitant arterial injury although rare can occur with penetrating or blunt cervical spine injury causing intimal tears or rupture of the vasa vasorum leading to intramural hematoma, traumatic dissections, stenosis or occlusion, pseudoaneurysms, or rarely transection. CT or MR angiogram is noninvasive and should be obtained in patients with a high clinical suspicion, neurological deficits, if the cervical fracture is extending into the carotid canal or foramen tranversarium and in patients with severe trauma such as facet dislocation, vertebral subluxation, or multiple fractures. Vertebral arterial injury tends to be more common than carotid arterial injury due to close proximity to the spine. Imaging findings are depicted as intimal flaps, segmental or focal narrowing, or occlusions on CT or MR angiograms.

Indication for Spine MRI

In patients with severe fractures, neurological deficits, significant pain, or high clinical suspicion based on the mechanism of injury, MRI of the spine should be obtained to evaluate for ligamentous injuries, traumatic disk herniation, spinal cord edema, cord contusion or compression, spinal cord transection, or prevertebral, intramedullary, or epidural hematoma. The utility of obtaining MRI in obtunded patients with negative spine CT findings is still debatable; however, recent evidence suggests that if an adequate neurological exam cannot be carried out in the first 24 h, MRI of the spine should be obtained, especially in high-speed trauma where ligamentous or soft tissue injury of the cervical spine is a possibility. The following sequences are usually obtained in trauma MRI, sagittal and axial T1-weighted images, sagittal and axial T2-weighted images, and sagittal gradient sequence.

Classification of Cervical Spine Fractures

Cervical spine fractures are classified based on the mechanism of injury and only the commonly encountered fractures will be discussed further [11, 12] (Tables 22.1, 22.2, 22.3, and 22.4).

Cervical Spine Fractures

Atlantooccipital Dissociation

Complete dislocation is fatal due to stretching injury of the brain stem. Subluxation is rare and can be missed on plain films. It should be suspected in patients with severe facial trauma, and the current methods used to determine subluxation are based on the distances between the occiput and axis which are as follows: Basion-axial interval (BAI) is the distance from the basion (inferior tip of the clivus) to a line drawn along the posterior body of C2, which should measure less than 12 mm. Vertical Basion-dens distance which should measure less than 12 mm (Fig. 22.2).

Table 22.1 Cervical injury by flexion mechanism

Mechanism	Submechanism	Fracture
Flexion	Flexion-distraction and rotational forces	Unilateral or bilateral facet dislocation, anterior subluxation
	Hyperflexion and compression	Flexion teardrop fracture
	Hyperflexion avulsion forces	Clay-shoveler's fracture
	Anterior compression	Wedge compression fracture

Table 22.2 Cervical injury by extension mechanism

Mechanism	Submechanism	Fracture
Extension	Hyperextension with distraction	Hangman's fracture
	Hyperextension with axial loading	Hyperextension sprain and fracture-dislocation
	Severe hyperextension	Lamina fracture
	Rotation and impaction	Pillar fracture
	Avulsion forces	Extension teardrop fracture
	Hyperextension and compression	Posterior arch of C1 fracture

Table 22.3 Cervical injury by axial loading

Mechanism	Submechanism	Fracture
Axial load	Burst compression	Jefferson fracture, Jefferson variants, and lateral mass fractures
	Vertical axial compression	Burst fractures

Table 22.4 Cervical injury by complex mechanism

Mechanism	Submechanism	Fracture
Complex	Severe extension or flexion with distraction and posterior translation	Atlantooccipital dissociation
	Severe flexion-extension, distraction, and rotational forces	Atlantoaxial instability
	Flexion or extension loading	Odontoid fracture

Occipital Condyle Fractures

These fractures are discussed with spine trauma due to the mechanism and their association with other cervical spine fractures. They occur from high-energy blunt trauma due to axial loading and lateral bending. Fractures of the occipital condyles are often undiagnosed on plain radiography and prevertebral soft tissue swelling may be the only radiographic marker (Fig. 22.3). These fractures may extend into the hypoglossal canal or the jugular foramen; therefore, clinical signs of injury to cranial nerves IX to XII may be found.

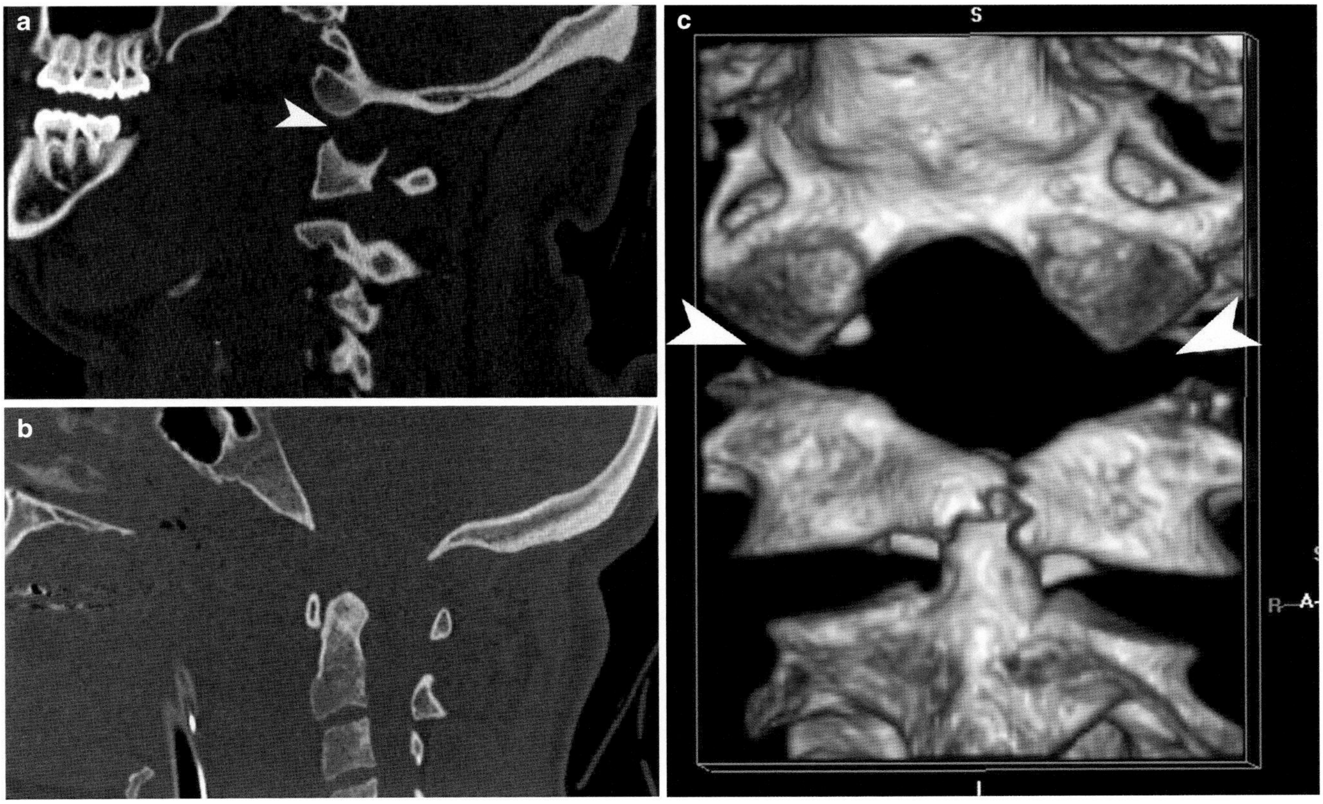

Fig. 22.2 Atlantooccipital dissociation. (**a**–**c**) Midline Sagittal CT reformation, parasagittal CT reformation, and 3D image shows widening to the atlantooccipital joint (*arrowheads*) and increased distance between the dens and the clivus

Anderson-Montesano divides occipital condyle fractures into three types (Table 22.5):

Jefferson Fracture

This occurs with axial loading injury with downward compression forces to C1, through the occipital condyles which can cause Jefferson fracture, Jefferson variants, or lateral mass fractures. The classic Jefferson fracture is a four-part fracture of the anterior and posterior arches (Fig. 22.4a). Jefferson variants are two- and three-part fractures (Fig. 22.4b) with the most common one being fracture of one anterior and two posterior arches. On frontal radiography, the presence of Jefferson fracture is implied by offset of the lateral masses of C1 relative to C2 and widening of the atlantodental interval. On MDCT with reformats, the fracture is easy to identify. These fractures can be unstable, if they are associated with disruption of the transverse atlantal ligament which fixes the dens to the anterior arch of C1 or when the lateral mass cumulative displacement is greater than 7 mm, if the atlanto-dens interval is greater than 5 mm or when they are associated with C2 fractures. Neurological compromise is infrequent as the fractures cause widening of the C1, thereby limiting cord compression. If the axial loading force is eccentric, a lateral mass

fracture may result. This fracture is often associated with fracture of the occipital condyle or articular process, and they are regarded as unstable fractures because the transverse atlantal ligament is often detached.

Dens Fracture

Anderson and D'Alonso classified dens fracture based on the location as types 1, 2, and 3 (Table 22.6). Type 1 fracture (Fig. 22.5a) is rare but stable. Type 2 (either acute or ununited) (Fig. 22.5b) and Type 3 fractures (Fig. 22.6) are considered unstable because they can result in atlantoaxial instability (since the ligaments, proximal fragment, C1, and occiput act as a single unit during motion).

Anomalies of Dens

The os terminale is an ossification center at the tip of the dens, which normally fuses by 12 years of age but may remain unfused in adulthood and simulate a type 1 fracture. The os odontoideum formation is debatable as some authors think it is congenital due to lack of fusion with the base of the dens or posttraumatic fracture of the synchondrosis before closure at

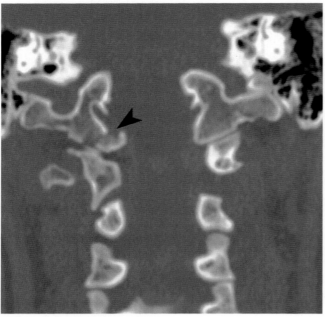

Fig. 22.3 Occipital condyle fracture. Coronal CT of the cervicothoracic junction shows minimal medially displaced oblique fracture (*arrowhead*) of the right occipital condyle

Table 22.5 Types of occipital condyle fractures

Types	Description
1	Comminuted impacted vertically oriented fracture without or with minimal displacement. Usually stable unless bilateral
2	More extensive skull base fracture extending into one or both the occipital condyles
3	Inferior medial avulsion fracture caused by a pull of the alar ligament with medial displacement of the fragment into the foramen magnum. Generally considered unstable since the contralateral alar ligament or tectorial ligament may be compromised and stressed resulting in partial or complete tear or if the degree of displacement is greater than 5 mm, if concomitant atlantooccipital dislocation is present, or if the fractures are bilateral

Table 22.6 Types of dens fracture

Types	Description
1	Rare oblique fracture involving the superolateral aspect of the dens from avulsion of the alar ligaments and are usually stable injuries
2	Most frequent unstable transverse fracture involving the base of the dens
3	Unstable fracture involving the base of the dens extending into the lateral masses and body of the axis. It has a better prognosis for healing because of the larger surface involved

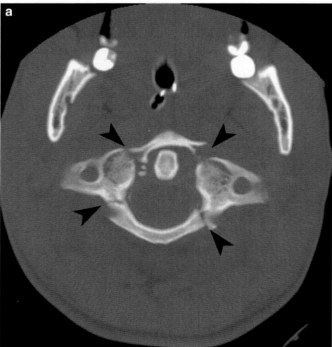
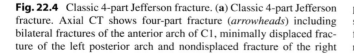
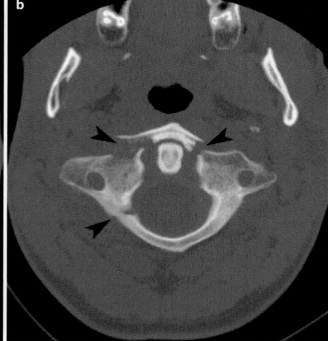

Fig. 22.4 Classic 4-part Jefferson fracture. (**a**) Classic 4-part Jefferson fracture. Axial CT shows four-part fracture (*arrowheads*) including bilateral fractures of the anterior arch of C1, minimally displaced fracture of the left posterior arch and nondisplaced fracture of the right posterior arch of C1. (**b**) 3-part Jefferson fracture variant. Axial CT shows three-part fracture (*arrowheads*) including displaced bilateral fractures of the anterior arch of C1 and nondisplaced fracture of the right posterior arch of C1

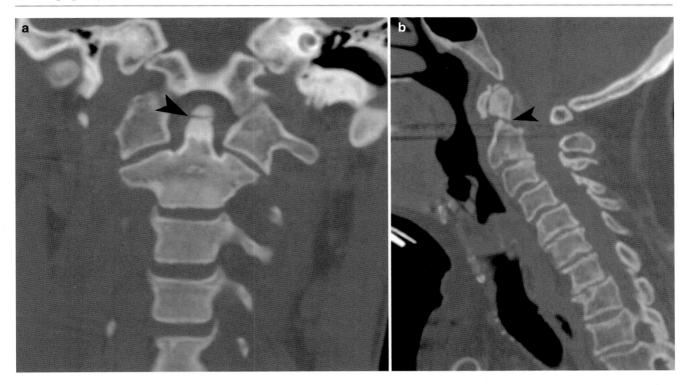

Fig. 22.5 Dens fracture. (**a**) Type 1 dens fracture. Coronal CT shows transverse fracture (*arrowhead*) through the tip of the dens. (**b**) Type 2 dens fracture. Sagittal CT shows oblique fracture (*arrowhead*) through the base of the dens, with mild anterior displacement and angulation of the superior dens

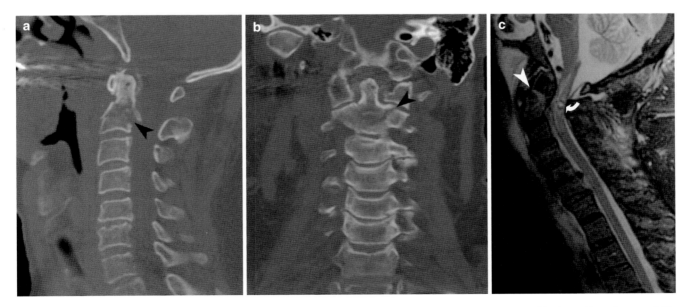

Fig. 22.6 Type 3 dens fracture. (**a**) Sagittal CT shows comminuted fracture (*arrowhead*) of the dens extending into the body with mild retropulsion of the superior dens into the spinal canal. Marked prevertebral soft tissue swelling is also noted. (**b**) Coronal CT shows the fracture (*arrowhead*) extending into the vertebral body and lateral mass of C2. (**c**) Sagittal MPGR MRI demonstrates fracture through the dens (*arrowhead*) with posterior displacement of the superior dens, spinal stenosis, cord edema (*curved arrow*), contusion, and hemorrhage

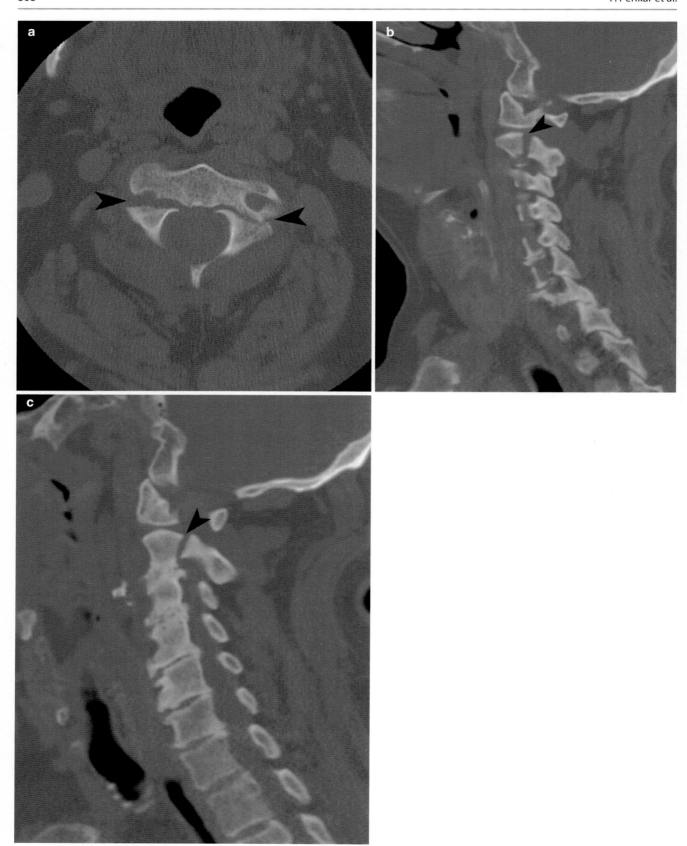

Fig. 22.7 Hangman's fracture. (**a**) Axial CT shows minimally displaced fracture (*arrowheads*) extending through the bilateral pars interarticularis of C2. (**b, c**) Parasagittal CT shows vertical fracture (*arrowhead*) through the C2 pars interarticularis

Table 22.7 Hangman's fracture classification

Types	Description
1	Normal C2/C3 disk space and less than 3 mm anterior translation of C2 on C3
2	Greater than 3 mm anterior translation, C2/C3 disk disruption, angulation of more than 10°, and significant disruption of the posterior longitudinal ligament and slight disruption of the anterior longitudinal ligament
3	Includes all the characteristics of type 2 plus unilateral or bilateral facet dislocation

Table 22.8 Types of rotatory fixation

Types	Description
1	Rotatory fixation without anterior displacement of the atlas
2	Rotatory fixation with anterior displacement of the C1 of 3–5 mm. Transverse ligament may be compromised
3	Rotatory fixation with more than 5 mm anterior displacement of C1 lateral masses, one greater than the other. Transverse and alar ligaments are compromised
4	Rotatory fixation with posterior displacement of the lateral masses of C1 on C2

age 5–6 years resulting in a large ossicle that is separated from the hypoplastic dens by a wide gap. It may be fixed to the arch of C1 or the clivus and may simulate a nonunited dens fracture or rarely result in atlantoaxial instability [8].

Hangman's Fracture

Bilateral pars interarticularis fracture at C2 is known as hangman's fracture and usually also involves the bilateral neural arches and the pedicles causing traumatic spondylolysis or spondylolisthesis (Fig. 22.7). They have been classified by Effindi and modified by Levine as follows (Table 22.7):

Atlantoaxial Instability

Atlantoaxial instability can be posttraumatic, congenital, or secondary to rheumatoid arthritis. There is excessive movement at the C1–C2 junction ranging from subluxation to dislocation due to excessive laxity or rupture of the transverse ligament with or without alar and tectorial membrane involvement. Instability can lead to compression of the spinal canal between the dens and posterior arch of C1 or vertebrobasilar artery insufficiency. There is widening of the atlanto-dens interval with asymmetrical distance between the lateral masses of C1 and dens, misalignment of the lateral masses of C1 and C2, and discontinuity of the spinolaminar line. Associated dens fracture is common.

In atlantoaxial rotatory subluxation, there is fixation of the atlantoaxial joint, so that C1–C2 joint moves as a single unit instead of rotating independently [13–15]. Atlantoaxial rotatory subluxation is divided into four subtypes according to Fielding and Hawkins [14] (Table 22.8). Types 3 and 4 are rare but have fatal consequences. Fixed rotatory subluxation is diagnosed if the distance from the dens to the C1 lateral mass on one side is persistently widened on all images compared to the other side when the head is imaged in the neutral, left, and right positions (Fig. 22.8).

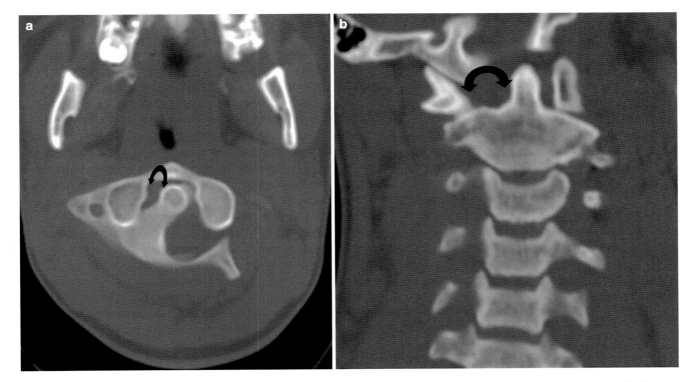

Fig. 22.8 Rotational subluxation. (**a**, **b**) Axial and coronal CT images show asymmetrical fixed widening (*curved arrows*) of the distance between the dens-lateral mass of C1 on the *right* when compared to the *left*. This is consistent with rotational subluxation

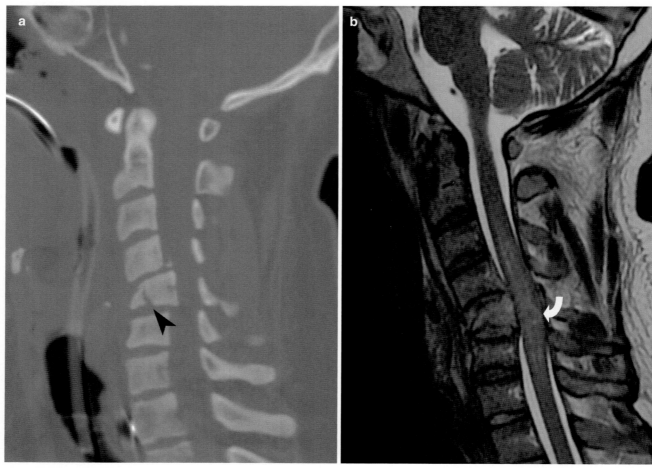

Fig. 22.9 Flexion teardrop fracture of C5. (**a**) Sagittal CT shows teardrop fracture (*arrowhead*) involving the anterior and inferior aspect of the C5 vertebral body with mild retropulsion of the posterior vertebral body into the spinal canal. Note the irregularity of the left posterior/ inferior corner of the C4 vertebral body with small adjacent bony fragment (*arrow*) consistent with a small corner fracture. (**b**) Sagittal T2-weighted MRI shows abnormal signal in the spinal cord (*curved arrow*) consistent with edema and hemorrhagic contusion

Flexion Teardrop Fracture

This is one of the most severe injuries of the cervical spine resulting from severe flexion and compression force injuries [8, 16]. This fracture most commonly occurs at C5–C6 and is characterized by a triangular teardrop fracture at the anterior-inferior aspect of the vertebral body with posterior displacement of the comminuted posterior vertebral body to varying degrees in the spinal canal, kyphosis, anterior subluxation, narrowing of the disk space, widening of the interspinous and interlaminar spaces, and disruption of the ligaments (Fig. 22.9). It can result in anterior cervical cord syndrome (quadriplegia, loss of pain, touch, and temperature with intact vibration, and proprioception).

Facet Dislocation

Unilateral interfacetal dislocation or unilateral locked facet results from flexion-distraction and rotation injury and usually occurs at C4–C5 and C5–C6 levels. It is characterized by

focal kyphosis and anterior subluxation by approximately 25 % of the vertebral body with the inferior articular facet of the superior vertebral body perched or locked anterior to superior facet of the inferior vertebral body or in the intervertebral foramen while the contralateral facet joint on the side of the rotational forces is fixed and acts as the pivot (Fig. 22.10). The spinous processes are malaligned at the level of the injury [13, 17]. There is concomitant injury of the posterior spinous ligamentous complex to varying degrees on the affected side (supraspinous and interspinous ligaments, posterior longitudinal ligament, annulus, ligamentum flavum, and facet joint capsule) and impaction fracture of the facets. Neurological deficits are rare and are of nerve root distribution.

Bilateral interfacetal dislocation results from more severe flexion-distraction injury. The dislocated facet joints may be perched or "jump" over one another to become locked. There is subluxation of the vertebral body by more than 50 %, and both the anterior and posterior ligamentous structures are disrupted at the site of the injury with fracture of the superior and inferior articular facets and disk extrusion (Fig. 22.11). There is a high degree of neurological deficits with this

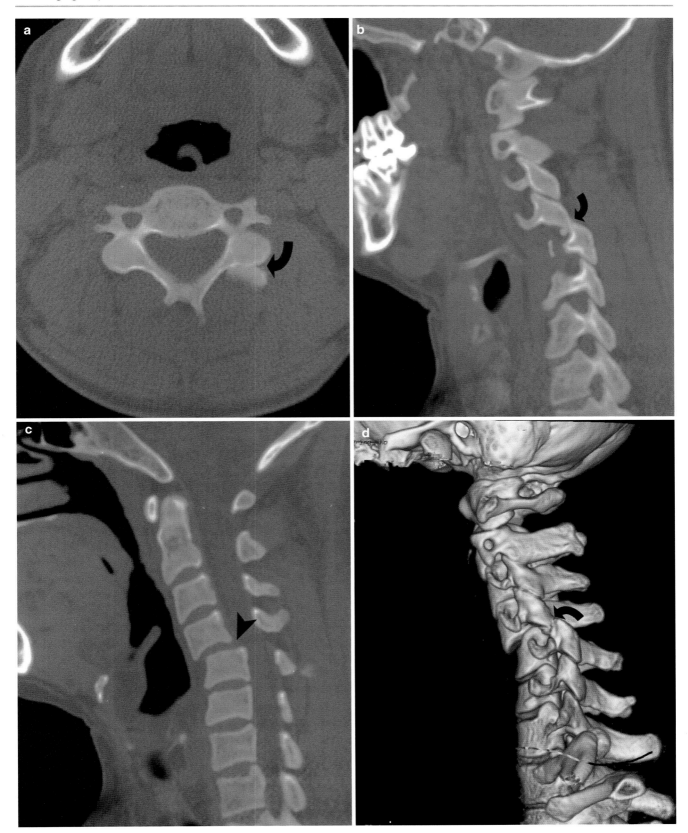

Fig. 22.10 Unilateral facet dislocation. (**a**) Axial CT shows reverse hamburger's bun sign (*curved arrow*); the left inferior articular facet of C4 is dislocated anterior to the superior articular facet of C5. (**b**) Left parasagittal CT shows unilateral left dislocated C4–5 facets (*curved arrow*). A small fracture fragment in the left C4–C5 interfacet joint space from superior articular process of C5 is also noted. (**c**) Midline sagittal CT shows grade 2 anterolisthesis (*arrowhead*) of C4 on C5. (**d**) Right parasagittal CT shows subluxed right C4–C5 facets (*arrowhead*)

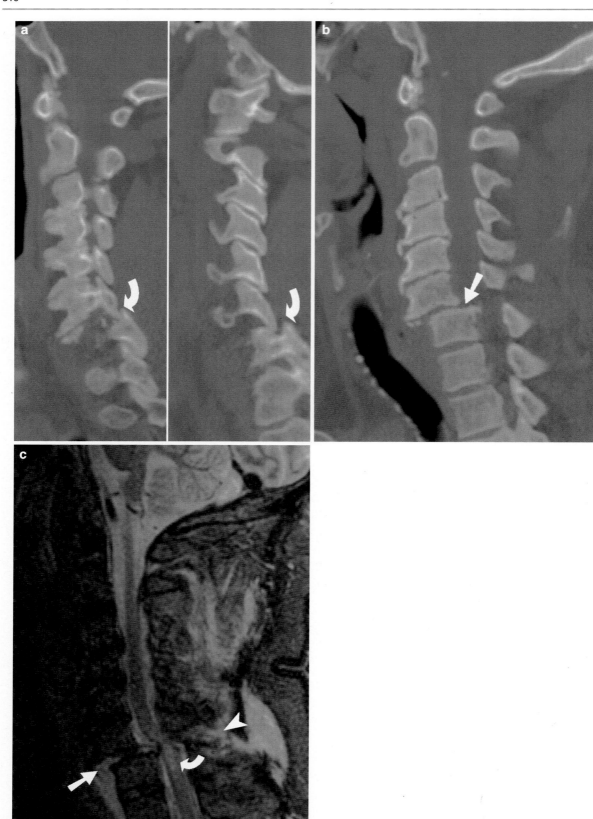

injury. The "reverse hamburger bun sign" refers to reversal of the normal articulating facet relationship with the rounded instead of the flat surfaces of the facets facing each other at the site of facet dislocation and the "naked facet sign" which refers to uncovered articulating facets processes with loss of the joint space.

Clay-Shoveler's Fracture

This is a stable fracture of the spinous processes of the lower cervical and upper thoracic vertebrae usually C6 to T1 from severe hyperflexion injury. There is sudden strenuous exertion of the paraspinal muscles, mainly the trapezius and rhomboid and the supraspinous ligaments causing avulsion of the spinous process (Fig. 22.12). A less common mechanism of injury is from direct trauma to the spinous process. The fracture is generally considered to be mechanically stable; however, if the fracture line extends to the lamina, there is a potential for spinal cord injuries.

Hyperextension Teardrop Fracture and Sprains

There is a corner avulsion fracture of the anteroinferior aspect of the C2 or C3 vertebral body by the anterior longitudinal ligament and tear of the annulus fibrosis from hyperextension injury (Fig. 22.13). Hyperextension sprains are seen in young adults with high-energy trauma, and fracture-dislocation occurs in elderly with underlying bone and joint diseases (ankylosing spondylitis, diffuse idiopathic skeletal hyperostosis (DISH), spondylosis, congenital spinal stenosis, and severe degenerative disk disease). Hyperextension sprains are soft tissue injuries occurring from blunt trauma to the face with resultant hyperextension of the cervical spine causing injury to the anterior column with intact tear or disruption of the longus colli, longus capitis, anterior longitudinal ligament, anterior annulus, detachment or tear of the intervertebral disk, anterior vertebral plate fracture, ligamentum flavum, and posterior longitudinal ligament [18, 19]. Momentary posterior dislocations may occur and reduce spontaneously but cause central cord syndrome (disproportionate greater neurological motor deficits in the upper extremities than in the lower extremities, variable sensory deficits below the level of the injury, and bladder dysfunction) due to compression of the spinal cord between the

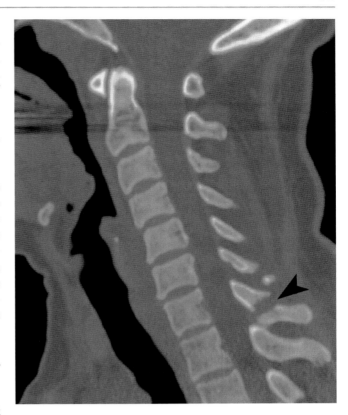

Fig. 22.12 Clay-shoveler's fracture. Sagittal CT shows displaced fracture (*arrowhead*) involving the posterior spinous processes of C7

posterior vertebral body and ligamentum flavum. Imaging findings may be subtle and show prevertebral soft tissue swelling, widening of the intervertebral disk space, and small avulsion fracture fragment arising from the anterior aspect of the inferior end plate of the dislocated vertebra (Figs. 22.14 and 22.15). In elderly patients with fracture-dislocation, there is posterior displacement of the vertebral body, fracture of the posterior elements, and facet joint disruption.

Pillar and Laminar Fractures

Pillar fracture is a type of articular facet impaction fracture from the suprajacent articular facet resulting from hyperextension and rotation injuries often extending into the transverse process or the lamina. Isolated lamina fractures are rare and are usually associated with other complex fractures and dislocations such as burst fractures,

Fig. 22.11 Bilateral facet dislocation. (**a**) Parasagittal right and left CT shows bilateral anteriorly dislocated facets (*curved arrows*) at C6–C7. Note is also made of small bony fractures in the right C6–C7 joint space from inferior and superior articular facets of C6 and C7, respectively. (**b**) Midline sagittal CT shows grade 2 anterolisthesis (*arrow*) of C6 on C7. The small bony fragments (*arrow*) are from the

fracture of the inferior end plate of C6. (**c**) Sagittal STIR MRI shows grade 2 anterolisthesis (*straight arrow*) at C6–C7, traumatic disk rupture, severe central canal stenosis, cord compression, and spinal cord compression (*curved arrow*) at this level. There is abnormal T2 hyperintensity consistent with anterior and posterior longitudinal ligaments and interspinous ligaments disruption (*arrowhead*)

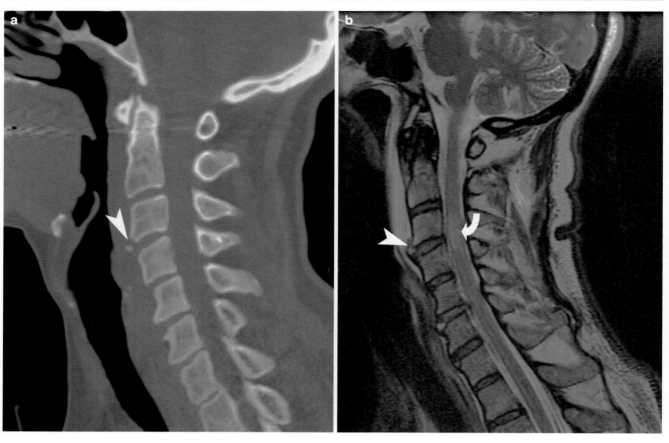

Fig. 22.13 Hyperextension teardrop fracture. (**a**) Sagittal CT reformation shows small displaced teardrop fracture (*arrowhead*) of the anterior and inferior aspect of the C3 vertebral body. (**b**) Sagittal T2 FSE MRI shows teardrop fracture with small tear (*arrowhead*) of the anterior longitudinal ligament and prevertebral edema. Associated spinal cord contusion (*curved arrow*) at the level of C3/C4

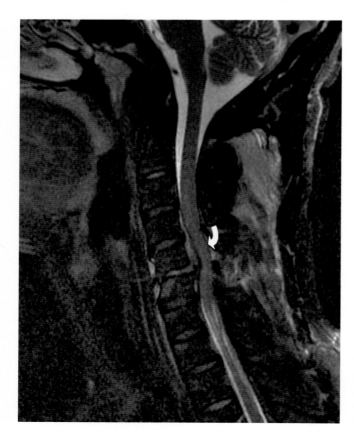

Fig. 22.14 Hyperextension injury. Sagittal T2-weighted FSE MRI shows mild kyphosis and grade 1 anterolisthesis of C5 on C6. Traumatic disk extrusion, severe central canal stenosis at C5–C6, and spinal cord contusion (*curved arrow*) from C4–C7 levels are also seen

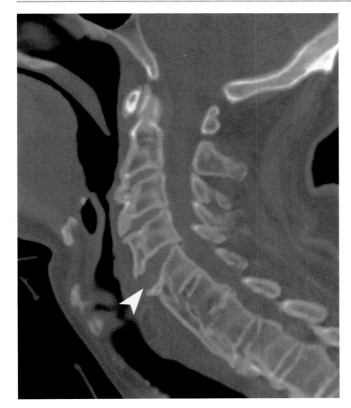

Fig. 22.15 Hyperextension injury in a patient with diffuse idiopathic spinal hyperostosis (DISH). Sagittal CT shows hyperextension injury, indicated by grade 1 retrolisthesis at C4–C5 with fracture through the anterior longitudinal ligament ossification (*arrowhead*) causing asymmetrical C4–C5 disk space widening

Table 22.9 Denis system of classification of compression fractures

Types	Description
A	Involves both the superior and inferior end plates
B	Involves only the superior end plate (most common type)
C	Involves only the inferior end plate (rare and usually occurs with pathological fractures)
D	Buckling or wedging of the anterior cortex with sparing of the superior and inferior end plates

height. The posterior cortex and posterior ligaments are intact; therefore, the fracture is considered to be stable [20]. Burst fracture is more common in the thoracolumbar spine but can also occur in the cervical spine and results from axial compression forces. It is characterized by comminuted vertical fracture of the vertebral body with anterior wedging, retropulsion of the bony fragments into spinal canal to varying degrees, and associated fractures of the posterior elements [21].

Thoracic and Lumbar Spine Fractures

Screening for thoracolumbar spine injuries has become easier with the advent of MDCT in polytrauma patients, in whom reformatted images of the thoracic and lumbar spine can be obtained from the chest-abdomen-pelvis scans. Recent data indicates that the reformatted spine images obtained from the body scans have practically replaced plain radiographs as they provide more information and also avoids additional radiation to the patient [2]. Dedicated spine CTs are reserved for cases where concurrent body imaging was not indicated. MRI of the lumbar and thoracic spine is obtained in patients with significant fractures and suspected cord or ligamentous injuries. Since the mechanism of trauma in both the thoracic and lumbar spine is similar, they will be discussed together.

Anterior and Lateral Wedge Compression Fractures

This is a common stable fracture due to axial loading and varying degrees of flexion forces [13]. There is buckling of the anterior cortex with involvement of the superior end plate and/or the inferior end plate causing a wedge-shaped vertebral body. The middle and posterior columns are intact. These fractures can occur at multiple levels in 20 % of the cases and can be further classified based on the Denis system of classification [22] which is based on the involvement of the vertebral plate (Table 22.9).

In lateral wedge compression fractures, the wedge deformity involves the lateral instead of the anterior cortex. They usually occur in the mid thoracic spine due to lateral flexion forces and are mostly insufficiency fractures.

pedicolaminar fracture-separation, and flexion teardrop fracture. They can be further divided into vertical fracture with compression of the vertebral body usually due to axial loading with or without rotation and transverse fractures which are avulsion fractures due to tear of the ligamentum flavum. Isolated laminar fractures are mechanically stable but neurological sequelae may result from fragments within the cervical spinal canal.

Posterior Arch of C1 Fracture

Isolated fracture of the posterior arch of C1 is due to hyperextension and compressive forces causing compression of the posterior arch of C1 between the occiput and the spinous process of C2. It is considered to be a stable fracture as there is lack of ligamentous involvement.

Wedge and Burst Compression Fracture

Wedge compression fracture is characterized by buckled anterior cortex with loss of the anterior vertebral body

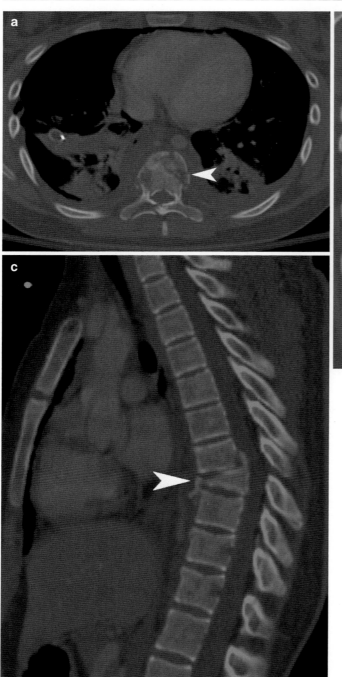

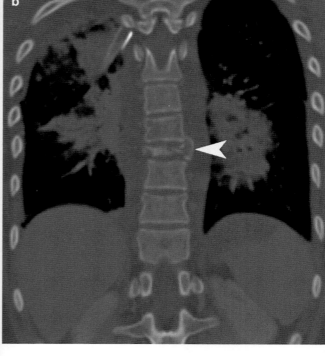

Fig. 22.16 Burst fracture with paraspinal hematoma. (**a**) Axial CT shows bilateral paraspinal hematoma adjacent to the T6 burst fracture (*arrowhead*). There are bilateral lower lobe pulmonary contusions. (**b**, **c**) Coronal and sagittal CT shows diffuse bilateral paraspinal hematoma due to burst fracture of T6 vertebral body (*arrowhead*). There is also fracture of the posteroinferior aspect of T5 vertebral body

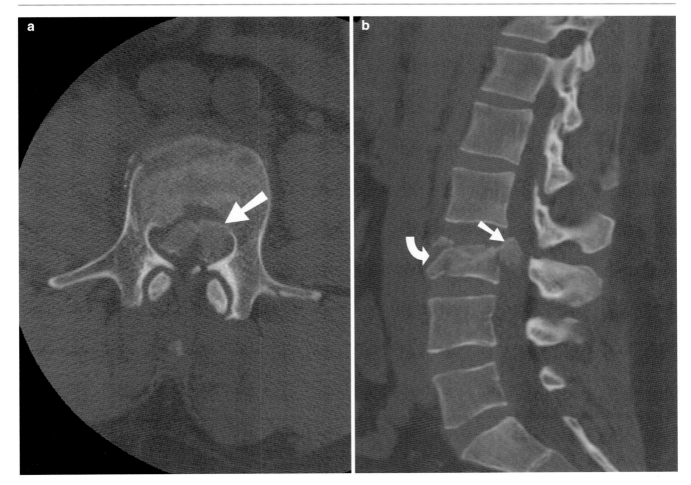

Fig. 22.17 Burst fracture. (**a**) Axial CT shows burst fracture of the L3 vertebral body with retropulsion of multiple bony fragments (*straight arrow*) into the spinal canal, causing severe spinal stenosis. (**b**) Sagittal CT shows similar findings of the L3 burst compression fracture (*curved arrow*) with significant loss of height and retropulsion (*straight arrow*)

Burst Fracture

Burst fractures occur from vertical compression forces resulting in comminuted fracture of the vertebral body [13, 23]. It involves both the superior and inferior vertebral end plates with loss of height and bowing deformity of the posterior cortex or retropulsion of the bony fragments to varying degrees into the spinal canal (Figs. 22.16, 22.17, and 22.18). They may be associated with concomitant facet fractures, and there is a high risk of neurological deficits. There may be associated bilateral calcaneal fractures due to mechanism of the injury; therefore, in patients with bilateral calcaneal fractures, the thoracic and lumbar spines need to be imaged for additional fractures.

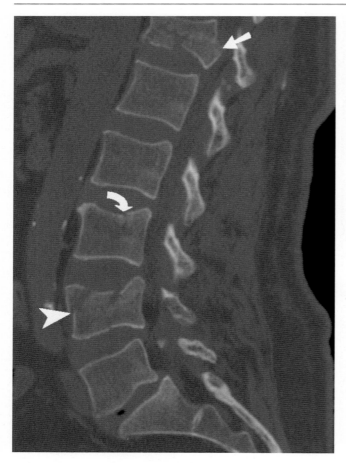

Fig. 22.18 Multiple vertebral body fractures. Sagittal CT shows burst fracture of T12 with retropulsion of the bony fragment (*straight arrow*) into the spinal canal. There is also superior end plate fracture of the L3 (*curved arrow*) and compression fracture of L4 vertebral bodies (*arrowhead*)

Chance Fracture

This is unstable horizontal fracture due to flexion-distraction impaction type of injury causing compression of the anterior vertebral body and distraction of the middle and posterior columns due to failure in tension of all the three columns (Fig. 22.19). The classic Chance fracture from seat belt trauma extends through the spinous process, lamina, pedicles, intervertebral disk space, posterior portion of the vertebral body or anterior wedging of the vertebral body and complex ligamentous involvement of the interspinous and supraspinous ligaments, posterior longitudinal ligament, posterior annulus, facet capsule, ligamentum flavum, and thoracodorsal fascia [13]. Fractures occur at the thoracolumbar junction or in the upper lumbar spine (T10 to L2). Neurological deficits depend on the severity of the fracture, but associated abdominal injuries (pancreatic, duodenal injuries) are common.

Other Miscellaneous Fractures

Fracture dislocations can occur from shearing distraction injuries or severe hyperflexion or hyperextension forces. They are characterized by ligamentous injuries with facet dislocation or posterior elements involvement depending on the mechanism [24]. These are unstable fractures with associated severe neurological deficits, dural tears, and abdominal injuries.

Transverse process and spinous process fractures can occur in isolation or in association with other fractures and typically occur at multiple levels. They are stable fractures; however, depending on the mechanism of injury, there may be associated trauma to the thoracic, abdominal, or pelvic structures.

Spine MRI

Ligamentous Injury

MRI of the spine is useful for imaging of the ligamentous structures such as the anterior and posterior longitudinal ligaments, interspinous and supraspinous ligaments, and ligamentum flavum. Ligamentous injuries are usually depicted as discontinuity or tears of the anterior or posterior longitudinal ligaments with or without associated hematoma [25]. Diffuse prevertebral soft tissue swelling or hematoma may be seen with disruption of the anterior longitudinal ligament (Fig. 22.13).

Traumatic Disk Herniation

This usually involves the cervical and thoracic spine and can occur in isolation or in association with fractures, which is more common. MRI findings are characterized by intervertebral disk hemorrhage or edema, end plate avulsions, narrowing or asymmetrical widening of the intervertebral disk space, tear of the annulus fibrosus, and disk herniations [26]. There is a high association of traumatic disk herniation with facet subluxation or dislocation, and therefore, preoperative MRI is recommended before facet reduction is attempted (Figs. 22.11 and 22.14).

Epidural Hematoma

Spinal epidural hematomas are extra-axial extradural in location and occur spontaneously or due to trauma. The source of hemorrhage is unclear but may originate from the epidural venous plexus, arterial origin, or vascular malformations.

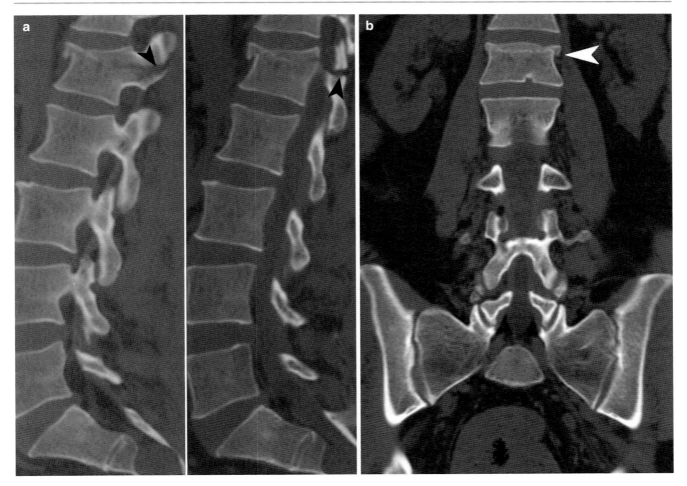

Fig. 22.19 Chance fracture. (**a**) Parasagittal CT reformations show the horizontal fracture of the L1 vertebral body extending through the posterior arch (*arrowheads*). (**b**): Coronal CT shows the horizontal fracture (*arrowhead*) through the L1 vertebral body

MRI is the modality of choice for evaluating the extent of the spinal epidural hematoma and the degree of cord compression (Fig. 22.20). The characteristic findings on the MRI depend on the age of the hemorrhage and vary accordingly on the T1- and T2-weighted images.

Spinal Cord Trauma

Spinal cord injury can result from direct or indirect trauma to the spinal cord. In patients with preexisting conditions such as spinal stenosis, ankylosing spondylitis, or rheumatoid arthritis, even minor trauma to the spine can lead to injury. MRI is the imaging method of choice when spinal cord injury is suspected. These findings may vary from intraspinal hematoma, cord edema, or contusion. Cord compression can result from epidural hematoma, traumatic disk herniation, or due to retropulsion of the bony fragments into the spinal canal. Spinal cord transection is rare. In acute cases, blood products are isointense to hyperintense on T1 and hypointense on T2 weighted due to deoxyhemoglobin and become hyperintense on T1 and T2 sequences, when the deoxyhemoglobin evolves into methemoglobin. Spinal cord edema is manifested as hyperintensity on T2-weighted sequences and cord swelling is seen as abnormal focal expansion of the cord, best seen on T1-weighted sequences [3]. Spinal cord transection occurs from facet dislocations and shearing injuries and seen as cord discontinuity or disruption on MRI. Diffusion-weighted MRI has recently been implemented in some centers to evaluate for spinal cord ischemia and the extent of axonal loss after spinal injury.

The term SCIWORA (spinal cord injury without radiological abnormality) is being used less commonly with the advent of MRI which aids in identification of spinal cord, soft tissue, and ligamentous injuries and so has now become a diagnosis of exclusion. The overall prognosis of patients with SCIWORA without any imaging findings is better than in patients with positive findings.

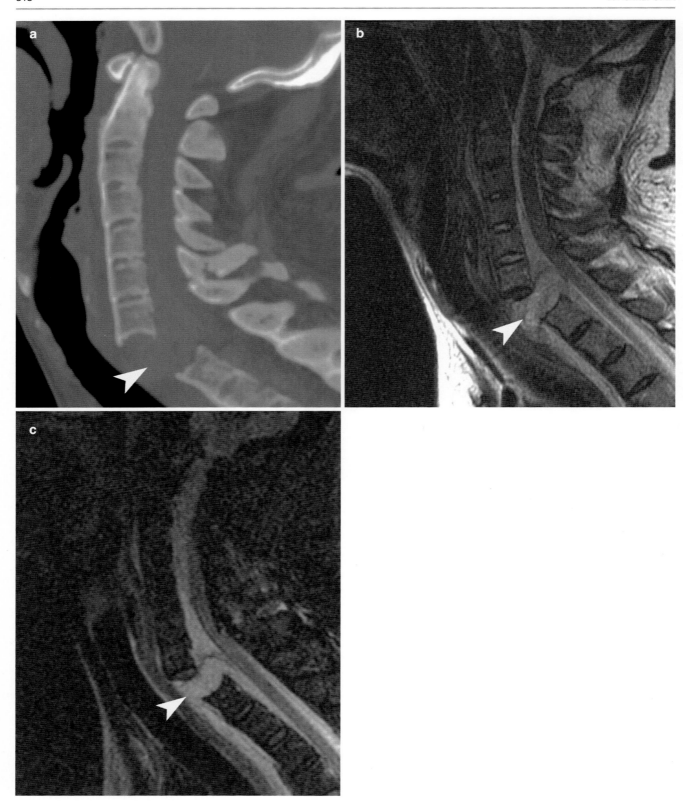

Fig. 22.20 Fracture distraction at C7–T1. (**a**) Sagittal CT shows complete fracture-distraction injury at C7–T1 with distraction and anterior displacement of the superior cervical vertebral column (*arrowhead*). Bridging syndesmophytes are seen at all levels, consistent with ankylosing spondylitis. (**b**, **c**) Sagittal T2 FSE and sagittal T2 STIR MRI images in addition show large intervertebral (*arrowhead*) and epidural hematoma, causing central canal stenosis and cord compression from the C6 to the T1 vertebral level

Conclusion

Imaging of a wide variety of spinal fractures is now possible with the use of multidetector CT and MR imaging which has essentially replaced radiography. Cross-sectional imaging is also more sensitive, accurate, and cost-effective in the long run. Current imaging guidelines recommend use of CT for initial assessment of suspected spine injury with MRI being reserved for soft tissue and spinal cord injuries, thereby decreasing the incidence of missed injuries and aiding in early diagnosis and management of spinal trauma.

References

1. National Spinal Cord Injury Statistical Center. Spinal cord injury: facts and figures at a glance. Available at www.spinalcord.uab.edu. Accessed on Mar 1, 2011.
2. Daffner RH, Hackney DB. ACR appropriateness criteria on suspected spine trauma. J Am Coll Radiol. 2007;4(11):762–75. doi:10.1016/j.jacr.2007.08.006.
3. Looby S, Flanders A. Spine trauma. Radiol Clin North Am. 2011;49(1):129–60.
4. Hoffman JR, Mower WR, Wolfson AB, Todd KH, Zucker MI. Validity of a set of clinical criteria to rule out injury to the cervical spine in patients with blunt trauma. National Emergency X-Radiography Utilization Study Group. N Engl J Med. 2000;343(2):94–9. doi:10.1056/NEJM20007133430203.
5. Stiell IG, Clement CM, Wells GA, Vandemheen KL, Clement CM, Lesiuk H, et al. The Canadian C-spine rule for radiography in alert and stable trauma patients. JAMA. 2001;286(15):1841–8. doi:10.1001/jama.286.15.1841.
6. Lange BB, Penkar P, Binder WD, Novelline RA. Are cervical spine radiograph examinations useful in patients with low clinical suspicion of cervical spine fracture? An experience with 254 cases. Emerg Radiol. 2010;17:191–3. doi:10.1007/s10140-009-0830-x.
7. Nunez DB, Ahmad AA, Coin CG, Leblang S, Becerra JL, Henry R, et al. Clearing the cervical spine in multiple trauma victims: a time-effective protocol using helical computed tomography. Emerg Radiol. 1994;1(6):273–8. doi:10.1007/BF02614949.
8. Blackmore CC, Ramsey SD, Mann FA, Deyo RA. Cervical spine screening with CT in trauma patients: a cost effectiveness analysis. Radiology. 1999;212(1):117–25.
9. Holmes JF, Akkinepalli R. Computed tomography versus plain radiography to screen for cervical spine injury: a meta-analysis. J Trauma. 2005;58(5):902–5. doi:10.1097/01.TA.0000162138.36519.2A.
10. Vandemark RM. Radiology of the cervical spine in trauma patients: practice pitfalls and recommendations for improving efficiency and communication. AJR Am J Roentgenol. 1990;155:465–72.
11. Weissledder R, Wittenberg J, Harisinghani MG. Primer of diagnostic imaging. Philadelphia: Mosby; 2002. p. 370–8.
12. Manaster BJ, May DA, Disler DG. The requisites, musculoskeletal imaging. Spine trauma. Elsevier Health Sciences 2002. p. 164–77.
13. Wheeless CR III, Nunley JA II, Urbaniak JR, Nasca R, Fitch B, Furey C, Musante D, Urquia D. Wheeless' textbook of orthopaedics. http://www.wheelessonline.com/. Accessed Mar 2011.
14. Fielding JW, Hawkins RJ. Atlanto-axial rotatory fixation. (Fixed rotatory subluxation of the atlanto-axial joint). J Bone Joint Surg Am. 1977;59:37–44.
15. Mirvis SE, Shanmuganathan K. Imaging of trauma and critical care, 2nd edition. Imaging of cervical spinal trauma. Saunders. p. 185–289.
16. Kim KS, Chen HH, Russel EJ, Rogers LF. Flexion tear drop fracture of the cervical spine. AJR Am J Roentgenol. 1989;152:319–26. 0361-803X/89/1522-0319.
17. Boyarsky I, Godorov G, Mueller B, Keenan MAE. Fractures of the cervical spine emedicine article 1267150. Updated 20 Oct 2009.
18. Schwartz ED, Flanders AE. Spinal trauma: imaging, diagnosis, and management. Philadelphia: Lippincott Williams & Wilkins; 2006. p. 130–5.
19. Rao SK, Wasyliw C, Nunez Jr DB. Spectrum of imaging findings in hyperextension injuries of the neck. Radiographics. 2005;25:1239–54.
20. Johan OO. Cervical trauma. In: van Goethem WM, vanden Hauwe L, Parizel PM, editors. Spinal imaging: diagnostic imaging of the spine and spinal cord. New York: Springer; 2007. p. 302.
21. Bohndorf K, Imhof H, Pope TL. Musculoskeletal imaging: a concise multimodality approach. New York: Stuttgart; 2001. p. 48.
22. Denis F. The three column spine and its significance in the classification of acute thoracolumbar spinal injuries. Spine. 1983; 8(8):817–31.
23. Bernstein MP, Mirvis SE, Shanmuganathan K. Chance-type fractures of the thoracolumbar spine: imaging analysis in 53 patients. AJR Am J Roentgenol. 2006;187:859–68.
24. Holdsworth F. Fractures, dislocations and fracture dislocations of the spine. J Bone Joint Surg Am. 1970;52:1534–51.
25. Schaefer DM, Flanders A, Northrup BE, Doan HT, Osterholm JL. Magnetic resonance imaging of acute cervical spine trauma. Correlation with severity of neurologic injury. Spine. 1989;14:1090–5.
26. Levitt MA, Flanders AE. Diagnostic capabilities of magnetic resonance imaging and computed tomography in acute cervical spinal column injury. Am J Emerg Med. 1991;9:131–5.
27. Stiell IG, Clement CM, McKnight RD, Brison R, Schull MJ, Rowe BH, et al. The Canadian C-spine rule versus the NEXUS low-risk criteria in patients with trauma. N Engl J Med. 2003;349:2510.

Imaging of Nontraumatic Mediastinal and Pulmonary Processes

Brett W. Carter and Victorine V. Muse

Introduction

Thoracic complaints including cough, shortness of breath, and pleuritic chest pain are common but nonspecific presenting symptoms in the emergency department, and as many as 5 % of visits are due to acute chest pain. Acute chest pain in the absence of trauma remains a diagnostic challenge because of extensive etiology that ranges from benign to potentially lethal. After cardiac and aortic etiologies are ruled out, three main categories of disease origin should be considered: mediastinum (including pulmonary vasculature only), lung, and pleura. Nontraumatic, noncardiac mediastinal processes which can present with chest symptoms include, but are not limited to, pulmonary embolism (technically lung but will be considered with mediastinum), esophageal perforation, mediastinitis, and abscess. Pulmonary pathology also tends to affect the pleural space so these two categories will be considered together. Pneumonia and pulmonary edema are the most common pulmonary diagnoses in the emergency room. It is equally important to delineate any associated complications including pulmonary abscess and empyema. Pneumothorax can also be nontraumatic in etiology and present with acute thoracic symptoms.

Imaging

Although accurate clinical history and physical examination are essential, diagnostic imaging continues to be indispensable in helping to navigate nonspecific thoracic signs and symptoms and reach a more refined assessment.

Chest Radiograph

The first radiological examination obtained on a patient with chest symptoms should be a good quality PA and lateral chest radiograph. Portable technique should be reserved for only those patients who are truly obtunded or too critical to transport to the radiology department. While a CXR is limited in its sensitivity and specificity, it is the most efficient way to quickly evaluate the patient and be able to categorize the management as a surgical issue which may need to be imminently addressed such as a pneumothorax or a non-life-threatening medical process such as pneumonia. Correlation with the patient's clinical history, immune status, and comorbidities is critical to the proper interpretation of the film.

Chest CT Scan

Chest CT can be helpful to further elucidate subtle findings seen on the chest radiograph. Contrast-enhanced examination should be obtained when possible so that contrast enhancement can better delineate mediastinal and vascular structures and help define and separate pleural and parenchymal processes. Pulmonary embolism protocol is a separate technique and needs to be specifically requested if this diagnosis is a consideration.

Ultrasound

Ultrasound has limited application in the lung and mediastinum but is very useful in delineating the pleural space as to the nature of the contained process. Directed ultrasound can also assist in guidance for diagnostic thoracentesis or drainage catheter placement.

B.W. Carter, MD
Department of Radiology, Baylor University Medical Center,
Dallas, TX, USA

V.V. Muse, MD (✉)
Department of Radiology, Massachusetts General Hospital,
Harvard Medical School,
Boston, MA, USA
e-mail: vmuse@partners.org

A. Singh (ed.), *Emergency Radiology*,
DOI 10.1007/978-1-4419-9592-6_23, © Springer Science+Business Media New York 2013

Mediastinum

Pulmonary Embolism

Acute pulmonary embolism (PE) is the third most common cause of cardiovascular death, with an average incidence in the USA of 1 per 1,000 persons. Approximately 300,000 patients die from PE each year. The most common signs and symptoms at the time of presentation include dyspnea, pleuritic chest pain, tachypnea, and tachycardia [1]. The classic clinical triad of chest pain, dyspnea, and hemoptysis is only seen in a minority of patients. Common risk factors for PE include acute medial illness, prolonged immobilization, malignancy, and orthopedic surgery.

The chest radiograph is usually the first imaging examination obtained in the evaluation of patients presenting with chest pain and can be used to detect other potential causes of symptoms mimicking PE, including pneumonia, pulmonary edema, and pneumothorax. Several classic radiographic signs of PE have been described, but are infrequently encountered. These include Westermark's sign, which is increased lucency of all or portion of a lung secondary to decreased vascular flow in the setting of obstructive PE. Hampton's hump is a peripheral, wedge-shaped opacity that may represent pulmonary infarction in the setting of PE [2].

Ventilation-perfusion scintigraphy is performed with the intravenous injection and inhalation of radiopharmaceuticals for the purpose of identifying PE. It is most valuable in the setting of a normal chest radiograph, as pulmonary parenchymal disease limits its sensitivity and specificity. The presence of a ventilation-perfusion mismatch, or a defect on the perfusion study only, is suggestive of PE. The Prospective Investigation of Pulmonary Embolism II (PIOPED II) interpretation scheme is used in the reporting of the ventilation-perfusion scan. The diagnostic categories include normal, very low probability, low probability, intermediate probability, and high probability. Many patients have scans between low and high probability and require additional testing for diagnosis [3].

Pulmonary angiography has traditionally been considered the gold standard examination to evaluate for PE. However, multidetector computed tomography (MDCT) with intravenous contrast has now surpassed angiography and is the primary modality utilized for diagnosis of PE in most institutions. Factors contributing to the effectiveness of CT over pulmonary angiography include widespread availability and fast scan times. Additionally, ventilation-perfusion scintigraphy and pulmonary angiography do not accurately demonstrate subsegmental PE. In addition to demonstrating PE within the main, lobar, and segmental PE, MDCT is more accurate in identifying PE affecting the subsegmental pulmonary arteries. In addition to identifying PE, CT can evaluate the remainder of the chest for abnormalities such as pneumonia, pulmonary edema, and pneumothorax. The most common finding on contrast-enhanced CT is hypodense filling defects within opacified pulmonary artery branches (Fig. 23.1) [4]. Saddle emboli, or pulmonary emboli bridging the main pulmonary arteries, may be seen. Abrupt vessel cutoff and complete occlusion may be identified. Cardiac dysfunction in the setting of massive acute PE may manifest as enlargement of the right atrium and ventricle, straightening of the interventricular septum, or bowing of the interventricular septum towards the left ventricle (Fig. 23.2) [5]. The most common finding within the lung parenchyma in patients with PE is atelectasis. Pulmonary infarction may be seen within the peripheral aspects of the lung parenchyma and typically manifests as wedge-shaped ground glass or mixed ground glass and solid opacities (Fig. 23.3). A thickened vessel may be seen extending to the margin of the opacity. Infarction is more common in patients with impaired collateral circulation and pulmonary venous hypertension. Pleural effusions may also be present [6].

Esophageal Perforation

Esophageal perforation is a potentially life-threatening phenomenon. The most common etiology of esophageal perforation is iatrogenic, usually associated with endoscopic instrumentation and thoracic surgery. The rate of perforation associated with endoscopy has been estimated at approximately 1 per 1,000. In one series, perforation was iatrogenic in 55 % of cases. Traumatic perforation is most common within the cervical portion of the thoracic esophagus, which is the narrowest portion. Other etiologies include spontaneous perforation (Boerhaave's syndrome) in 15 %, foreign body in 14 %, and blunt or penetrating trauma in 10 %. Underlying esophageal disease, such as esophagitis or malignancy, appears to place patients at an increased risk of rupture [7].

Boerhaave's syndrome or spontaneous esophageal perforation is a rare phenomenon, affecting approximately one per 6,000 patients [7]. Perforation is typically due to an episode of violent vomiting. In this scenario, the posterior esophagus ruptures, usually near the crus of the left hemidiaphragm. The most common clinical symptoms include history of vomiting, chest pain, and fever. Subcutaneous emphysema may be present on physical examination [7, 8]. The role of conventional chest radiography in the assessment of esophageal perforation is limited, and initial radiographs may be normal. The most common abnormalities are characterized as indirect signs of esophageal perforation and include pneumomediastinum, pneumothorax, and pleural effusion (Fig. 23.4) [7, 8].

Pneumomediastinum may appear as visualization of the white pleural line adjacent to the mediastinum, areas of radiolucency in the soft tissues, and focal air collections within the mediastinum and retrosternal region. The "continuous diaphragm sign," a linear collection of air along the diaphragm, and "V sign" of Naclerio, a collection of air along the left paraspinal region above the left hemidiaphragm, are

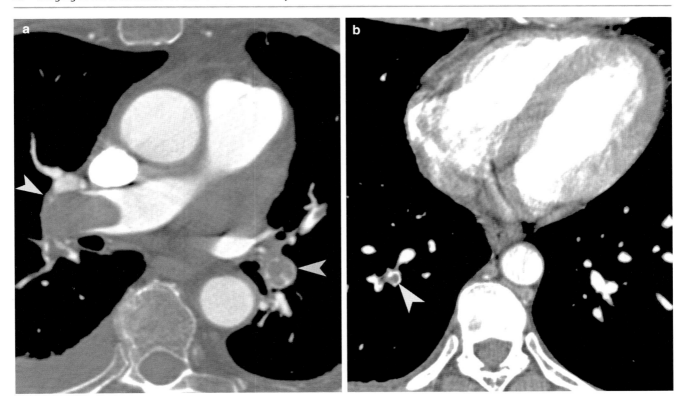

Fig. 23.1 Pulmonary embolism. (**a, b**) Axial CT images show filling defects (*arrowheads*) within the right and left pulmonary arteries, as well as segmental pulmonary arterial branch in right lower lobe

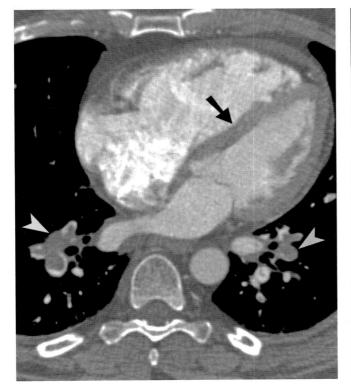

Fig. 23.2 Pulmonary embolism. Axial CT image shows extensive pulmonary emboli (*arrowheads*) within the lower lobes. Straightening of the interventricular septum (*arrow*) is consistent with right cardiac dysfunction

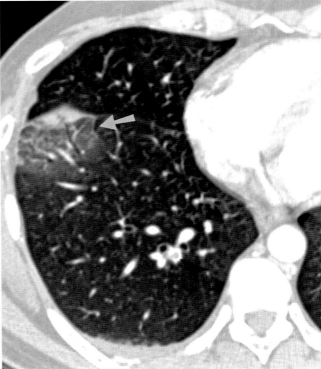

Fig. 23.3 Pulmonary embolism and infarction. Axial CT image demonstrates a mixed ground-glass and solid opacity within the right lower lobe along the major interlobar fissure. This opacity represents pulmonary infarction (*arrow*) in this patient with pulmonary emboli (*arrowhead*)

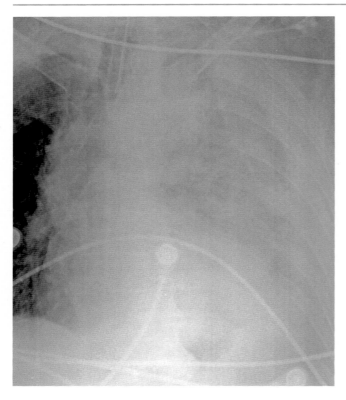

Fig. 23.4 Boerhaave's syndrome. Frontal chest radiograph demonstrates a left pleural effusion and near-complete opacification of the left hemithorax in this patient with Boerhaave's syndrome

well-described signs of pneumomediastinum that are rarely seen. CT is definitive in demonstrating the presence of pneumomediastinum, pneumothorax, and pleural effusion complicating esophageal perforation.

If oral contrast material is used at the time of CT imaging, extravasation of contrast from the esophageal lumen into the mediastinum or pleura may be present (Fig. 23.5). Esophagography had previously been considered the initial examination of choice in the evaluation of uncomplicated esophageal disease. In the event of esophageal perforation, esophagography should be performed with water-soluble contrast material, which is rapidly absorbed by the mediastinum. However, water-soluble contrast material should not enter the tracheobronchial tree, as its hyperosmolar composition may result in pulmonary edema. Contrast esophagography may demonstrate extravasation of intraluminal contrast material into the mediastinum or pleura (Fig. 23.6). However, false-negative results may be encountered 10 % of the time [7].

Mediastinitis and Abscess

Acute mediastinitis, or infection of the mediastinum, may be caused by esophageal perforation, tracheobronchial injury, or direct extension from adjacent structures affected by infectious organisms. Hematogenous spread of infection is uncommon. The most common etiology of acute mediastinitis

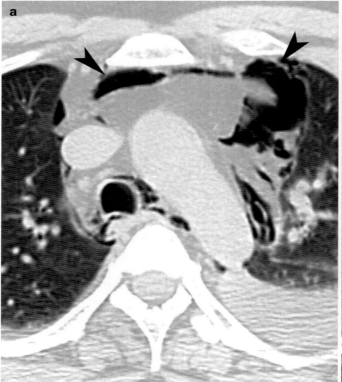

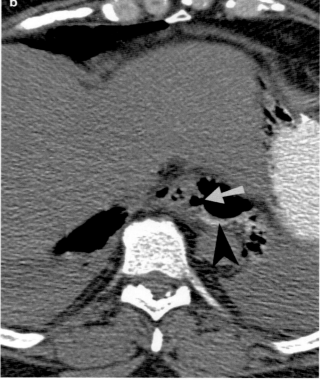

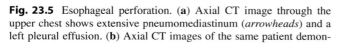

Fig. 23.5 Esophageal perforation. (**a**) Axial CT image through the upper chest shows extensive pneumomediastinum (*arrowheads*) and a left pleural effusion. (**b**) Axial CT images of the same patient demonstrate a defect (*arrow*) within the left lateral wall of the distal thoracic esophagus. An extraluminal collection of air and contrast material (*arrowhead*) is present to the left of the esophageal wall defect.

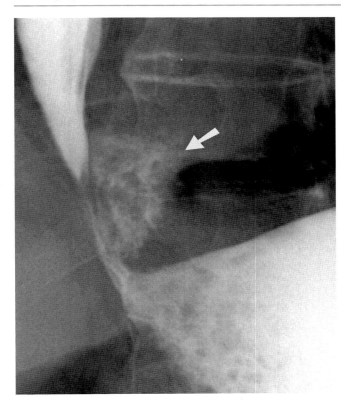

Fig. 23.6 Boerhaave's syndrome. A magnified image from an esophagram shows leakage of contrast material (*arrow*) from the distal thoracic esophageal lumen into the left hemithorax in this patient with Boerhaave's syndrome

is esophageal perforation, with approximately 1 % of patients developing mediastinitis and mediastinal abscess. Additional etiologies include postoperative infection following thoracic surgery for coronary artery bypass grafting, cardiac valve replacement, sampling of mediastinal lymph nodes, and pulmonary resection [7]. Signs and symptoms at the time of presentation are nonspecific and may be confused for those associated with myocardial infarction, acute aortic syndrome (including aortic dissection, intramural hematoma, and penetrating atherosclerotic ulcer), and pulmonary embolism. Early diagnosis and treatment are critical for patient survival.

The most common abnormalities identified on chest radiography include widening of the superior mediastinum (Fig. 23.7) and loss of the normal mediastinal contours. Pneumomediastinum may be present. In the absence of these findings, the initial chest radiograph may be normal. In cases of esophageal perforation, contrast esophagography may demonstrate extravasation of intraluminal contrast material into the mediastinum or pleura. CT is definitive in demonstrating mediastinal widening and increased attenuation of the mediastinal fat, both of which are secondary to edema and inflammatory changes. Pneumomediastinum may be seen (Fig. 23.7). CT is excellent for visualization of potentially drainable fluid collections such as abscesses and may be used to guide percutaneous drainage. Concomitant acute

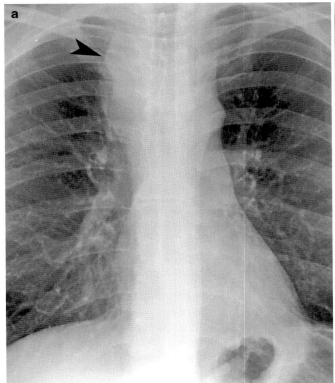
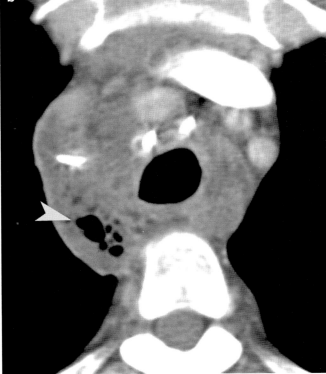

Fig. 23.7 Mediastinitis. (**a**) Frontal chest radiograph demonstrates widening (*black arrowhead*) of the superior mediastinum. (**b**) Axial CT image of the same patient shows extensive inflammatory stranding and edema within the mediastinum. Pneumomediastinum (*white arrowhead*) is also present in this patient with mediastinitis

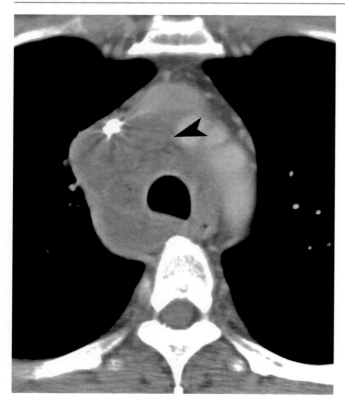

Fig. 23.8 Mediastinal abscess. Axial CT demonstrates inflammatory stranding and low density with in the mediastinum (*arrowhead*), consistent with abscess

abnormalities of the lung parenchyma, such as bronchopneumonia, lobar pneumonia, abscess, and empyema, may be identified (Fig. 23.8). Secondary signs of mediastinal infection, including mediastinal lymphadenopthy, pleural effusions, and pericardial effusions, may also be identified. In patients with acute mediastinitis secondary to esophageal perforation, thickening of the esophageal wall, pneumothorax and pleural effusion, extravasation of intraluminal contrast material, and abscesses may be present. In patients with acute mediastinitis following thoracic surgery, CT is excellent for visualization of sternal dehiscence and pleuromediastinal fistulas [7].

Lungs and Pleura

Pneumonia

There are over four million cases of pneumonia each year in the USA with one million hospitalizations a year. Pulmonary infections are the eighth leading cause of death in the USA and are the most common cause of infection-related mortality [9]. Pneumonias can be classified into main four clinical groups: community acquired, aspiration, healthcare associated, and hospital acquired. Cough, fever, and dyspnea are the usual presenting symptoms, but 50 % of patients also complain of pleuritic chest pain. Even with advances in current medical techniques, the specific etiology can be determined in only 50–70 % of cases [10].

Definitive diagnosis requires confirmation of pulmonary findings by imaging. ATS recommendations include PA and lateral chest radiographs which increase the sensitivity of the exam; portable technique should be reserved for truly obtunded patients. The main radiological patterns of lobar pneumonia, bronchopneumonia, and interstitial pneumonia are recognized with sufficient frequency and correlate enough with different causative organisms in enough cases, so their recognition is useful diagnostically [10] . CT is used to further characterize a complex pneumonia, visualize a process not seen on chest radiograph (Fig. 23.9a, b), and look for complications such as abscess or empyema [11].

Community-acquired pneumonia (CAP) is the most common cause of pulmonary infection in both immunocompromised and immunocompetent patients presenting to the emergency room [10]. *Streptococcus pneumonia*e, the most common bacterial cause, typically demonstrates a lobar pattern of consolidation (Fig. 23.10); air bronchograms are common, and pleural effusions are uncommon.

Staphylococcus aureus is a less common cause of CAP and usually is seen in debilitated patients. A multifocal lobar and bronchopneumonia pattern primarily in the lower lobes with pleural effusions can be seen on the CXR (Fig. 23.11a), and the presence of associated pneumatoceles and/or abscesses better seen on CT scan (Fig. 23.11b) may suggest this diagnosis. Atypical infections including *Mycoplasma pneumoniae* (Figs. 23.12 and 23.13) have an asymmetric patchy bilateral interstitial and alveolar pattern which sometimes can be hard to confirm by chest radiograph. CT findings include patchy ground-glass opacities, centrilobular nodules, and septal thickening: pleural effusions are uncommon. Viral pneumonias have a similar pattern and are becoming a much more common cause of CAP [9].

Aspiration pneumonia has a more distinct pattern on chest radiograph (Fig. 23.14). It occurs in the dependent portion of the lower lobes, favoring the right lung because of the straight orientation of the right mainstem bronchus with respect to the trachea. In supine patients, the aspirated material collects in the posterior segments of the upper lobes and superior segments of the lower lobes. Pleural effusions are common (Fig. 23.15b). Anaerobic organisms are the etiology of the resultant pneumonia 90 % of the time [11].

Pulmonary Abscess and Empyema

A lung abscess represents a localized infection that undergoes tissue destruction and necrosis. They are most common in mixed anaerobic infections, so should be suspected in patients at risk for aspiration. Multiple abscesses can also be seen in septic emboli. The chest radiograph may

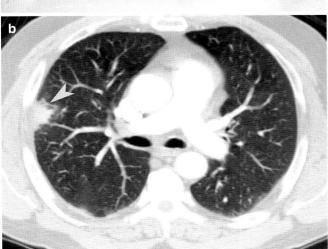

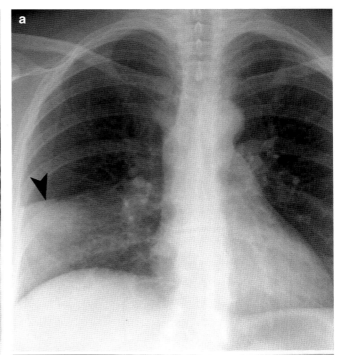

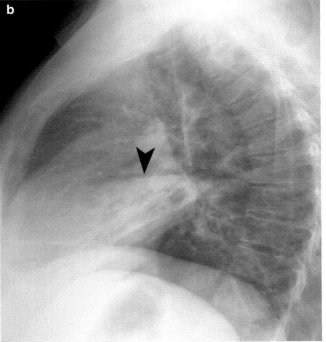

Fig. 23.9 Pneumonia. (**a**) Frontal chest radiograph shows a peripheral opacity (*arrowhead*) in the anterior segment of the right upper lobe. (**b**) Axial CT scan confirms a peripheral pneumonia (*arrowhead*) in the right upper lobe

Fig. 23.10 Right middle lobe pneumonia. (**a**) Frontal radiograph of the chest demonstrates classic right middle lobe pneumonia (*arrowhead*) with ill definition of the right heart border. (**b**) The *right middle lobe* pneumonia (*arrowhead*) is seen projecting over the heart on the lateral view

demonstrate an air-fluid level indicating communication with the tracheobronchial tree. CT scan can better delineate the abscess (Fig. 23.15) which typically manifests a smooth internal wall and develops within and is adjacent to parenchymal consolidation, an imaging feature which can help differentiate it from a cavitary neoplasm [11].

Most pleural effusions associated with pneumonia are sterile sympathetic effusions. Empyemas develop when the pleural space becomes infected, usually from direct extension of a pulmonary parenchymal source. An empyema can also exhibit an air-fluid level, but since the fluid conforms to the pleural space,

the air-fluid level is longer on the lateral view (Fig. 23.16a). Contrast-enhanced CT scan demonstrated adjacent compressed lung as well as the "split pleura" sign of thickened inflamed visceral and parietal pleura which is seen in over half of patients

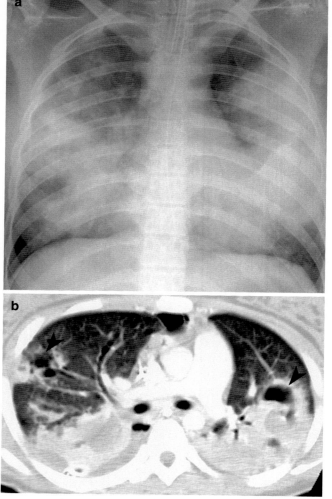

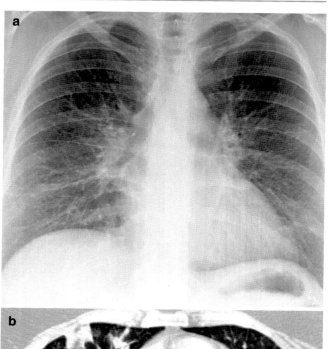

Fig. 23.11 Bronchopneumonia. (**a**) Plain radiograph of the chest demonstrates bilateral multifocal bronchopneumonia. (**b**) Axial CT demonstrates pneumatoceles (*arrowheads*) associated with the pneumonic process

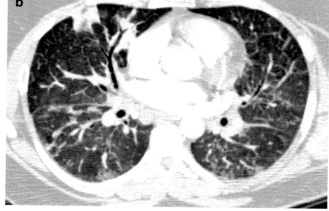

Fig. 23.12 *Mycoplasma pneumonia.* (**a**) Chest radiograph shows atypical *Mycoplasma pneumoniae* with bilateral patchy interstitial opacities. (**b**) Axial CT shows bilateral asymmetric septal thickening and ground-glass nodules. Note the absence of pleural effusions

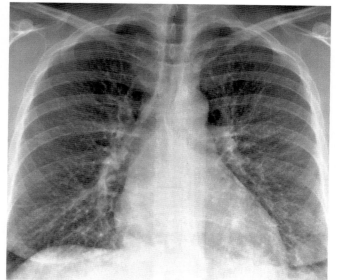

Fig. 23.13 Viral pneumonia. Chest radiograph shows bilateral central interstitial prominence along with some left lower lobe subsegmental air-space disease

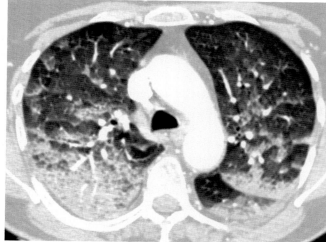

Fig. 23.14 Aspiration pneumonia. Axial CT demonstrates bilateral dependent confluent consolidation, greater on the right

Fig. 23.15 Pulmonary abscess. Axial CT shows right upper lobe pulmonary abscess (*arrowhead*) which developed in a focus of consolidation

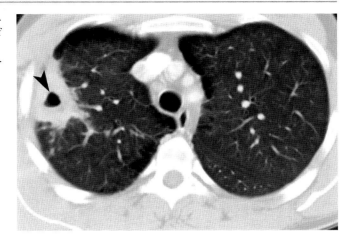

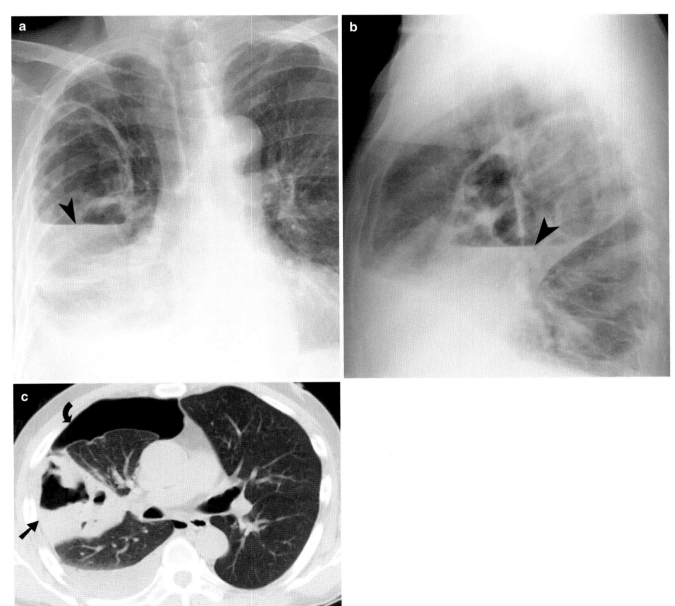

Fig. 23.16 Empyema. (**a**, **b**). Plain radiograph demonstrates empyema of the right pleural space with air-fluid levels (*arrowheads*). (**c**) Axial CT demonstrates empyema (*straight arrow*) in the oblique fissure with the complication of pneumothorax (*curved arrow*)

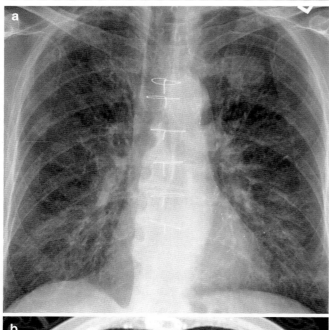

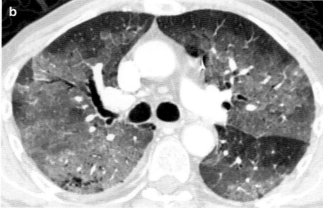

Fig. 23.17 Pulmonary edema. (**a**) Plain radiograph demonstrates diffuse bilaterally symmetrical central interstitial prominence. (**b**) Axial CT demonstrates bilateral ground-glass opacities

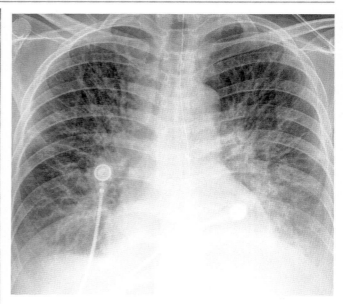

Fig. 23.18 Pulmonary edema. Plain radiograph demonstrates cardiomegaly with bilateral interstitial as well as alveolar edema and bilateral pleural effusions

Chest radiographs can be very nonspecific and tend to be the ones ordered with portable technique which further decreases their sensitivity. In cardiogenic edema, cardiomegaly with a widened vascular pedicle, bilateral symmetric septal thickening, coalescing alveolar opacities, and bilateral pleural effusions are common manifestations delineated on chest radiograph (Fig. 23.17a). Peribronchial cuffing and perihilar prominence are also present and may be a differentiating factor from a noncardiogenic cause [13]. CT scan can delineate further the septal thickening; air-space edema on CT can be ground glass or frankly consolidative (Fig. 23.17b). Pulmonary edema tends to be symmetric except in cases where the patient has severe underlying emphysema. Noncardiogenic pulmonary edema tends to be less "wet" looking with no widened vascular pedicle or peribronchial cuffing minimal septal lines, a lack of pleural effusions, and a more patchy air-space appearance with air bronchograms (Fig. 23.18) [14].

with empyema (Fig. 23.16b). Chest ultrasound combined with CT scan helps define the nature of fluid collections in the pleural space and better delineate the phase of empyema: exudative, fibropurulent, or organized, which will direct patient management as to drainage or more invasive surgical procedures [12].

Pneumothorax

Nontraumatic pneumothorax can be attributed to one of two categories: primary spontaneous or secondary to complications of underlying lung disease.

Primary spontaneous pneumothaces occur most commonly in young, tall, thin males without predisposing factors, although rupture of small bleb or bullae and smoking are thought to play roles. Secondary causes include COPD, metastatic disease, infection, and cystic lung disease [15]. Pneumomediastinum can cause pneumothorax but not vice versa.

Pulmonary Edema

Pulmonary edema can either be cardiogenic or noncardiogenic in etiology and although they have distinct causes, they can be indistinguishable by imaging so clinical correlation is critical. The majority of cases presenting to the emergency room are cardiogenic in nature due to heart failure. Noncardiogenic causes to consider include pneumonia, sepsis, inhalation injury, and aspiration of gastric contents [13].

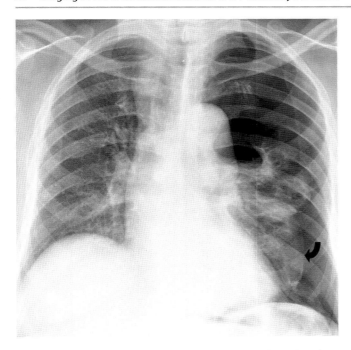

Fig. 23.19 Tension pneumothorax. Plain radiograph of the chest demonstrates visceral pleural line (*curved arrow*) with a left-sided tension pneumothorax. There is flattening of the left dome of diaphragm and partial collapse of the lung centrally with mediastinal shift

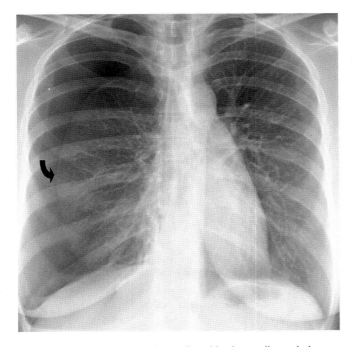

Fig. 23.20 Tension pneumothorax. Portable chest radiograph demonstrates large right-sided tension pneumothorax (*curved arrow*) with mediastinal shift to the left side

An upright chest radiograph in most cases can confirm the presence of a pneumothorax by demonstrating the absence of lung markings from the edge of the visceral pleura to the chest wall (Fig. 23.19). In supine patients, a deep sulcus sign can develop as air layers out anteriorly and projects as an area of increased lucency that outlines the costophrenic sulcus [16]. Expiratory views have no additional diagnostic value and are not needed, although lateral views can sometimes be helpful if it is uncertain whether a pneumothorax is present. Tension pneumothorax occurs if intrapleural pressure increases to a point where gas exchange and cardiac function become compromised. Radiographically, this manifests as contralateral mediastinal shift and diaphragmatic depression (Fig. 23.20), both of which should resolve with decompression. CT can be used to detect patients with small pneumothorax (less than 15 %) as well as to further elucidate the possible underlying cause such as blebs, bullae, or pulmonary disease.

Teaching Points

1. Chest radiograph should be the first imaging modality used in the assessment of nontraumatic thoracic emergencies.
2. The most common CT finding of PE is hypodense filling defects within opacified pulmonary artery branches. Abrupt cutoff and complete occlusion may also be seen.
3. The most common findings of esophageal perforation on chest radiograph and CT include pneumomediastinum, pneumothorax, and pleural effusion. If oral contrast material is administered, extravasation of contrast into the mediastinum or pleura may be seen.
4. The radiographic pattern of pneumonia in CAP may help suggest a causative organism to better tailor treatment; CT is helpful to define subtle cases or detect superimposed complications.
5. Pneumothorax may present in nontraumatic causes and can be usually diagnosed by chest radiograph.

References

1. Tapson VF. Acute pulmonary embolism. N Engl J Med. 2008;358:1037–52.
2. Coche EE, Verschuren F, Hainaut P, et al. Pulmonary embolism findings on chest radiographs and multislice spiral CT. Eur Radiol. 2004;14:1241–8.
3. Stein PD, Woodard PK, Weg JG, Wakefield TW, Tapson VF, Sostman HD, et al. Diagnostic pathways in acute pulmonary embolism: recommendations of the PIOPED II Investigators. Radiology. 2007;242(1):15–21.
4. Han D, Lee KS, Franquet T, et al. Thrombotic and nonthrombotic pulmonary arterial embolism: spectrum of imaging findings. Radiographics. 2003;23:1521–39.
5. Wittram C, Maher MM, Yoo AJ, Kalra MK, Shepard JA, McLoud TC. CT angiography of pulmonary embolism: diagnostic criteria and causes of misdiagnosis. Radiographics. 2004;24(5):1219–38.
6. Coche EE, Müller NL, Kim KI, Wiggs BR, Mayo JR. Acute pulmonary embolism: ancillary findings at spiral CT. Radiology. 1998;207(3):753–8.

7. Giménez A, Franquet T, Erasmus JJ, Martínez S, Estrada P. Thoracic complications of esophageal disorders. Radiographics. 2002;22:S247–58.

8. Hingston CD, Saayman AG, Frost PJ, Wise MP. Boerhaave's syndrome – rapidly evolving pleural effusion; a radiographic clue. Minerva Anestesiol. 2010;76(10):865–7.

9. Nair GB, Niederman MS. Community-acquired pneumonia: an unfinished battle. Med Clin North Am. 2011;95:1143–61.

10. Tarver RD, Teague SD, Heitkamp DE, Conces DW. Radiology of community-acquired pneumonia. Radiol Clin North Am. 2005; 43(3):497–512.

11. Waite S, Jeudy J, White CS. Acute lung infections in normal and immunocompromised hosts. Radiol Clin North Am. 2006;44:295–315.

12. Heffner JE, Klein JS, Hampson C. Diagnostic utility and clinical application of imaging for pleural space infections. Chest. 2010; 137:467–79.

13. Ware LB, Matthay MA. Acute pulmonary edema. N Engl J Med. 2005;353:2788–96.

14. Glueker T, Capasso P, Schnyder P, Gudinchet F, et al. Clinical and radiologic features of pulmonary edema. Radiographics. 1999;19: 1507–31.

15. Luh S. Diagnosis and treatment of primary spontaneous pneumothorax. J Zhejiang Univ Sci B. 2010;11(10):735–44.

16. Jeudy J, Waite S, White CS. Nontraumatic thoracic emergencies. Radiol Clin North Am. 2006;44:273–93.

Neil Patel, Ajay Singh, and Sridhar Shankar

Thorax injury remains the third most common type of injury in trauma patients [1]. With the number of trauma cases on the increase, the incidence of injuries to the thorax is proportionally increasing. The overall mortality rate of thoracic trauma is approximately 10 % and is highest in patients with cardiac or tracheobronchial-esophageal injuries [1]. More than two-thirds of cases of trauma in developed countries are caused by motor vehicle collisions. The remaining cases are the result of falls or blows from blunt objects [2].

Historically, plain radiographs have been the imaging modality of choice because of their low cost and their ability to be done quickly. While they may be useful for the evaluation of many traumatic injuries including large pneumothoraces or fractures, CT has been shown to change the management in 20 % of trauma cases [3]. Specifically, thoracic CT has shown improved accuracy over conventional radiography in the diagnosis of pneumothorax, subtle fractures, hemopericardium, detailed lung parenchymal injury, and both mediastinal hemorrhage and direct vascular injury, among other injuries. Furthermore, it is not uncommon for a plain radiograph to identify a possible injury that needs further evaluation with CT whether it be for surgical planning or to definitively assess the degree of the injury [4].

Injuries to the Pleural Space

The pleural space is defined as the space between the visceral pleura and the parietal pleura. In a healthy patient, this is a potential space that is not well visualized on radiograph

or CT. When either the visceral pleura, parietal pleura, or possibly both are interrupted, the potential space can expand, most commonly with blood or air in the setting of trauma.

Pneumothorax

When air fills the pleural space, a pneumothorax results. The most common clinical presentation of this is shortness of breath with decreased breath sounds. They may be caused by ruptured alveoli which would allow air to enter the space from the visceral aspect or by external trauma to the chest which would allow air to enter from the parietal aspect [5].

On chest radiograph, the visceral white line is visible, along with peripheral lack of lung markings (Fig. 24.1). Although, pneumothorax is often accentuated on expiratory film, the British Thoracic Society does not recommend its routine. A lateral radiograph should be performed if the frontal view is negative for pneumothorax and there is high clinical suspicion of pneumothorax. The air in the pleural space tends to accumulate anteromedially on supine radiograph. A 2 cm or more rim of air is equivalent to approximately 50 % of the hemithorax. Deep sulcus sign refers to the presence of air lucency between diaphragm and spine, resulting in prominence of costodiaphragmatic space. Tension pneumothorax is characterized by progressive flattening of the ipsilateral diaphragm and shift of mediastinum to the opposite side.

The early diagnosis of a small pneumothorax can become clinically important especially if the patient is going to be mechanically ventilated as this can expand the pleural space leading to greater mass effect and mediastinal shift. This, in turn, can cause decreased blood return to the heart more likely from the loss of negative intrapleural pressure rather than the presence of positive intrapleural pressure [6]. Large, symptomatic pneumothoraces are usually treated with chest tube (24 Fr) or smaller caliber image-guided catheter (6–12 F). Smaller pneumothorax may be conservatively

N. Patel, MD • S. Shankar, MD, MBA
Department of Radiology, University of Tennessee,
Memphis, TN, USA

A. Singh, MD (✉)
Department of Radiology, Massachusetts General Hospital,
Harvard Medical School, 10 Museum Way,
524, Boston, MA 02141, USA
e-mail: asingh1@partners.org

A. Singh (ed.), *Emergency Radiology*,
DOI 10.1007/978-1-4419-9592-6_24, © Springer Science+Business Media New York 2013

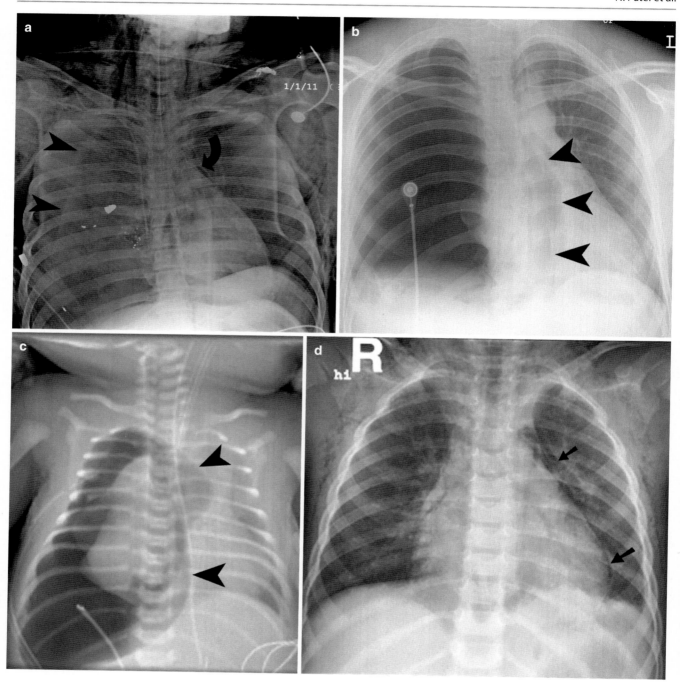

Fig. 24.1 (**a**) Pneumomediastinum and pneumothorax. Single frontal chest radiograph from a trauma patient after a gunshot wound reveals air between the epicardium and the pleura on the *left* (*curved arrow*). Pneumothorax on the *right* with collapsed lateral lung margin (*arrowheads*) and loss of peripheral lung markings. The ballistic fragment can be seen within the right mid lung. Extensive subcutaneous emphysema is present. (**b**) Tension pneumothorax. Frontal radiograph shows relative lucency and loss of lung markings within the right hemithorax with shift of mediastinum to the *left*. The medial margin of the right tension pneumothorax is seen crossing the midline (*arrowheads*). (**c**) Tension pneumothorax. In this pediatric patient, there is a large lucency in the right hemithorax with loss of lung markings. There is associated shift of the mediastinal structures, including the heart to the *left*. Medial margin of the enlarged pleural cavity crosses the midline (*arrowheads*). (**d**) Pneumomediastinum. Frontal radiograph shows air outlining the heart (*arrows*) as well as extensive subcutaneous emphysema. (**e**) Pneumomediastinum and pneumopericardium. Frontal radiograph reveals are outline structures in the upper mediastinum outlined by air (*black arrow*). Pneumopericardium is best seen outlining the left ventricle (*white arrow*). (**f**) Pneumomediastinum. Lateral radiograph shows the pneumomediastinum (*arrow*) as a large lucent area posterior to the sternum and surrounding the heart

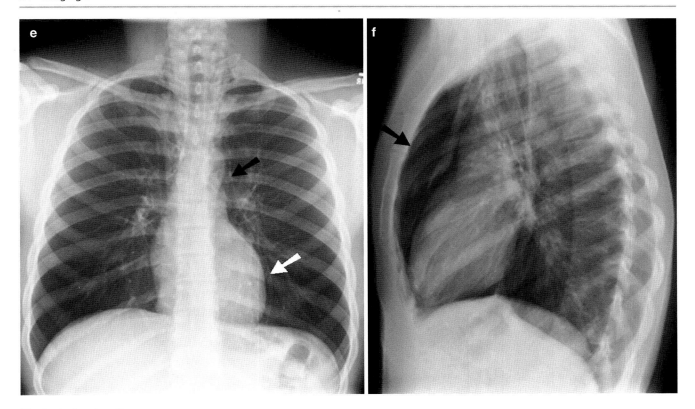

Fig. 24.1 (continued)

monitored with serial radiographs, provided the patient is not breathless. If the patient is breathless, a chest tube or catheter drainage should be performed irrespective of the size of pneumothorax.

Hemothorax

When blood fills the pleural space, a hemothorax results and occurs in approximately 50 % of major thoracic trauma victims [7]. Blood may originate from injury to the lung, chest wall, heart, great vessels, or abdominal organs. Although, bleeding from venous structures is often self-limiting secondary to the low pressure, hemorrhage from high-pressure arterial sources such as the internal mammary, intercostal, or subclavian arteries can cause rapid mass effect on the mediastinum.

CT can accurately identify a small hemothorax more readily than plain radiographs. On plain radiographs, the density of the pleural fluid is difficult to determine but with the use of CT, a density of 30–70 HU suggests blood with greater than 90 HU indicative of acute blood (Fig. 24.2) [6]. Of note, hemorrhage of extrapleural origin is usually associated with rib fractures.

Injuries to the Lung Parenchyma

Pulmonary Contusion

Pulmonary contusion is seen in 17–70 % of trauma patients and represents the most common injury to the lung parenchyma [8]. Contusions result from the direct transmission of energy through adjacent solid structures and thus are usually found along the ribs, sternum, and vertebral bodies. They may be unilateral or bilateral, focal, multifocal, or diffuse depending on the mechanism of injury. Pathologically, the opacification of the lung is caused by hemorrhage and edema filling the alveoli which originates from damage and resultant leak from the alveolar-capillary membrane [9]. Radiographically, this is seen as peripheral focal ground-glass opacities or patchy consolidative opacities that are distributed along a bronchopulmonary segmental anatomy (Fig. 24.3a) [6].

Plain radiograph tends to underestimate the size of pulmonary contusion and lag behind the clinical presentation by up to 6 h. The appearance of pulmonary opacities greater than 24 h after initial injury should suggest other possible diagnoses like pneumonia or fat embolism [7]. Resolution of contusions is within 24–48 h and is complete between 3 and 10 days.

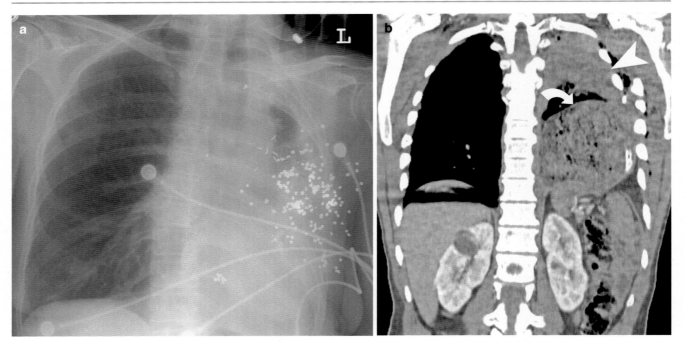

Fig. 24.2 (**a**) Hemothorax after gunshot injury. Frontal radiograph shows multiple shotgun pellets within the left hemithorax and a large hemorrhagic left pleural fluid collection. (**b**) Hemothorax and diaphrag-matic rupture. Coronal CT reformation demonstrates left hemothorax (*arrowhead*) with left rib fractures and left diaphragmatic hernia (*curved arrow*)

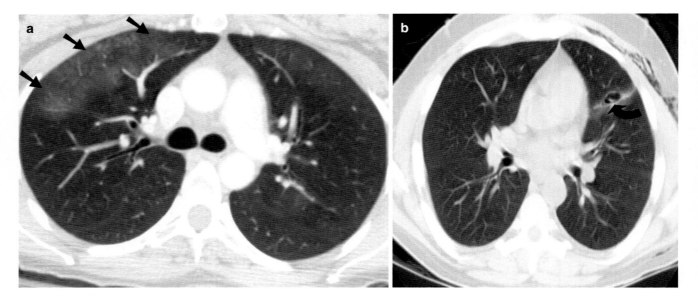

Fig. 24.3 (**a**) Pulmonary contusion. Axial CT shows non-segmental distribution of ground-glass opacification (*arrows*) in the right upper lobe, indicative of contusion. (**b**) Pneumatocele. Axial CT shows a pneumatocele (*curved arrow*) with adjacent hemorrhage in this patient who suffered a knife stab injury to the left anterior chest wall. The cav-ity is formed due to retraction of the edges of the lacerated lung. (**c**) Lung laceration. Coronal CT shows the linear pulmonary laceration (*arrows*) following the bullet path through the left lung as a central lucent area with adjacent hemorrhage. Subcutaneous emphysema is also present

Fig. 24.3 (continued)

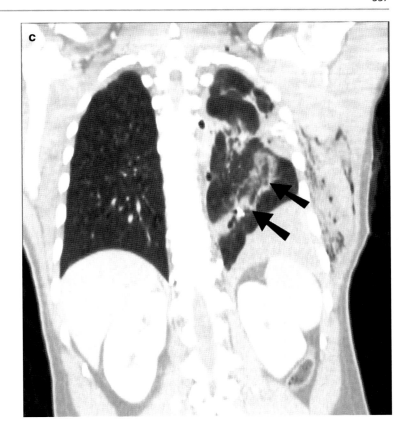

Pulmonary Laceration

Pulmonary lacerations are less common than contusions and result from disruption of the lung parenchyma, most commonly from penetrating trauma. The result is formation of a cavity within the lung as the surrounding parenchyma pulls back from the laceration itself (Fig. 24.3b, c). Because of this, they are more common in younger patients who have more optimal lung elasticity [10].

The formed cavity from the laceration may contain air, blood, or a combination of the two and the terms pneumatocele, hematocele, and hematopneumocele correlate to the contents of the cavity.

CT is more sensitive than radiograph in the evaluation of pulmonary laceration. Pulmonary lacerations are usually more difficult to diagnose on plain radiographs, often due to the presence of surrounding contusion. They become more apparent as the densities from contusion clears up. The pulmonary laceration classification by Wagner et al. is based on the mode of injury and the imaging indication (Table 24.1).

Traumatic Lung Herniation

A segment of the peripheral lung rarely can herniate outside the confines of the thoracic cavity either as the result of blunt

Table 24.1 Classification of pulmonary laceration

Type 1 laceration	They are the most common laceration and are seen within the deep lung parenchyma. They tend to be large and result from direct compressive force to the lung.
Type 2 laceration	They occur in paraspinal region and are caused by a sudden blow to the lower thorax, resulting in shift of the lower lobes across the spine.
Type 3 laceratio	They occur when the lung is torn by penetrating ribs and are thus usually seen in the lung periphery.
Type 4 laceration	It occurs when the lung tears away from an adhesion.

or penetrating thoracic trauma. The anterior thorax is often the site of herniation because of a general lack of support (Fig. 24.4). Surgical reduction of intercostal lung hernia is recommended because of the potential for incarceration or strangulation. This potential risk is much greater in mechanically ventilated patients.

Injuries to the Airways

Injury to the tracheobronchial tree is rarely seen in clinical practice, because up to 78 % of the patients die before arriving at the hospital [10]. The majority of these cases occur

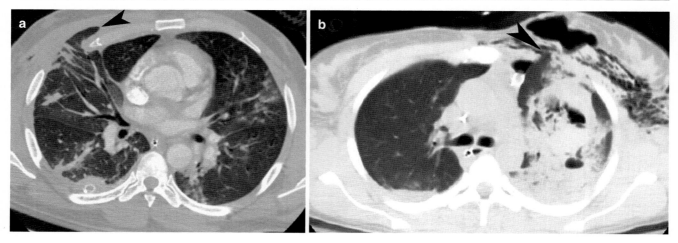

Fig. 24.4 (**a**) Lung herniation. Axial CT shows anterior herniation (*arrowhead*) of a portion of the right upper lobe, between consecutive ribs. An area of ground-glass density likely representing pulmonary contusion can be seen in the posterior left upper lobe. A chest tube is noted in the posterior right hemithorax. (**b**) Lung herniation. Axial CT shows herniation (*arrowhead*) of the medial portion of the left upper lobe into the adjacent anterior chest wall. Subcutaneous emphysema, pulmonary hemorrhage, and a pneumatocele are also present on the *right side*. There is a small left anterior pneumothorax present

during deceleration when the airways may be compressed against the sternum or spine or when elevated thoracic pressure from compression occurs in the setting of a closed glottis. Anatomically, the thoracic trachea is more commonly affected than the cervical trachea and the right main stem bronchus is more commonly injured than the left. CT is an important tool for early diagnosis as up to 68 % of injuries are not accurately diagnosed [11].

Clinically, these patients may present with respiratory distress, cough, and hemoptysis among other symptoms. These symptoms are more common in the setting of bronchial injuries as opposed to tracheal injuries.

Bronchial lacerations are more common than tracheal lacerations because the bronchial walls are not as strong as the tracheal walls. The common imaging manifestations of bronchial injuries include pneumomediastinum and pneumothorax, and bronchial lacerations should be considered when a pneumothorax persists even in the presence of a chest tube and suction. The "fallen lung" sign is seen when bronchial lacerations cause the ipsilateral lung to fall away from the hilum. This sign represents the most specific radiographic sign for tracheobronchial rupture [6].

Tracheal lacerations usually occur at the junction of the cartilaginous and membranous portions. Pneumomediastinum is the most common finding in the setting of tracheal lacerations (Fig. 24.5).

The Macklin effect, which can be seen in up to 40 % of blunt chest trauma patients, involves alveolar rupture, with air dissection along the bronchovascular sheaths and spreading into the mediastinum. In 70–100 % of cases, overdistention or herniation of an endotracheal balloon reveals tracheal laceration [7]. Tracheal laceration should

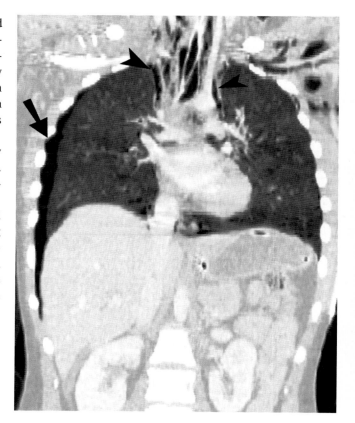

Fig. 24.5 Tracheal laceration. Chest coronal reformation in a patient with tracheal laceration demonstrates pneumothorax (*arrow*) and pneumomediastinum (*arrowheads*)

always be emergently confirmed with laryngoscopy or fiberoptic bronchoscopy. The potential complications include airway obstruction, pneumonia, bronchiectasis, abscess, and empyema.

Cardiac Injuries

Injuries to the heart usually result from motor vehicle collisions and may range from cardiac contusion to frank rupture of the heart. Some of the earliest signs of injury are an abnormal EKG or elevated cardiac enzymes. Chest wall contusions or fractured ribs suggest adequate force to cause cardiac injury. Many of these patients are cardiovascularly asymptomatic, especially those with myocardial contusions and small pericardial tears. Pericardial tears are usually due to direct trauma or from increased intra-abdominal pressure. The most common site of pericardial injury is the left side of the pericardium, parallel to the phrenic nerve [12].

The imaging findings may include contrast material extravasation into the pericardium/mediastinum or pneumomediastinum. The patients with penetrating trauma may present with pneumopericardium (Fig. 24.6). Injury to the valves and chambers typically occur in the patients with preexisting cardiac disease. The right chambers are more commonly involved, and the aortic and mitral valves are the most commonly injured valves [12].

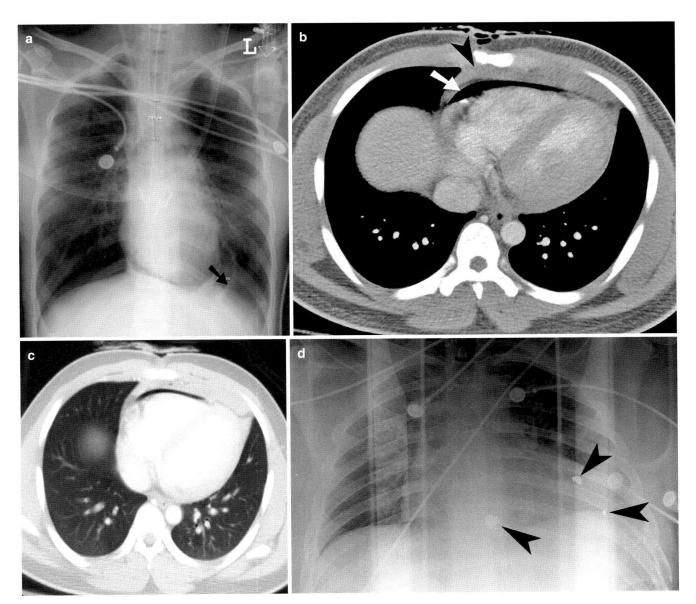

Fig. 24.6 (a) Pneumopericardium. Frontal radiograph shows air around the ventricles and displacing the parietal pericardium (*arrow*). (b, c) Pneumopericardium. Contrast-enhanced axial CT in a 16-year-old male stab victim shows air outlining the right ventricle (*arrow*) with retrosteral hemorrhage (*arrowhead*). (d) Cardiac injury from gunshot wound. Frontal chest radiograph shows three bullet fragments (*arrowheads*) overlying the cardiopericardial silhouette. (e) Hemopericardium. Axial contrast-enhanced CT shows a high-density pericardial effusion representing hemopericardium (*arrow*) in this gunshot wound patient. Bullet fragments can be seen in the left ventricle wall (*black arrowhead*) and pericardial space (*white arrowhead*). Adjacent pulmonary hemorrhage (*curved white arrow*) is also identified

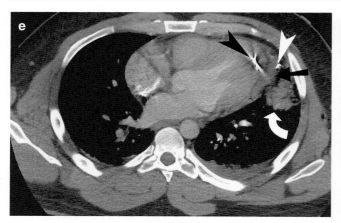

Fig. 24.6 (continued)

Aortic Injury

The danger of rapid exsanguination remains a constant risk among patients who initially survive traumatic aortic injury. With progressively rapid transport to trauma centers, there are an increasing number of patients with aortic injury making it to the emergency department alive [13]. The most common theory proposed for aortic injury suggests that aortic injury is a combination of rapid decelerations and compression, producing rotational and shearing forces as well as transverse laceration at the vulnerable portions of the aorta [8]. Thoracic aorta injuries typically occur at the sites of aortic attachment, including (in descending order of frequency) the proximal descending aorta, aortic arch, aortic root, and distal descending aorta at the aortic hiatus.

Contrast CT angiogram involves the IV administration of 120–150 ml of contrast at 5 ml/s followed by the initiation of the scan when the density in the descending thoracic aorta is at least 150 HU. The study should assess the presence, location, and extent of the mediastinal hemorrhage and aortic injury as well as any injury to adjacent vessels. Periaortic hematoma formation from rupture of the vasa vasorum can be seen on CT but is not always present. CT may also diagnose associated pseudoaneurysms, changes in the aortic contour or diameter, intimal flap consistent with dissection, thrombus, and active extravasation (Fig. 24.7). The aortic contour is often distorted by tearing of the wall and compression from the adjacent pseudoaneurysm or hematoma.

In most cases, the aortic injury presents as a pseudoaneurysm that projects anteriorly or anteromedially from the aortic lumen at the level of the left pulmonary artery. In addition, there is typically a surrounding collar of mediastinal blood [7].

Active extravasation is seen radiographically as any area of contrast outside the vascular lumen. If active extravasation is present, angiography is the next step to try and control the bleeding via coiling or other interventional methods.

Transesophageal echocardiography (TEE) has sensitivity much lower than that of CT for the distal ascending aorta as

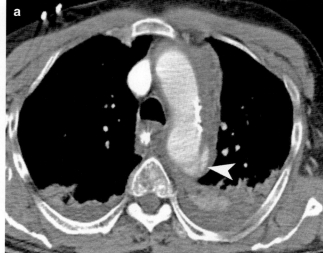

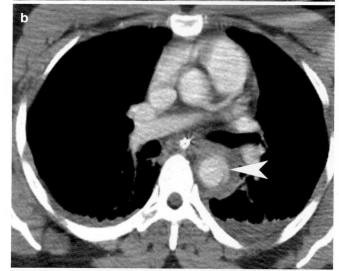

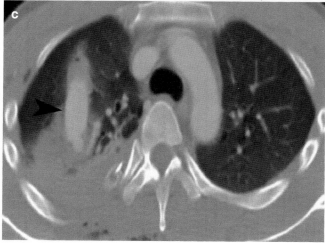

Fig. 24.7 (**a**) Aortic injury. Axial CT with contrast at the level of the aortic arch shows a focal extravasation of contrast (*arrowhead*) at the level of the posterior aortic arch with hemorrhage seen tracking anteriorly. (**b**) Aortic transection. Contrast-enhanced axial CT shows irregularity of the descending thoracic aorta with contrast leaking (*arrowhead*) outside the vessel. (**c**) Pseudoaneurysm of pulmonary artery branch in the right upper lobe. Axial CT shows a focal tubular contrast collection (*arrowhead*) with a saccular outpouching seen posteriorly

well as the proximal aortic branches. TEE does offer a good alternative for patients who are too unstable to travel to the CT scanner [14]. Thoracic angiography is still commonly used because it has high sensitivity and specificity but relatively low morbidity. The major drawbacks of angiography include higher cost, invasiveness, and nonavailability in a timely fashion [7]. As a result, angiography is used for further investigation based on initial CT results.

Magnetic resonance imaging (MRI) is currently not commonly used in the everyday imaging of patients with suspected aortic injury because of its cost, difficulty in developing adequate protocols, and problems with having life support equipment in the presence of a strong magnetic field; rather, it is reserved for problem solving in difficult situations.

Injuries to the Diaphragm

Diaphragmatic Injury

Injuries to the diaphragm are uncommon with a prevalence of 0.16–5 % in trauma patients [7]. Injuries are most commonly caused by a sudden increase in intra-abdominal or intrathoracic pressure against a fixed diaphragm. Motor vehicle accidents are responsible for up to 90 % of traumatic diaphragmatic injuries [15]. The left hemidiaphragm is more commonly injured compared to the right. Associated injury to the abdominal organs such as the spleen, kidneys, and liver are relatively common in trauma patients. In addition, coinciding thoracic injuries such as pneumothorax,

hemothorax, and lung contusions are often seen. Displaced lower rib fractures should particularly increase the concern for possible left hemidiaphragm tears.

Diagnosis of diaphragm injuries based on imaging can be difficult especially if herniation of abdominal contents is not present. Plain radiographs are normal or nonspecific in 25–50 % of cases [15]. Radiographic signs suggestive of rupture include elevation of the hemidiaphragm, distortion of diaphragmatic contour, and contralateral displacement of the heart and mediastinum. Presence of abdominal contents within the thorax is diagnostic for diaphragm rupture (Fig. 24.7).

CT is the mainstay for diagnosis because of its accuracy, speed, and cost (Table 24.2) (Fig. 24.8). The sagittal and coronal reconstructions are especially valuable in diagnosing diaphragmatic rupture and should be carefully scrutinized in every trauma case. Other modalities used to augment diagnosis include ultrasound and MRI. Ultrasound is specifically helpful in evaluating the right hemidiaphragm as the liver acts as an acoustic window.

Table 24.2 CT findings in diaphragmatic rupture

1. Collar sign – The collar sign is produced by a waist-like constriction of herniated viscera at the site of herniation
2. Dependent viscera sign – The dependent viscera sign results from the abdominal viscera falling dependently against the posterior chest wall through the diaphragmatic tear
3. Diaphragmatic thickening due to hemorrhage
4. Peridiaphragmatic contrast material extravasation

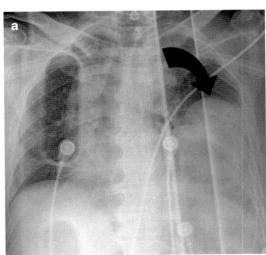 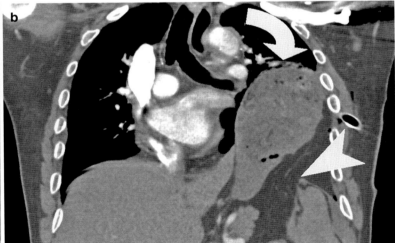

Fig. 24.8 (**a**) Diaphragmatic injury. Plain radiograph shows significantly elevated left hemidiaphragm (*curved arrow*) with elevation of gastric air bubble in a motor vehicle trauma victim. (**b**, **c**) Herniated stomach (*curved arrow*) is seen above the level of the diaphragm in this coronal reformatted image. There is a large left diaphragmatic defect (*arrowhead*). (**d**) Chest CT scout film in a gunshot victim shows the gastric air bubble (*straight arrow*) well above the expected level of the left hemidiaphragm. (**e**) AP radiograph in a trauma patient demonstrates a raised left hemidiaphragm with bilateral chest tubes, and endotracheal and NG tubes (*curved arrow*) in place. (**f**) Coronal CT reformat in the same patient shows the large stomach herniation (*arrow*) through a diaphragmatic defect, bullet fragment (*arrowhead*), and left hemothorax

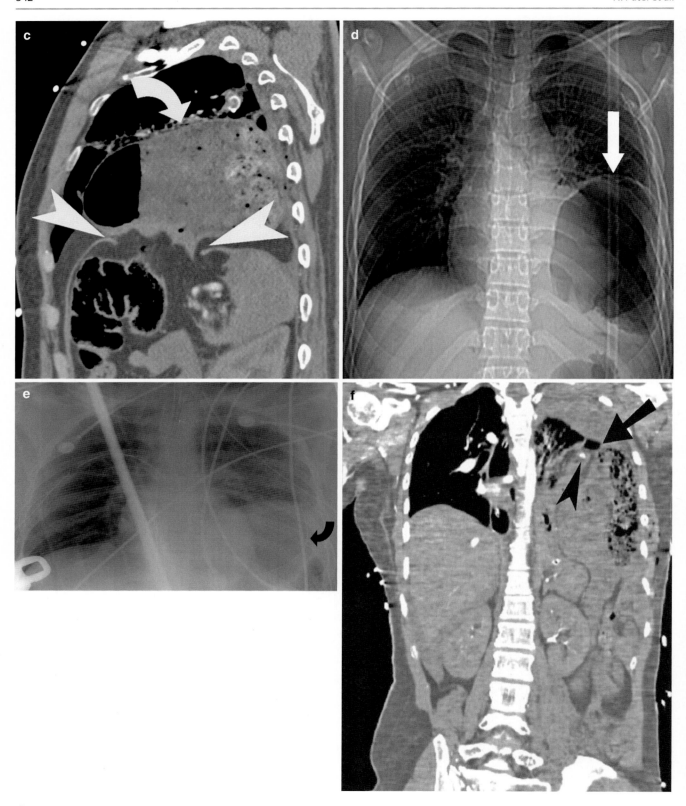

Fig. 24.8 (continued)

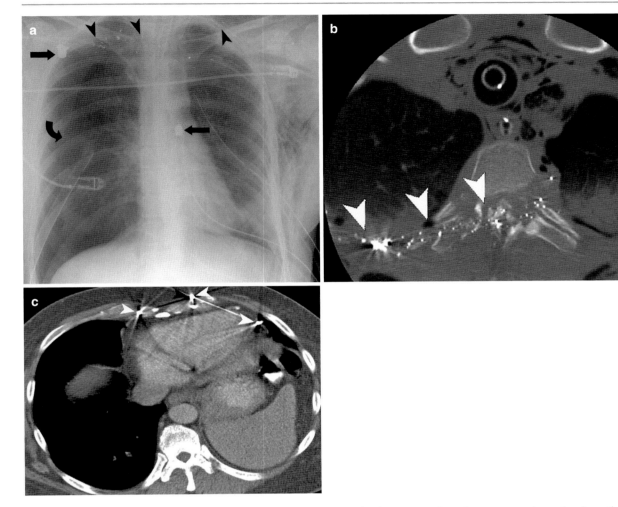

Fig. 24.9 (**a**) Gunshot injury to spinal canal. Right-sided pneumothorax (*curved arrow*) with chest tubes in place bilaterally. Bullets (*straight arrows*) are seen over the right upper chest and left paramediastinal locations. Small shrapnels (*arrowheads*) indicate the track of the bullet in the right and left upper chest. (**b**) Spinal cord injury. Axial CT scan in the same patient demonstrates shrapnels along the bullet track (*arrowheads*) passing through the spinal canal. Note also the pneumomediastinum, subcutaneous emphysema, endotracheal tube, and nasogastric tubes. (**c**) Gunshot injury to chest wall. Multiple shotgun pellets (*arrowheads*) are seen in the anterior chest wall and the pericardium

Injuries to the Chest Wall

Rib fractures are the most common skeletal injury in chest trauma and occur in approximately 50 % of patients. While single rib fractures are rarely life threatening, multiple rib fractures have been associated with increased morbidity and mortality probably because of their coexistence with more severe thoracic injury [4]. Double fractures in three or more ribs can lead to "flail chest" and is clinically significant because it can impair respiratory mechanics, promote atelectasis, and impair pulmonary drainage. Fracture of the first three ribs is considered to be high-energy trauma because these ribs are well protected. Some common complications of rib fractures are pneumothorax, hemothorax, extrapleural hematoma, and lung contusions (Fig. 24.9).

Sternal fractures are usually the result of deceleration injuries or direct anterior chest trauma. Displaced sternal fractures and those with associated joint disruption frequently occur with cardiac and spinal injuries. Sternal fractures are best seen on sagittal CT images and should be suspected by the presence of an anterior mediastinal hemorrhage.

Sternoclavicular dislocations are not common but are clinically important because of injury to the mediastinal blood vessels, trachea, and esophagus secondary to posterior dislocations. Anterior dislocations usually result from anterior blows to the shoulders, for example, from a seat-belt injury, and posterior dislocations result from posterior blows.

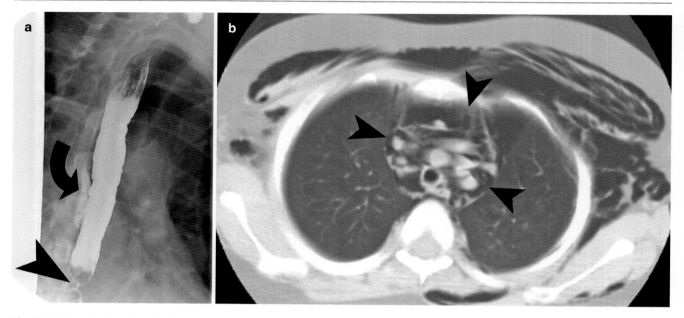

Fig. 24.10 (a) Esophageal perforation. Water-soluble contrast swallow demonstrates esophageal perforation in the mid posterior aspect of the esophagus (*curved arrow*) with impacted food located just proximal to a distal stricture (*arrowhead*). (b) Pneumomediastinum. Post-contrast axial CT demonstrates pneumomediastinum (*arrowheads*). Subcutaneous emphysema is present as well

Injuries to the Esophagus

Injuries to the esophagus are much more common with penetrating thoracic trauma. Distal esophageal tears usually occur along the left side [6]. CT findings in the setting of esophageal rupture may include pneumomediastinum, mediastinitis, hydropneumothorax, or leakage of orally administered contrast into the mediastinal or pleural space (Fig. 24.10). Water-soluble contrast esophagram or flexible esophagoscopy is usually the next step in investigating esophageal rupture.

Conclusions

Thoracic trauma continues to constitute a large percentage of life threatening injuries in overall trauma patients, the number of which is on the rise. Because a variety and combination of injuries to the intrathoracic contents can lead to complications and possible death, efficient diagnosis is of the utmost importance. Multidetector CT remains the primary modality to quickly and accurately diagnose these injuries; it has increased sensitivity over chest radiography and allows for a more complete analysis.

References

1. The American College of Surgeons Committee on Trauma Leadership. In: Clark DE, Fantus RJ, editors. National Trauma Data Bank (NTDB) annual report 2007. Chicago: American College of Surgeons; 2007. p. 1–64.
2. Report on injuries in America: all unintentional injuries. 2005. Available at http://www.nsc.org/library/report_table_1.htm. Accessed 9 Dec 2007.
3. Omert L, Yeaney WW, Protetch J. Efficacy of thoracic computerized tomography in blunt chest trauma. Am Surg. 2001;67:660–4.
4. Livingston DH, Haurer CJ. Trauma to the chest wall and lung. In: Moore EE, Feliciano DV, Mattox KL, editors. Trauma. 5th ed. Philadelphia: McGraw-Hill; 2004. p. 507–37.
5. Miller LA. Chest wall, lung, and pleural space trauma. Radiol Clin North Am. 2006;44:213–24.
6. Kaewlai R, Avery LL, Asrani AV, Novelline RA. Multidetector CT of blunt thoracic trauma. Radiographics. 2008;28(6):1555–70.
7. Mirvis SE, Kathirkamanathan S. Imaging in trauma and critical care. 2nd ed. New York: Saunders; 2003. p. 297–367.
8. Wagner RB, Crawford Jr WO, Schimpf PP. Classification of parenchymal injuries of the lung. Radiology. 1988;167:77–82.
9. Green R. Lung alterations in thoracic trauma. J Thorac Imaging. 1987;2:1.
10. Goodman LR, Putman CE. The SICU chest radiograph after massive blunt trauma. Radiol Clin North Am. 1981;19:111.
11. Halttunen PE, Kostianen SA, Meurala HG. Bronchial rupture cause by chest trauma. Scand J Thorac Cardiovasc Surg. 1984;18:141.
12. Fulda G, Brathwaite CE, Rodriguez A, Turney SZ, Dunham CM, Cowley RA. Blunt traumatic rupture of the heart and pericardium: a ten-year experience (1979–1989). J Trauma. 1991;31:167–73.
13. Stark P. Traumatic ruptures of the thoracic aorta: a review. Crit Rev Diagn Imaging. 1984;21:221.
14. Read RA, Moore EE, Moore FA, et al. Intravascular ultrasonography for the diagnosis of traumatic aortic disruption: a case report. Surgery. 1993;114:624.
15. Kearney PA, Rouhana SW, Burney RE. Blunt rupture of the diaphragm: mechanism, diagnosis, and treatment. Ann Emerg Med. 1986;18:438.

Ajay Singh and Chris Heinis

The emergency room has evolved over the years, and the practice has become increasingly complicated, commonly turning them into mini ICUs. During rapid assessment and stabilization of the patients in acute setting, there is often need to intubate the respiratory failure patients and provide intravenous fluid during resuscitation. With the growing volume of septic patients managed in the ED, central venous pressure monitoring has become more commonplace. This has led to the ED physicians placing more central line than ever. In this controlled chaos environment, the physicians are frequently exposed to anatomic variations which can lead to errors in line placement. Since image guidance is not routinely used during placement, the line or an endotracheal tube can be commonly malpositioned. However, we rely heavily on radiology to help confirm that the line or tube is where it should be without inadvertent damage to the surrounding tissue.

Endotracheal Tube

Once an endotracheal tube has been positioned, it is critical to evaluate its position on the chest radiograph. The endotracheal tube tip should be approximately 3–7 cm from the carina or at the level of the aortic arch. Flexion or extension of the chest can cause movement of the endotracheal tube by approximately 2–4 cm in either direction [1]. Ideally, when the neck is flexed, the endotracheal tube is 3 cm from the carina; conversely, when the neck is extended, the endotracheal tube should be 7 cm from the carina. Malpositioning

A. Singh, MD (✉)
Department of Radiology, Massachusetts General Hospital,
Harvard Medical School,
10 Museum Way, # 524, Boston, MA 02141, USA
e-mail: asingh1@partners.org

C. Heinis, MD
Department of Emergency Radiology, University of Massachusetts
Memorial Medical Center,
Worcester, MA, USA

[2] of the tube can occur in approximately 10–20 % of endotracheal intubations. Low placement of the endotracheal tube can cause bronchial intubation or carinal irritation.

The carina is not always well seen on a portable radiograph of the chest. In these scenarios, other landmarks may be useful in determining the position of the endotracheal tube. In 95 % of the cases (Fig. 25.1) [3], the positioning is proper when an endotracheal tube is 3.4–5 cm above the tangential line to the caudal edge of the aortic arch. Even when the carina is not visible, the endotracheal tube positioning can be confirmed if the tip ends at the level of T3 or T4 vertebral body. Goodman et al. found that carina projects over T5, T6, or T7 in 95 % of the patients [4]. The endotracheal tube's diameter should be anywhere between one-half to

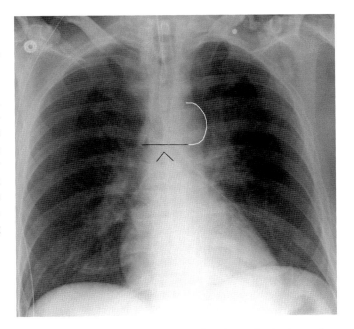

Fig. 25.1 Positioning of endotracheal tube when carina is obscured on a radiograph. Schematic representation of the left aortic arch outline which when extended horizontally at its inferior limit gives the landmark where the endotracheal tube should be placed. There is a nasogastric tube tip seen in the left bronchial tree

A. Singh (ed.), *Emergency Radiology*,
DOI 10.1007/978-1-4419-9592-6_25, © Springer Science+Business Media New York 2013

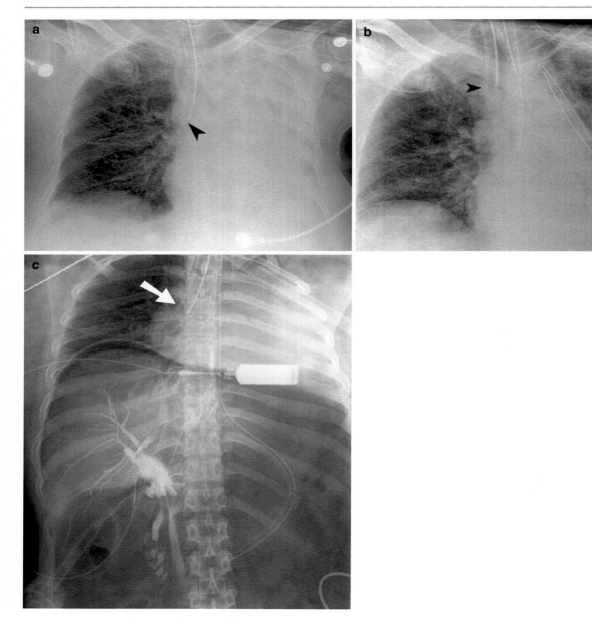

Fig. 25.2 Bronchial intubation. (**a**) Portable chest radiograph demonstrates the tip of the endotracheal tube (*arrowhead*) extending into the right main bronchus. There is lack of aeration in the left hemithorax with collapse of the left lung. (**b**) Follow-up chest x-ray after repositioning of the endotracheal tube into the trachea demonstrates reexpan-sion of the left lung. A left-sided chest tube was surgically placed based on the clinician's interpretation of the chest radiograph. (**c**) Intraoperative radiograph of the chest and abdomen, obtained during laparoscopic cholecystectomy, demonstrates right main bronchial intubation (*arrow*) with secondary collapse of the left lung

two-thirds the width of the trachea. The radiolucency within the tracheal cuff should be confined to the lumen of the trachea, without distending it.

The radiographic findings of a right main stem bronchial intubation include hyperinflation of the right lung, atelectasis of the left lung, and atelectasis of the right upper lobe (with a right lower lobe intubation) (Fig. 25.2). Repositioning of the endotracheal tube in the trachea leads to rapid reexpansion of the collapsed lung in patients where inadvertent main stem bronchial incubation was performed.

Other complications of endotracheal intubation include pneumothorax, tracheal rupture, tracheal stenosis (secondary to ischemia), and esophageal intubation (Fig. 25.3). The balloon cuff of the endotracheal tube should fill but not distend the lumen of the trachea. The ratio of balloon cuff diameter to tracheal diameter of more than 150 % is a predictor of tracheal damage [5].

The imaging findings of esophageal intubation include endotracheal tube cuff diameter more than that of the trachea, distention of the bowel lumen, and presence of air

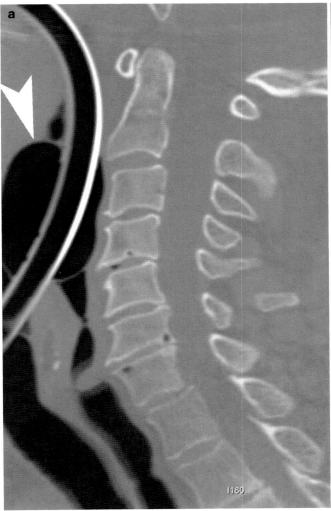
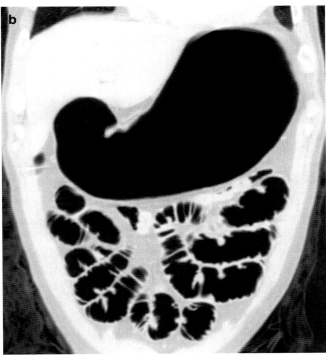

Fig. 25.3 High placed endotracheal tube. (**a**) Sagittal CT reformation demonstrates the cuff (*arrowhead*) of the endotracheal tube inflated in the hypopharynx. The upper esophagus is outlined by air from the endotracheal tube. (**b**) Coronal CT reformation of the abdomen demonstrates gaseous distention of the stomach and small bowel loops due to air leaking from the endotracheal tube

column in the esophagus. If an esophageal intubation is suspected, then a chest radiograph should be done after rotating the head to the right side and turning the patient to the right side by 25°. This obliquity results in esophageal air column projecting separate from the tracheal air column.

Tracheostomy Tube

Tracheostomy tube is used for long-term ventilation or in patients with laryngeal obstruction. Its caliber should be two-thirds the caliber of the trachea. It should be inserted at the level of the third tracheal cartilage with the tip placed above the level of the carina. It is not unusual to see pneumomediastinum and subcutaneous emphysema after placement

of a tracheostomy tube. The complications include tracheal perforation, fistulous communication between trachea and esophagus, and malpositioning (Fig. 25.4).

Nasogastric Feeding

Nasogastric tube is widely used to decompress the acidic gastric contents and reduce aspiration risk. It is recognized by the presence of a radiopaque line traversing the entire tube length. The side port of the nasogastric tube is approximately 8 cm from the tip. Ideal location of the nasogastric tube is in the stomach with the side port below the gastroesophageal junction. If the side holes of the tube are located in the distal esophagus, it can lead to aspiration pneumonia.

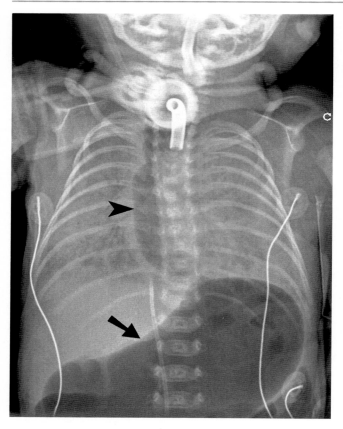

Fig. 25.4 Abnormal tracheostomy tube positioning. Plain radiograph of the chest and upper abdomen demonstrates marked distention of the esophagus (*arrowheads*) and stomach (*arrow*) due to leakage of air from the tracheostomy tube into the upper gastrointestinal tract

A feeding tube is recognized by the presence of a linear radiopaque tungsten band at the tip of the tube. It is ideally place in the distal duodenum and is used for enteric feeding without the risk of gastroesophageal reflux. Placement of the tip distal to the gastric pylorus reduces the risk of aspiration.

The enteric tubes may be coiled in the pharynx, esophagus, or stomach. The may be malpositioned into the bronchial tree, mediastinum, or pleural space (Fig. 25.5). If the post feeding tube or nasogastric tube placement radiograph shows placement in the tracheobronchial tree, the tube should be withdrawn and a follow-up radiograph obtained to rule out a pneumothorax [6]. Rare complications include esophageal perforation and swallowing of entire enteric tube.

G and GJ Tubes

G and J tubes are widely used for long-term enteric feeding, often used in patients with failure to thrive, risk of aspiration, swallowing dysfunction. There are an increasing number of these tubes placed by interventional radiologist because of the advantage of their placement without the need for general anesthesia. There is 5 % major complication rate associated with G-tube placement [7]. The complications include colonic perforation, tube dislodgement, tube migration, peritonitis, abscess formation, septicemia, tube site insertion infection, and GI bleeding (Fig. 25.6).

Central Venous Catheters

More than five million central venous catheters are placed by physicians in the USA, most often by surgeons and anesthesiologist, without image guidance [8]. While tunneled catheters are most often placed by surgeons or interventional radiologists, nontunelled catheters are most commonly placed by the surgeons and anesthesiologists. In 1999, interventional radiologists accounted for 20 % of the tunneled and 15 % of the nontunelled catheters placed in Medicare patients [9].

The subclavian vein is separated from the subclavian artery by anterior scalenus muscle. The subclavian vein is separated from the pleura of the lung apex by only 5 mm. The needle placement at the time of subclavian central venous catheter insertion should be in inward and slightly upward direction (from the mid clavicle, aiming toward the sternoclavicular joint).

Imaging plays an important role in documenting correct position of the central venous line tip as between 10 and 30 % of the catheters placed without imaging guidance are in suboptimal position. The right tracheobronchial angle is the best anatomic landmark to delineate the border of the superior vena cava and right atrium junction. The optimal position of central line tip is in the superior vena cava, adjacent to the cavoatrial junction. If the central venous line tip is placed too high from the cavoatrial junction, the tip may be above the venous valves or may be outside the vascular lumen. The valves are found in the subclavian vein and internal jugular vein, approximately 2.5 cm from their confluence to form the brachiocephalic vein. The placement of the catheter tip above the valves can lead to inaccurate measurement of central venous pressures (most commonly elevated pressures).

Although there is tendency among interventional radiologist to place the catheter tip in the upper right atrium, the FDA disagrees with this practice because of the potential for cardiac-related complications. According to 1989 FDA precautionary statement related to central venous catheter, the catheter tip should not be placed in the heart.

A chest radiograph should be obtained in every patient where subclavian venous catheter placement was attempted, irrespective of whether it was successful or not. Despite the presence of venous canals, central venous catheter may extend up the internal jugular vein or less commonly into the

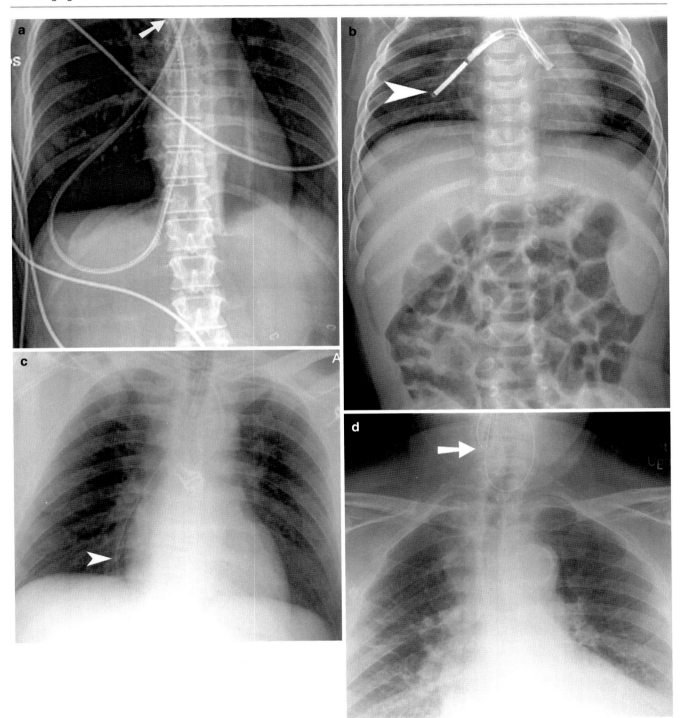

Fig. 25.5 Abnormal nasogastric and feeding tube positions. (**a**) Plain radiograph demonstrates a feeding tube (*arrow*) extending through the right main bronchus and penetrating into the pleural space. (**b**) Plain radiograph demonstrating feeding tube extending coiled in the left main bronchus and the tip (*arrowhead*) extending into the right main bronchus. (**c**) Plain radiograph demonstrating nasogastric tube (*arrowhead*) extending into the right lower lobe bronchus. (**d**) Plain radiograph demonstrating coiling of the nasogastric tube (*arrow*) in the hypopharynx. (**e**) Plain radiograph of the abdomen demonstrating tip of the feeding tube in the stomach on the first study and in the distending colon (*arrow*) on the second study. The patient had swallowed the feeding tube between the two studies

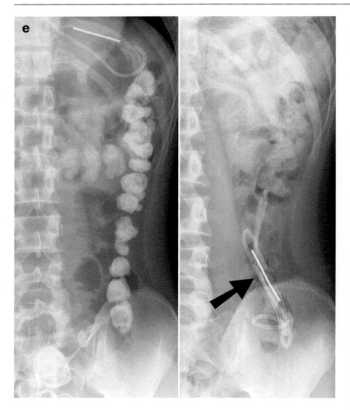

Fig. 25.5 (continued)

contralateral brachiocephalic, subclavian, internal jugular, or azygous veins. The most common location of a misplaced subclavian central line is the ipsilateral internal jugular vein (Fig. 25.7) [6]. Central venous catheter tip of which is located within the internal jugular vein should not be used, as there is a risk of thrombosis and vascular rupture. The extension of a left-sided central line into the right brachiocephalic vein can be seen, especially in patients where the left brachiocephalic vein is higher and more horizontally located. Right-sided central line placement does not usually extend to the left brachiocephalic vein as the right brachiocephalic vein course is more in line with the superior vena cava. A central venous catheter placed into the azygous vein can be best identified on the lateral view, as the catheter courses posteriorly at the level of the superior vena cava.

Central venous catheter tip located in the mediastinum and pleural space can result in infusion of the IV fluid into the mediastinal space or pleural cavity (Figs. 25.8 and 25.9). Rapid accumulation of pleural effusion is a clue to the diagnoses of pleural placement of the central line.

The complications of central venous line placement include arterial placement (Fig. 25.10), vascular perforation, SVC syndrome, catheter break, and infection.

Uncommon locations of the catheter tip include pericardiophrenic vein, internal mammary vein, superior intercostal vein, left superior accessory vein, axillary vein, or left-sided superior vena cava (Figs. 25.11 and 25.12). Left-sided superior vena cava is seen in 0.3 % of the control population and will lead to placement of the left-sided central line along the left superior mediastinum, coursing posterior to the heart (coronary sinus), into the right atrium.

The placement of the catheter tip in the heart can lead to arrhythmia, myocardial rupture, and pericardial tamponade. Pneumothorax is seen in approximately 5 % of patients after central line or port placement and is most commonly seen after subclavian rather than internal jugular line placement (Fig. 25.13). The majority of the pneumothorax from central venous line placement is asymptomatic and resolve spontaneously. Symptomatic or enlarging pneumothorax requires treatment with a pigtail drainage catheter.

Infections associated with central venous line catheters are most commonly related to staphylococcus species. The presence of sepsis usually mandates removal of the catheter and treatment with antibiotics. The single most common cause of catheter dysfunction is formation of a fibrin sheath, made up of eosinophilic material and inflammatory cells at the catheter tip. It is often associated with thrombus and functions as a one-way valve which allows the catheter to be flushed but not aspirated. The treatment of a fibrin sheath is tissue plasminogen activator infusion into the catheter, which if not successful can be treated with catheter exchange over an Amplatz guidewire. The sheath can sometimes be removed using a loop snare or balloon angioplasty.

Catheter breakage can lead to embolization of the catheter fragment into the right atrium, right ventricle, or pulmonary circulation. These catheter fragments can be retrieved percutaneously using a snare (Fig. 25.14).

Long-term venous central venous access can lead to thrombosis and venous stenosis. The risk of thrombosis is less in patients with Broviak and Hickman catheters.

Subcutaneous Ports and Tunneled Catheters

A subcutaneous port most often used is the Port-A-Cath. It is often used for repeated access of the venous system and is most often used either in oncology or in cystic fibrosis patients. Typical port is located subcutaneously in the anterior chest wall and is connected to the central vein by tubing which typically enters the thorax via the internal jugular vein. The complications include thrombosis of the port/tubing, disconnection of the tubing from the port, upward retraction of the tubing, infection, and fibrin sheath formation (Fig. 25.15).

Tunneled catheters offer a benefit over nontunneled versions. Tunneled catheters can be used for hemodialysis and other longer duration vascular access. If the internal jugular vein is punctured more than 3–4 cm above the clavicle, the tunneled catheter has high chance of kinking and occlusion.

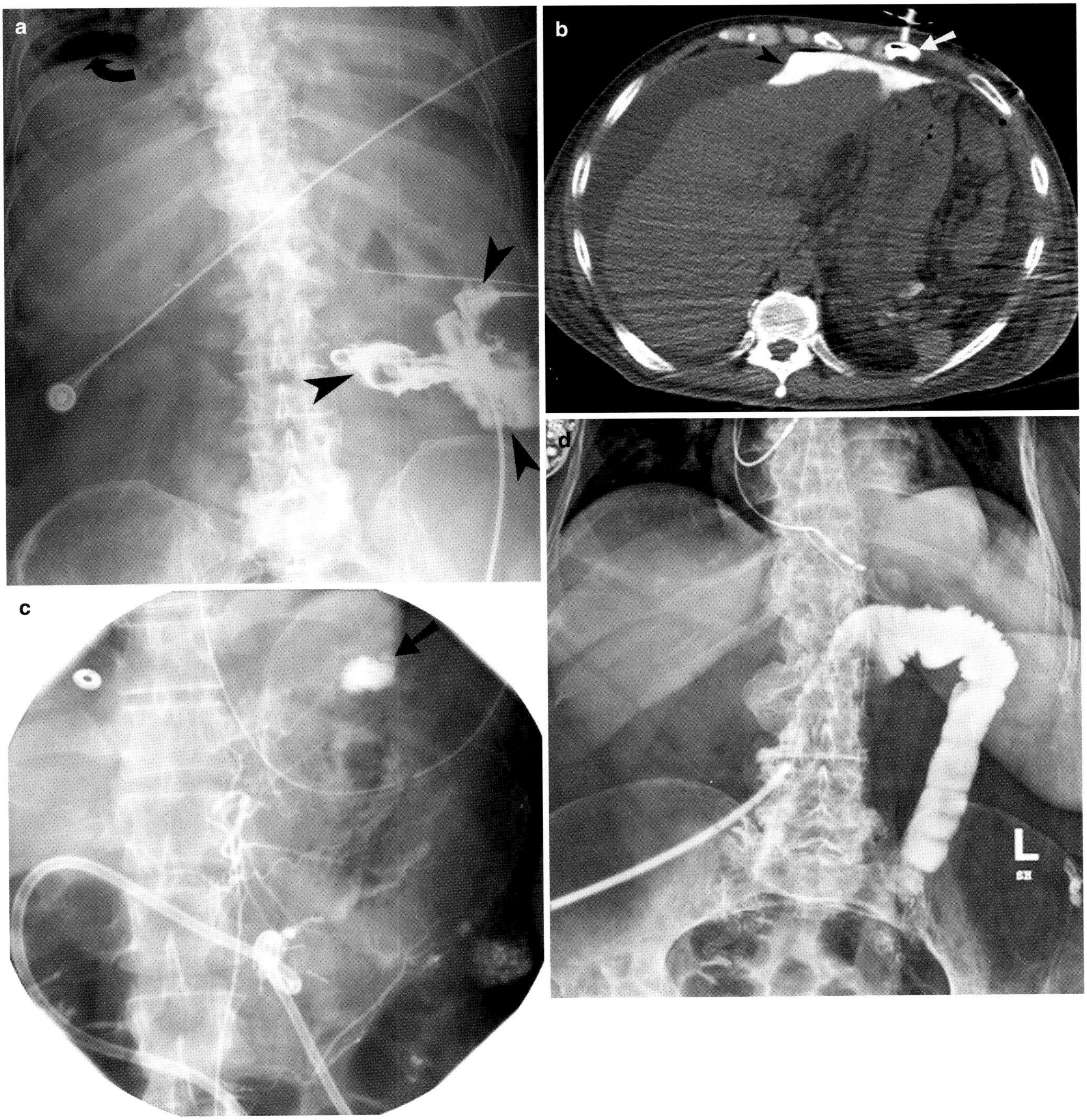

Fig. 25.6 G-tube malposition. (**a**) Tube injection study demonstrating the G tube located outside the stomach. There is contrast extravasation outside the bowel loops (*arrowheads*). There is free air (*curved arrow*) under the right dome of diaphragm. (**b**) Noncontrast CT after tube injection demonstrates the G tube (*arrow*) located in the left anterior abdominal wall. The contrast (*arrowhead*) injected through the G tube is present within the peritoneal cavity, anterior to the left lobe of the liver and the stomach. (**c**) Left gastric arteriogram demonstrates active arterial bleeding (*arrow*) after gastrojejunostomy tube insertion. (**d**) G-tube injection study demonstrates opacification of the colonic lumen from inadvertent colonic perforation

When the patient moves from supine to upright position, the tunneled central venous catheter has a tendency to migrate cranially by several centimeters. In female population, the downward pull on the tunneled catheter or the port by breast can exaggerate cranial migration of the catheter tip.

Intra-aortic Balloon Pump

The use of intra-aortic balloon pump has increased in recent times for treatment of low cardiac output in patients with

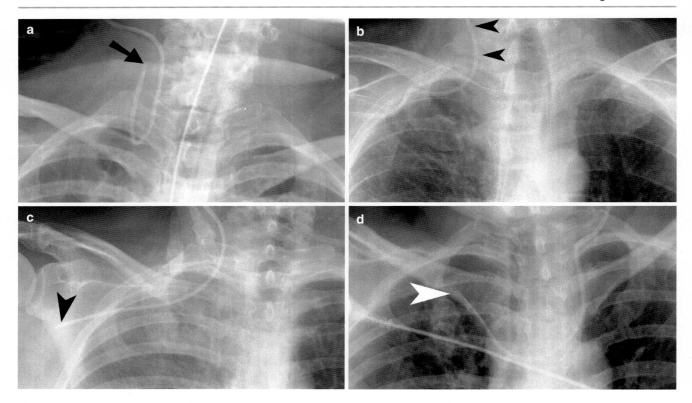

Fig. 25.7 Abnormal central venous line positions. Plain radiograph of the upper chest demonstrates: (**a**) Right internal jugular venous line tip (*arrow*) coiled in the internal jugular vein. (**b**) Right subclavian venous line extending up, into the right internal jugular vein (*arrowheads*). (**c**) Right internal jugular venous line extending into the right axillary vein (*arrowhead*). (**d**) Left internal jugular venous line extending into the right subclavian vein (*arrowhead*)

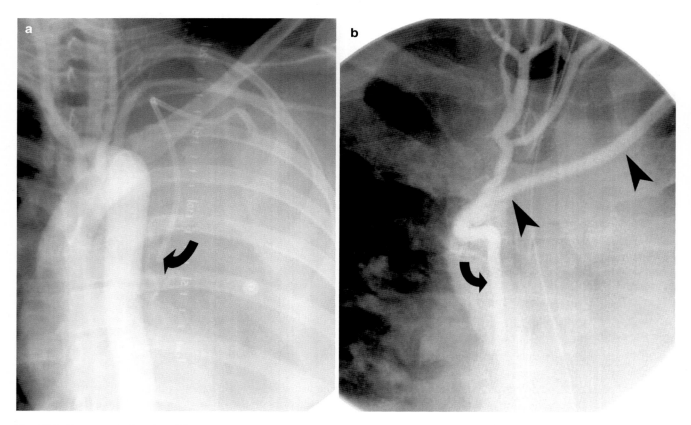

Fig. 25.8 Extravascular location of lines. (**a**) Aortogram study demonstrates left-sided Port-A-Cath tip (*curved arrow*) located in the left pleural space. The large left pleural effusion was produced by inadvertent usage of the left Port-A-Cath. (**b**) Venogram study through the left hemodialysis catheter (*arrowheads*) demonstrates opacification of the azygous vein (*curved arrow*)

Fig. 25.9 Extravascular location of venous line. Plain radiograph of the chest (*left image*) demonstrates left-sided subclavian venous line tip (*arrowhead*) projecting beyond the right margin of the superior vena cava. There is moderate-size pleural effusion seen on the right due to infusion of saline through the central line. CT venogram (*right image*) demonstrates extension of the tip of the left subclavian venous line (*arrowhead*) beyond the margin of the superior vena cava

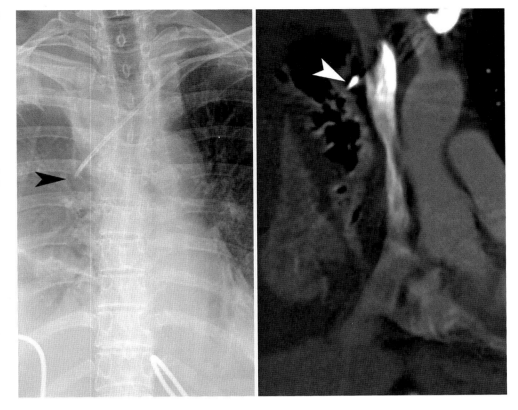

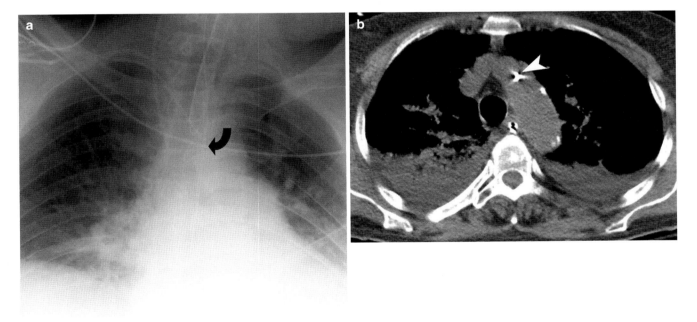

Fig. 25.10 Arterial location of central venous lines. (**a**) Plain radiograph of the chest demonstrates right subclavian line (*curved arrow*) extending across the midline to the left side. (**b**) Noncontrast CT of the chest confirms the arterial location of the central line (*arrowhead*)

congestive heart failure. It inflates in diastole, increasing the coronary artery blood flow as well as peripheral vascular flow. It deflates in systole, decreasing the left ventricular afterload.

The tip of the intra-aortic balloon pump should be 1 cm distal to the origin of the left subclavian artery (Fig. 25.16a). The radiopaque tip marker should be at the level of the carina. If the tip is too proximally placed in the aortic arch, it can

Fig. 25.11 Central venous line extending into the left superior intercostal vein. Plain radiograph (*left image*) and coronal CT (*right image*) reformation demonstrate left internal jugular venous line (*arrowhead*) extending into the left superior intercostal vein

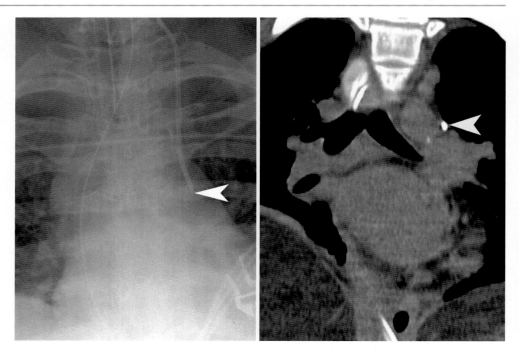

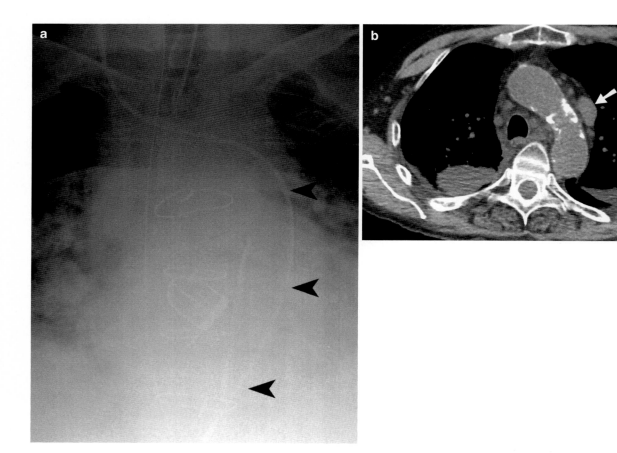

Fig. 25.12 Central line in left-sided superior vena cava. (**a**) Portable radiograph of the chest demonstrates right-sided internal jugular venous line (*arrowheads*) extending into left-sided superior vena cava and cor-onary sinus arrowheads. (**b**) Axial CT of the chest demonstrates a left-sided superior vena cava (*arrow*). There is no right-sided superior vena cava

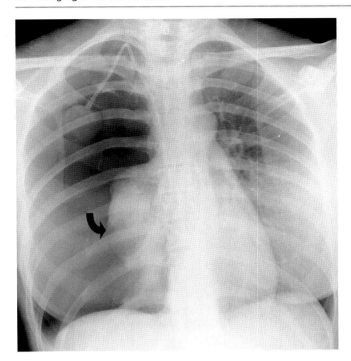

Fig. 25.13 Tension pneumothorax after Port-A-Cath placement. Plain radiograph of the chest demonstrates large right-sided pneumothorax with complete collapse of the right lung (*arrow*) due to visceral pleural puncture at the time of right Port-A-Cath placement

occlude the branches of the aortic arch. If the tip is too distally placed, then the IABP may not be effective enough in increasing coronary blood flow.

The complications of intra-aortic balloon pump include aortic dissection, aortic wall laceration, embolic phenomenon, vascular insufficiency in the catheterized length, hemolysis, and improper positioning (Fig. 25.16b).

Swan-Ganz Catheter

Swan-Ganz catheter is used to measure the pulmonary artery wedge pressure, which is useful in evaluating end-diastolic left ventricular pressure and pulmonary capillary hydrostatic pressure. Swan-Ganz catheter is helpful in distinguishing cardiogenic from noncardiogenic pulmonary edema. When the pressure is not being measured, the Swan-Ganz catheter is positioned in the right or left pulmonary artery (Fig. 25.17). The catheter wedges into the distal pulmonary artery segment when the balloon is inflated, thereby giving the pulmonary artery wedge pressure. The balloon of the Swan-Ganz catheter should be kept deflated, unless pulmonary artery wedge pressure reading is required.

The complications of a Swan-Ganz catheter placement include cardiac arrhythmia, pulmonary infarction, intracardiac knotting, balloon rupture, pseudoaneurysm formation, and rupture of the pulmonary artery.

Fig. 25.14 Fractured central venous line. PA and lateral views of the chest demonstrate fractured central venous line tubing (*arrowheads*) located in the right ventricle. This was taken out using a snare

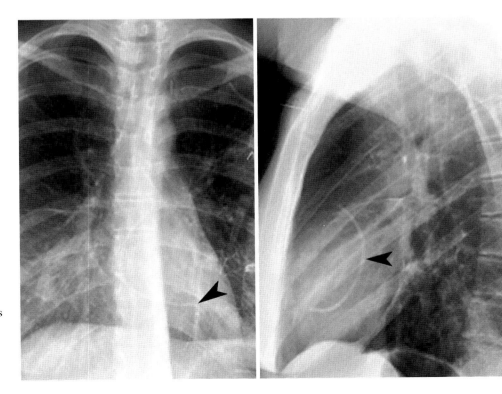

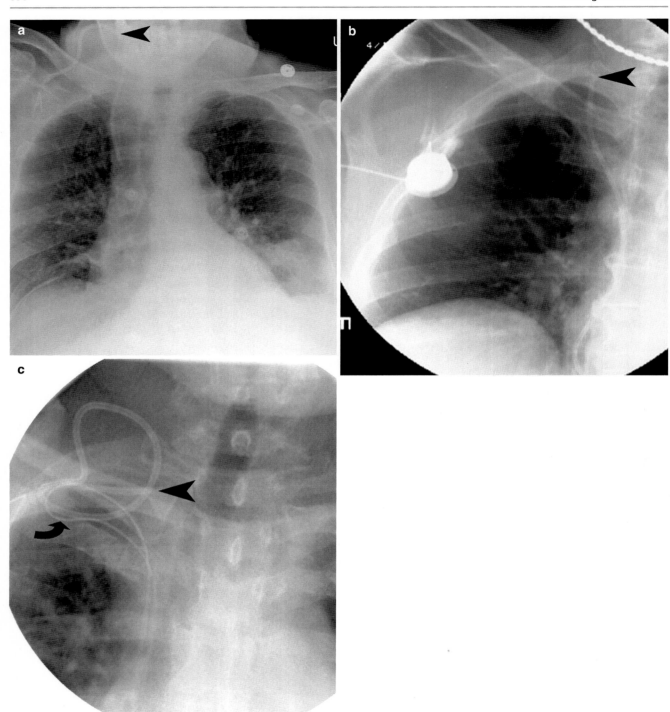

Fig. 25.15 Port-A-Cath abnormalities. (**a**) Plain radiograph of the chest demonstrates abnormally high loop (*arrowhead*) of the Port-A-Cath tubing. (**b**) Plain radiograph of the chest demonstrates separation of the port from the tubing (*arrowhead*). (**c**) Scout film of the upper chest demonstrates retraction of the right Port-A-Cath tubing (*arrowhead*) into the right subclavian vein. The spot film also demonstrates snare (*arrow*) which was used to pull the tip of the tubing back into the superior vena cava

Fig. 25.16 Intra-aortic balloon pump. (**a**) The *left-sided* image demonstrates normal position of intra-aortic balloon pump (*arrowhead*), just below the aortic arch. The *right-sided* image demonstrates an abnormally high location of an intra-aortic balloon pump tip, extending into the left subclavian artery (*arrowhead*). (**b**) Axial contrast-enhanced CT scan study of the upper abdomen demonstrates wedge-shaped splenic infarct (*arrow*), secondary to the intra-aortic balloon pump (*arrowhead*) seen adjacent to the origin of the celiac artery

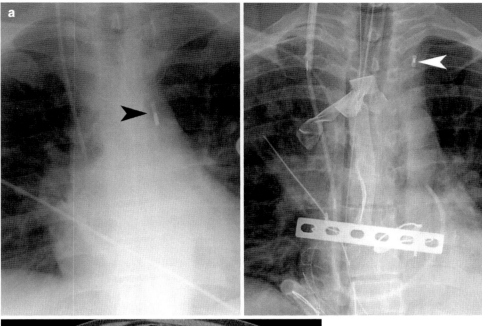

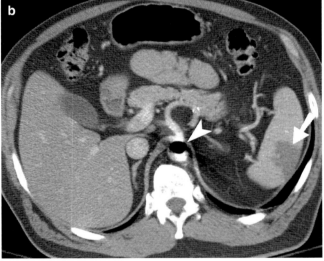

Fig. 25.17 Swan-Ganz catheter. (**a**) *Left-sided* image demonstrates Swan-Ganz catheter tip (*curved arrow*) in the right main pulmonary artery. The radiograph on the right demonstrates the tip of the Swan-Ganz catheter (*straight arrow*) into the interlobar artery branch of the right pulmonary artery. (**b**) Plain radiograph of the chest demonstrates Swan-Ganz catheter tip (*arrowhead*) coiled in the outflow tract of the right ventricle. (**c**) Pulmonary arteriogram before and after coil placement. The image on the *top* demonstrates a pseudoaneurysm (*arrow*) secondary to Swan-Ganz catheter placement in the past, supplied by the right middle lobe artery. The image at the *bottom* demonstrates placement of tornado coils into the arterial feeder of the pseudoaneurysm

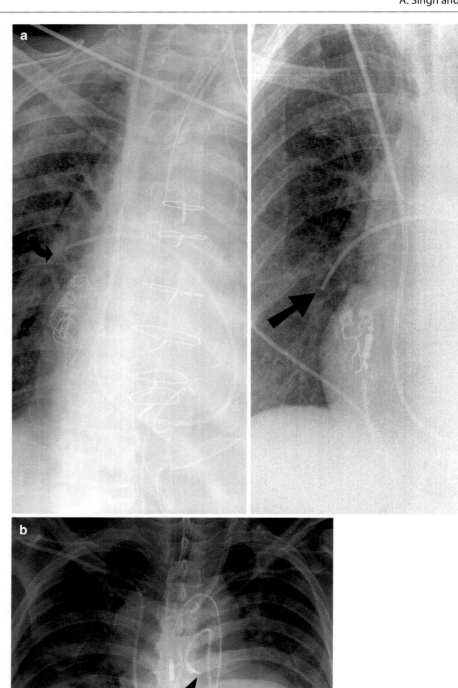

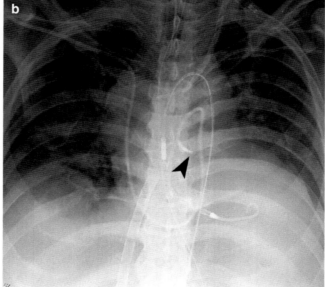

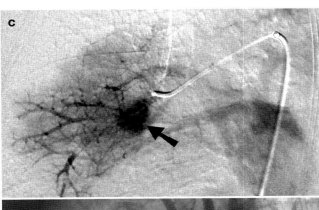

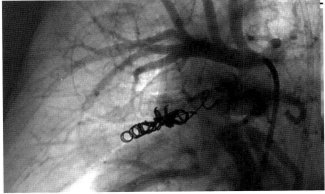

Fig. 25.17 (continued)

References

1. Goodman LR, Conrardy PA, Laing F. Radiographic evaluation of endotracheal tube position. Am J Roentgenol. 1976;127:433–4.
2. Stauffer JL, Olson DE, Petty TL. Complications and consequences of endotracheal intubation and tracheostomy: a prospective study of 150 critically ill adult patients. Am J Med. 1981;70:65–76.
3. Pappas JN, Goodman PC. Predicting proper endotracheal tube placement in underexposed radiographs: tangent line of the aortic arch. Am J Roentgenol. 1999;173:1357–9.
4. Goodman LR, Conrardy PA, Laing F, Singer MM. Radiographic evaluation of endotracheal tube position. Am J Roentgenol. 1976; 127:433–4.
5. Price DB. Tubes in the alimentary and respiratory tracts: appearances on CT scans of the head and neck. Am J Roentgenol. 1991;156: 1047–51.
6. Aronchick JM, Miller Jr WT. Tubes and lines in intensive care setting. Semin Roentgenol. 1997;32:102–16.
7. Friedman JN, Ahmed S, Connolly B, Chait P, Mahant S. Complications associated with image-guided gastrostomy and gastrojejunostomy tubes in children. Pediatrics. 2004;114(2):458–61.
8. McGee DC, Gould MK. Preventing complications of central venous catheterization. N Engl J Med. 2003;348:1123–33.
9. Reeves AR, Seshadri R, Trerotola SO. Recent trends in central venous catheter placement: a comparison of interventional radiology with other specialties. J Vasc Interv Radiol. 2001;12(10): 1211–4.

Imaging of Pediatric Emergencies

26

John J. Krol, Paul F. von Herrmann, Harigovinda R. Challa, and Johanne E. Dillon

Introduction

The diagnosis and management of pediatric patients in the emergency department has unique challenges that often require a different approach by the clinician than with an adult patient. Although children may develop many of the same illnesses as adults, certain life-threatening diagnoses are seen more often in the pediatric population. An immature immune system, small body size, and developmental anomalies are several factors that can place children at an increased risk for specific diseases. This chapter will focus on the imaging evaluation of diagnoses that occur more often or with a unique appearance in the pediatric population.

Neurology

Acute Disseminated Encephalomyelitis (ADEM)

Acute disseminated encephalomyelitis is a diagnostic challenge both to the clinician and the radiologist owing to its similarity in presentation with other diseases, specifically multiple sclerosis (MS). The disease is an acute demyelinating process (often preceded by a viral illness or vaccination) predominantly affecting the white matter, deep gray matter, brain stem, and spinal cord with an estimated mortality rate as high as 5 % [1]. Because of the confusing and severe presentations of patients, imaging is frequently obtained for further evaluation.

Magnetic resonance imaging (MRI) of the head is the preferred modality for evaluation of the majority of patients with symptoms suggestive of ADEM, and further evaluation with MRI of the spine is often performed as well. The limited literature available comparing the sensitivity of computed tomography (CT) to MRI suggests that MRI is far superior both in sensitivity and specificity compared to CT [2]. CT may be performed initially to exclude neurosurgical emergencies, but CT will often underestimate the extent of disease and may not appropriately characterize the condition. On MRI, the imaging findings of ADEM are similar to other demyelinating disorders and typically include focally increased signal in the white matter on T2-weighted sequences, mild enhancement on postcontrast sequences, and restricted diffusion in acute lesions (Fig. 26.1). The distribution of lesions is variable, though certain patterns of involvement may help favor the diagnosis of ADEM over MS. The thalamus (30–40 %), basal ganglia (30–40 %), cerebellum (30–40 %), and brain stem (45–55 %) are affected more frequently in ADEM than MS, and the periventricular white matter and corpus callosum are frequently spared [3, 4].

Treatment includes admission for administration of intravenous steroids and for some patients, intravenous immunoglobulin. The majority of patients will improve clinically with mild residual impairment in 57–90 % of patients [1]. Disease relapses are possible.

Intracranial Complications of Acute Otitis Media and Sinusitis

Due to the high prevalence of viral infections and the small diameter of draining pathways for the middle ear cavity and sinuses, children are at increased risk for developing acute otitis media (AOM) and acute sinusitis. In rare cases, the infection can extend intracranially. Meningitis, intracranial abscesses, and septic thrombosis of intracranial venous structures may result. Patients with known or suspected sinusitis or AOM presenting with sudden worsening of headache, visual symptoms, seizures, or neurologic deficits may necessitate imaging for further evaluation.

J.J. Krol, MD (✉) • P.F. von Herrmann, MD
Department of Radiology, University of Kentucky,
800 Rose Street, HX-307B, Lexington, KY 40536-0293, USA
e-mail: johnjkrol@uky.edu

H.R. Challa, MD • J.E. Dillon, MD
Division of Pediatric Radiology, University of Kentucky,
Lexington, KY, USA

A. Singh (ed.), *Emergency Radiology*,
DOI 10.1007/978-1-4419-9592-6_26, © Springer Science+Business Media New York 2013

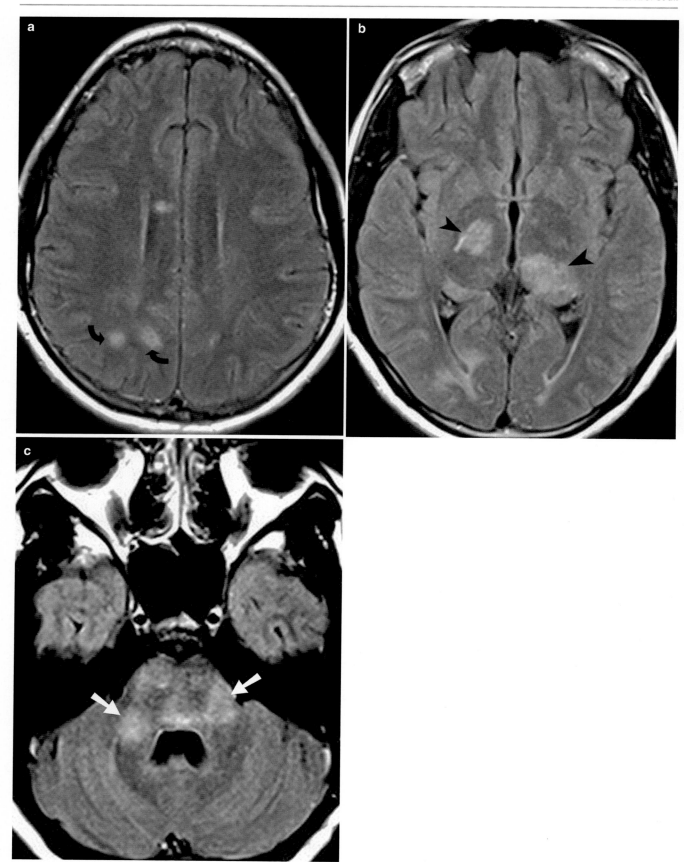

Fig. 26.1 ADEM. (**a–c**) Axial FLAIR sequence images in a 4-year-old girl demonstrate increased signal in the bilateral subcortical white matter (*curved arrows*), bilateral thalami (*arrowheads*), and middle cerebellar peduncle (*straight arrows*) involvement

Fig. 26.2 Frontal sinusitis with subdural empyema. (**a**) Axial CT images of an 11-year-old boy exhibits opacification of the right maxillary (*arrow*) and frontal sinuses (*arrowhead*). (**b**) Axial post-gadolinium T1-weighted image demonstrates oval abscess (*arrow*) with meningeal enhancement in the interhemispheric fissure

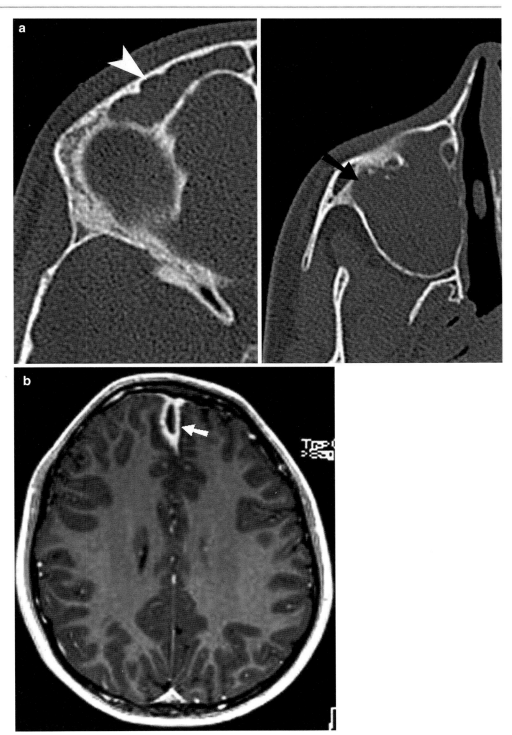

MRI of the head with contrast is the examination of choice to evaluate for intracranial spread of infection. The specificity of MRI is superior in evaluation for meningitis and intracranial abscesses and in differentiating dural reaction from extra-axial or intra-axial abscess. Early in the process, meningeal inflammation may be the first abnormality present, which typically appears as meningeal enhancement on both CT and MRI. As an extra-axial abscess develops, the appearance is typically a fluid collection with high T2 signal intensity and low T1 signal intensity on MRI and usually higher attenuation relative to cerebrospinal fluid (CSF) on CT (Fig. 26.2). Abscess on either modality generally

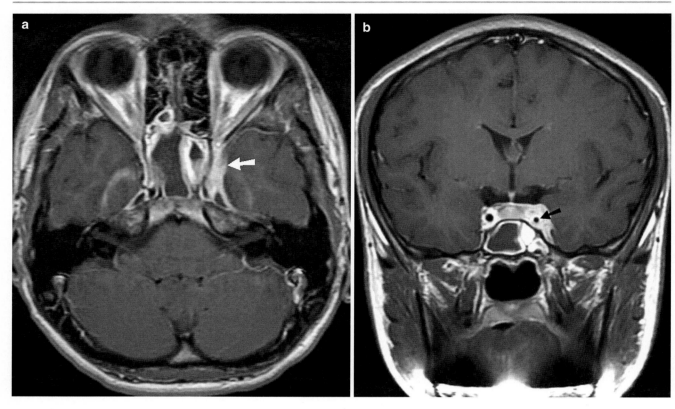

Fig. 26.3 Cavernous sinus thrombosis. (**a, b**) Axial and coronal T1-weighted post-gadolinium demonstrates enhancement and enlargement of the left cavernous sinus (*white arrow*) in a patient with marked mucosal enhancement of the adjacent sphenoid sinus. Note the diminished caliber of the left internal carotid artery (*black arrow*) relative to the right side due to mass effect

demonstrates peripheral enhancement on postcontrast images. Dural venous or cavernous sinus thrombosis are often challenging with either CT or MRI, though thrombosis is best established on postcontrast images on either a CT or MR venogram examination appearing as a filling defect in the venous structure. Venous congestion may result from septic venous thrombosis and vasogenic and cytotoxic cerebral edema, sometimes with associated susceptibility artifact (representing hemorrhage) or restricted diffusion, may be seen in the parenchyma drained by the thrombosed dural venous sinus (Fig. 26.3) [5]. Cerebritis typically manifests as focally decreased attenuation on CT and increased T2 signal intensity in the brain parenchyma on MRI. As the process progresses to abscess formation, either modality will demonstrate progressive peripheral enhancement on postcontrast imaging along with surrounding vasogenic edema. Intracranial abscesses often exhibit restricted diffusion on MRI.

Intravenous antibiotics are indicated for intracranial spread of infection. Treatment of intracranial abscess typically involves surgical drainage. Septic thrombosis of the dural venous sinuses and cavernous sinus is managed with intravenous antibiotics and surgical drainage of the adjacent infectious source.

Orbital Infection: Subperiosteal Abscess and Orbital Cellulitis

Infection in the orbit constitutes an ophthalmologic emergency. Whether as a result of sinusitis or periorbital cellulitis extending across the orbital septum, this constitutes an emergency as the infection can cause blindness and spread intracranially. Imaging may be performed to determine the extent of the infection, to localize an abscess or for surgical planning.

CT of the orbits is often the first imaging modality ordered because it is quick, accessible, and has a high sensitivity and specificity; however, according to the 2009 American College of Radiology (ACR) Appropriateness Criteria, contrast-enhanced MRI is recognized as a first-line imaging test to evaluate orbital infections. With periorbital cellulitis invading the orbit, the infection typically invades medially as the orbital septum is thinner in its medial portion. Orbital cellulitis will be seen on CT as obliteration of fat planes and soft tissue enhancement if contrast is administered. On MRI, the infection will demonstrate low T1 signal intensity, high T2 signal intensity and soft tissue enhancement. In regards to subperiosteal abscess, the findings at CT generally include an extraconal fluid collection adjacent to an opacified sinus. Early orbital abscesses may not demonstrate peripheral

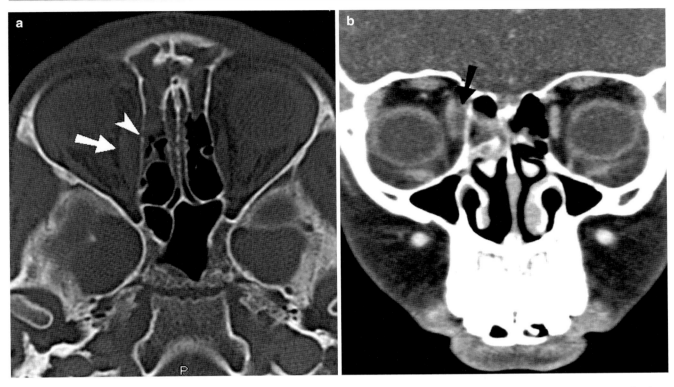

Fig. 26.4 Subperiosteal abscess. (**a**, **b**) Axial and coronal CT image demonstrates ethmoidal and frontal sinusitis with right extraconal subperiosteal abscess (*arrow*), adjacent to the medial rectus muscle. There is breech identified in the right lamina papyracea (*arrowhead*)

enhancement on contrast-enhanced examinations on CT (Fig. 26.4) [6]. On MRI, subperiosteal abscesses have low T1 signal intensity, high T2 signal intensity, often peripherally enhance and often restrict diffusion (Fig. 26.5). When contrast is administered, both MRI and CT are acceptable in diagnosing superior ophthalmic venous thrombosis.

Treatment for orbital cellulitis is intravenous antibiotics. Subperiosteal abscess typically warrants surgical intervention especially when there is visual acuity loss or paralysis of extraocular muscles.

Transverse Myelitis

One of the more neurologically devastating diagnoses is transverse myelitis, which is defined as demyelination across the spinal cord that can occur at any level. Back pain and sensory deficits are common presenting symptoms. In addition to CSF analysis, imaging is often warranted to support the diagnosis and define its extent, as well as to exclude a mass in the spinal column that could produce similar symptoms but would have a different treatment.

MRI of the spine with contrast is the examination of choice in patients with suspected transverse myelitis, and MRI of the head is often also obtained. Affected portions of the spinal cord characteristically have increased signal on T2-weighted images and typically span at least two-thirds of the spinal cord in transverse dimensions (Fig. 26.6). There

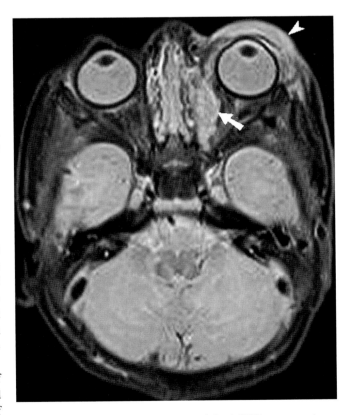

Fig. 26.5 Subperiosteal abscess. T2-weighted STIR sequence in an 8-day-old demonstrates subperiosteal abscess (*short white arrow*) along medial wall of the left orbit, secondary to ethmoidal sinusitis. There is left-sided proptosis with preseptal edema (*arrowhead*)

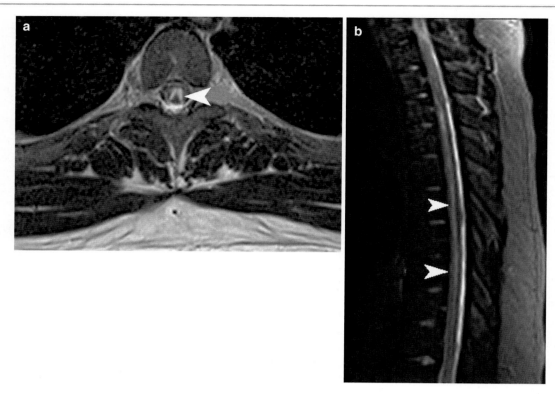

Fig. 26.6 Transverse myelitis. (**a**, **b**) Axial and sagittal T2-weighted images of the thoracic spine demonstrate multiple foci of abnormal increased signal (*arrowheads*) extending transversely through the spinal cord in an acutely paraplegic 18-year-old male

may be edema resulting in expansion of the cord. Contrast enhancement, usually peripherally around the lesion, may be seen in a significant percentage of patients [7].

Treatment generally includes intravenous steroids, though some patients may also receive plasmapheresis. Prognosis is variable with approximately one-third of patients fully recovering and one-third of patients regaining minimal to no function.

Ventriculoperitoneal Shunt Malfunction

Ventriculoperitoneal (VP) shunts are usually placed to treat hydrocephalus. Shunting malfunction may manifest with either increased or decreased ventricle size with accompanying changes in intracranial pressure. Radiologically important causes of shunt malfunction include shunt valve malfunction, infection, tubing discontinuity, and loculated CSF accumulation in the peritoneal cavity (CSF pseudocyst), each of which are treated differently. Radiologic evaluation is usually indicated to confirm a change in size of the ventricles, evaluate for other intracranial abnormalities as well as to identify potential underlying mechanisms of disease.

VP shunt radiographic series usually includes images of the skull, neck, chest, and abdomen. If a discontinuity of the catheter exists at the level of the reservoir, a soft tissue mass may be seen within the scalp, representing a CSF leak into the scalp; however, most reservoirs are radiolucent, and radiolucency should not be confused with discontinuity in this location. Discontinuity, if present, will often be easily identified along the other portions of the tubing (Fig. 26.7). Within the abdomen, a new dense region located near the shunt tip is strongly suggestive of a CSF pseudocyst. This finding can be confirmed with ultrasound by demonstration of an anechoic to hypoechoic structure in the peritoneum without internal blood flow.

To assess interval change in size of ventricles, either CT or MRI may be utilized and comparison to prior examinations is helpful to assess for subtle changes from the patient's baseline examination. Considering the priority of limiting ionizing radiation in children and the regularity that children with shunts require advanced imaging of the brain, "rapid MRI" examinations have been developed at many institutions. Rapid MRI provides assessment of ventricular size equivalent to CT and is reasonable for excluding other intracranial causes of symptoms. The time commitment is much shorter than with routine MRI examinations. Rapid MRI examinations typically consist of T2-weighted images in the axial, sagittal, and coronal planes and typically require 5–10 min to acquire. In the absence of comparison studies, large ventricles and transependymal flow of CSF, seen as hypoattenuation on CT and high T2 signal intensity on MRI, in the periventricular white matter may suggest recent increase in ventricle size and pressure, though these are

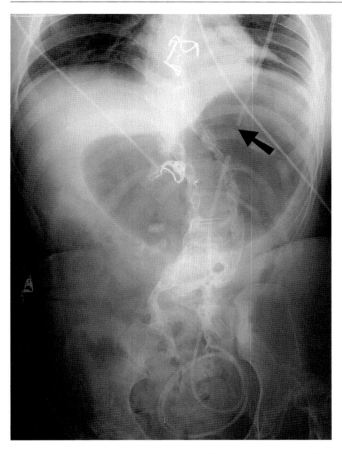

Fig. 26.7 Shunt catheter fragmentation. Abdominal radiograph in a patient with VP shunt malfunction shows fragmentation of the intra-abdominal portion of the shunt catheter (*arrow*)

nonspecific findings. Slit-like appearance of the ventricles may suggest overshunting in the absence of comparison examinations (Fig. 26.8) [8].

The main finding in the setting of ventriculitis on imaging is the abnormal appearance of CSF. On MRI, the infected CSF within the ventricles may retain signal characteristics on FLAIR and be relatively increased in signal to CSF on T1. On CT, infected CSF in the ventricles appears increased in attenuation relative to the rest of the CSF. The adjacent periventricular white matter usually appears edematous, with low attenuation on CT and high T2 signal on MRI.

Treatment of VP shunt malfunction is tailored to the specific cause of the malfunction, though most complications require neurosurgical procedures.

Chest

Bronchiolitis

Bronchiolitis is an infection of the smaller airways, which produces thick secretions that can obstruct the airways. Chest radiography may be performed to support the diagnosis and

to exclude other potential etiologies such as superimposed pneumonia.

The characteristic imaging findings of bronchiolitis result from thick secretions within the airways, which cause a combination of air trapping and atelectasis (Fig. 26.9). Air trapping results in a combination of focally and globally hyperexpanded lungs, which result in flattened diaphragms on both frontal and lateral radiographic views. Patchy atelectasis often results in streaky perihilar opacities, although it may present as larger portions of collapsed lung. Peribronchial thickening is typically present due to airway inflammation.

Treatment is generally supportive, though antiviral medication is used in severe cases of respiratory syncytial virus (RSV) infections.

Round Pneumonia

Pneumonia is common in the pediatric population, causing 13 % of infectious illnesses in children under the age of 2 years, with its incidence decreasing with increasing age [9, 10]. Chest radiography is the primary radiologic examination for the evaluation of pediatric pulmonary infections.

Bacterial pneumonia in children produces pulmonary consolidation(s) with air bronchograms that may be similar in appearance to infections in adults. The pediatric lung differs from the adult lung in the number of microscopic communicating channels between alveoli, called the pores of Kohn and channels of Lambert. The decreased number of these communications between alveoli prohibits the spread of exudates between adjacent alveoli [11]. The result is that some pediatric patients with pneumonia will present with well-defined, rounded airspace consolidations termed "round pneumonia" (Fig. 26.10).

The appearance of round pneumonia may be disconcerting because its shape may mimic a mass. If a diagnosis of round pneumonia is not definitive, a follow-up chest radiograph may be considered in approximately 6 weeks to evaluate for resolution.

Abdominal

Ingested Foreign Body

Due to the tendency for young children to place objects in their mouth, both accidentally and purposefully ingested foreign bodies are a relatively common occurrence in the pediatric population. The overall significance of the ingested foreign body depends on its nature [12]. Most small objects, however, will pass harmlessly through the gastrointestinal tract.

Radiographic evaluation of suspected foreign body ingestion may include a neck and chest radiograph to evaluate the esophagus and airways as well as an abdominal radiograph

Fig. 26.8 Overshunting after shunt placement. Post-shunt placement baseline CT and follow-up rapid MR in an 11-year-old female shows marked decrease in the size of the lateral ventricles on follow-up imaging. The overshunting was believed to be the cause of the patient's acute episode of vomiting and headache

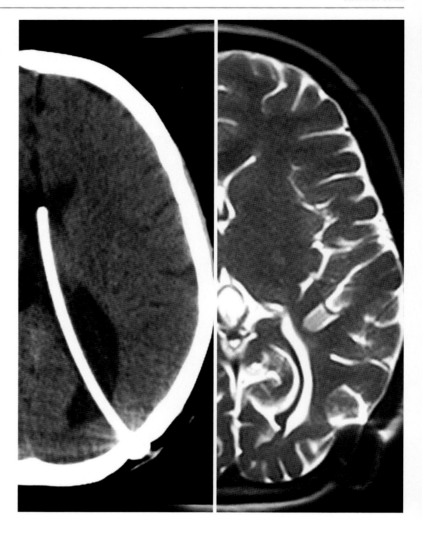

to assess the remainder of the gastrointestinal tract. Some plastics and naturally occurring objects, such as wood, are radiolucent and may be radiographically undetectable. Most glass and metallic foreign bodies, excluding thin aluminum objects, are conspicuous (Fig. 26.11).

Management will depend on the object that has been ingested and its potential for harm. Obstruction and a high risk of perforation may be managed with endoscopy or surgery depending on the location of the foreign body. Smaller objects may warrant serial radiographs to assess distal progression. Batteries, particularly the disk varieties, may leak their contents and are therefore followed closely, with a low threshold for intervention. Magnets are unique in their ability to attract each other in adjacent segments of bowel, poten-

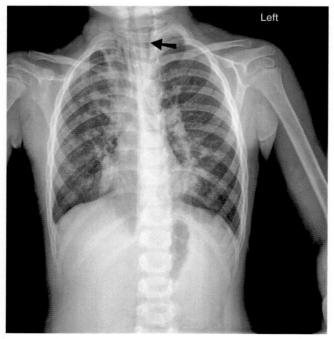

Fig. 26.9 Bronchiolitis and pneumomediastinum. Frontal chest radiograph in a patient with RSV infection demonstrates a combination of bilateral perihilar atelectasis and hyperexpanded lungs. Note the presence of pneumomediastinum (*arrow*) with gas tracking up the neck soft tissues

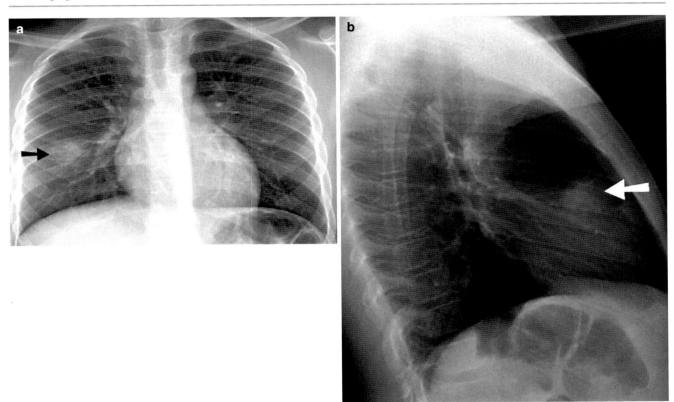

Fig. 26.10 Round pneumonia. (**a**, **b**) Frontal and lateral chest radiographs demonstrate a round consolidation in the right middle lobe (*arrows*)

tially causing focal pressure necrosis which may result in perforation and sepsis.

Intussusception

Intussusception is one of the most common and important causes of an acute abdomen in the pediatric population, occurring most frequently at the ileocecal valve. The history and physical examination in patients with an intussusception is often nonspecific. The clinical threshold to proceed to imaging workup is low because of the potential for adverse outcome associated with failing to diagnose and treat an intussusception.

The initial imaging workup for a child with suspected intussusception is an abdominal ultrasound noting that when abdominal radiographs are performed, the bowel gas pattern may be abnormal and nonspecific. Ultrasound is estimated to have a 97.9 % sensitivity, a 97.8 % specificity, and a 99.7 % negative predictive value (Fig. 26.12) [13]. Dilated, fluid-filled small bowel may be seen, suggesting obstruction. The intussusception will appear as a round mass with the imaging characteristics of its contents: Bowel wall is hypoechoic with a hyperechoic mucosa, but the appearance of the wall of the intussusceptum may be relatively hypoechoic due to congestion and edema. The mesentery

contains fat, which is hyperechoic relative to bowel, and lymph nodes, which are oval and hypoechoic relative to fat. The classic bowel-within-bowel appearance of an intussusception is best appreciated on images obtained transverse to the bowel lumen.

The treatment of intussusception is dependent on the patient's clinical status. If the patient presents relatively early in the process, air contrast or water-soluble contrast enema reduction may be attempted with high success rates. Patients who appear septic warrant surgical consultation [14].

Malrotation with Midgut Volvulus

The small and large bowel has ligamentous attachments, which tether it in place. In the case of malrotated bowel, these attachments are often absent. The bowel is therefore free to move and rotate, potentially on its axis, with resulting obstruction and vascular compromise. Volvulus is most commonly seen in the first few days of life, although any young child with bilious vomiting warrants consideration of this diagnosis. If not recognized and treated promptly, the bowel supplied by the superior mesenteric vessels will infarct and bowel necrosis will ensue.

The initial test of choice in an infant younger than 6 weeks of age with bilious vomiting is the abdominal radiograph,

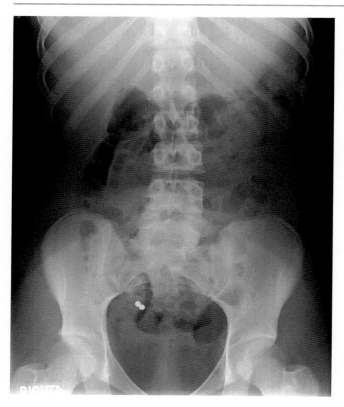

Fig. 26.11 Ingested metallic foreign bodies. Frontal radiograph of the abdomen and pelvis demonstrates two radiodense objects in the right lower quadrant. These were known to be batteries and when distal progression halted, surgery was performed and the batteries were found in the lumen of the appendix

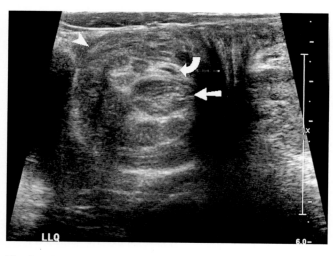

Fig. 26.12 Intussusception. Abdominal ultrasound of the descending colon demonstrates centrally located hypoechoic bowel (*straight arrow*) within the descending colon (*arrowhead*). Note the hyperechoic mesenteric fat (*curved arrow*) with internal hypoechoic lymph nodes associated with the intussusceptum

which is used to evaluate for obstruction and to determine if the obstruction is proximal or distal. If there are findings suspicious for proximal obstruction, upper GI fluoroscopy is

then performed in order to evaluate the anatomy, and specifically, the position of the ligament of Treitz. In malrotation with midgut volvulus, enteric contrast will empty into the proximal duodenum; however, instead of crossing the midline to the left and into the third portion of the duodenum, contrast will be descending inferiorly on the right. As small quantities of oral contrast advance through the proximal small bowel, a corkscrew configuration may be evident representing the bowel having been twisted upon its axis in a midgut volvulus [15] (Fig. 26.13).

Prompt surgical intervention is indicated; the classic intervention is the Ladd procedure.

Hypertrophic Pyloric Stenosis

While hypertrophic pyloric stenosis does not necessarily represent a true surgical emergency, it is a commonly encountered problem in the emergency department due to its striking presentation and potential to lead to dehydration. Clinical suspicion of the hypertrophic pyloric stenosis generally merits ultrasound workup as this is nearly 100 % sensitive and specific for the purpose of confirming or excluding hypertrophic pyloric stenosis [16].

Pyloric ultrasound is the preferred imaging test for an older infant (greater than 6 weeks) with a new onset of nonbilious vomiting. The length of the pyloric channel is measured in the longitudinal plane, while the pyloric muscle diameter is best obtained in the transverse plane relative to the pylorus. The upper limit of normal for thickness of the muscularis is approximately 3 mm (Fig. 26.14). The pyloric channel length is typically also reported for purpose of surgical planning [17]. Failure to demonstrate passage of gastric contents through the pylorus and into the duodenum during the examination further supports the diagnosis.

Surgical treatment consists of pyloromyotomy; long-term prognosis is excellent.

Musculoskeletal

Septic Arthritis and Transient Synovitis

One of the most common pediatric musculoskeletal surgical emergencies is septic arthritis. A clinically similar condition, transient synovitis, is characterized by sterile joint fluid and synovial inflammation that may mimic the imaging features of septic arthritis. In both septic arthritis and transient synovitis, there is almost always a joint effusion present, and there may be accompanying warmth and erythema. It may not be possible to reliably examine the hip joint in some patients, especially when the patient is

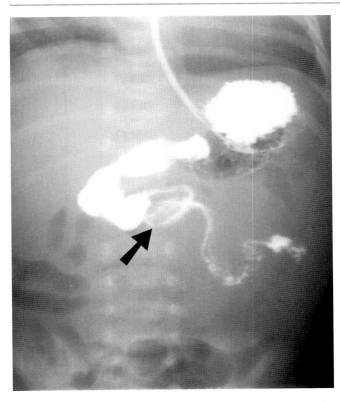

Fig. 26.13 Midgut volvulus. Frontal radiograph from an upper GI series demonstrates the proximal small bowel in a corkscrew pattern (*arrow*)

unable to tolerate movement of the joint. For this reason, the hip joint often receives more imaging consideration than other joints.

The predominant imaging findings in both transient synovitis and septic arthritis are joint effusion and synovial enhancement. Effusion is often easily identified in most joints, but small hip effusions may be occult both clinically and radiographically. Hip ultrasound is often performed initially. The affected side will demonstrate a hip joint capsule with increased fluid, which can vary in echogenicity from anechoic to hyperechoic (Fig. 26.15). Sonographic comparison to the unaffected side should always be made. If clinically indicated, an MRI with contrast may be obtained. The typical MRI findings of both septic arthritis and transient synovitis are a joint effusion with high T2 signal intensity and low T1 signal intensity and synovial enhancement on T1-weighted post-gadolinium images. On MRI, if there is abnormal bone marrow signal and enhancement in the bones adjacent to the affected joint, these findings favor the diagnosis of septic arthritis (Fig. 26.16) [18]. If septic arthritis is clinically suspected, joint fluid analysis should be obtained.

Septic arthritis warrants prompt surgical exploration, debridement, and treatment with intravenous antibiotics. Transient synovitis is usually self-limiting and does not necessitate surgical intervention.

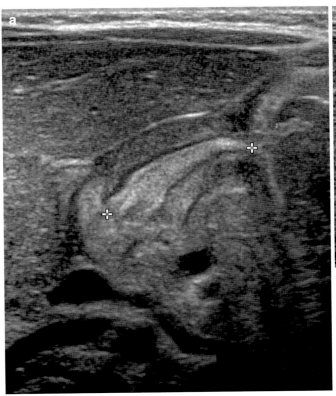

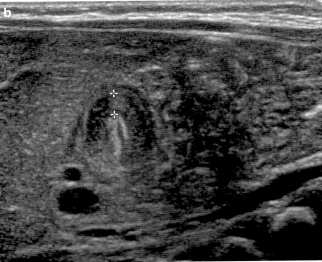

Fig. 26.14 Hypertrophic pyloric stenosis. (**a, b**) Longitudinal and transverse grayscale ultrasonographic images of the pylorus in a child with projectile vomiting demonstrating a pylorus measuring 3.5 mm in thickness and a pyloric channel measuring 2 cm in length

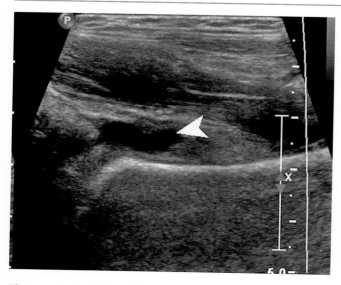

Fig. 26.15 Hip effusion. Grayscale ultrasound evaluation of the right and left hips in a 4-year-old girl with acute pain and refusal to walk on the left leg demonstrates a left hip effusion (*arrowhead*)

Teaching Points

- ADEM is best diagnosed by combining clinical, radiological, and laboratory information.
- MRI of the head with contrast is the imaging test of choice when evaluating for intracranial spread of sinus or middle ear infections due to its better specificity compared to CT as well as its lack of ionizing radiation.
- MRI of the orbits with contrast is considered by the ACR to be the best initial imaging examination for evaluation of pediatric orbital infections for its detailed information of the patient's abnormalities and its lack of ionizing radiation.
- Patients with acute onset of severe neurologic deficits and back pain in the absence of trauma warrant MRI evaluation with contrast owing to its ability to define the location and extent of the abnormality as well as to evaluate for mass lesions that may produce similar symptoms.
- To assess the brain and ventricles of pediatric patients with VP shunts, order rapid MRI examinations when

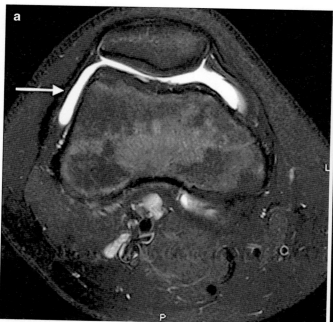

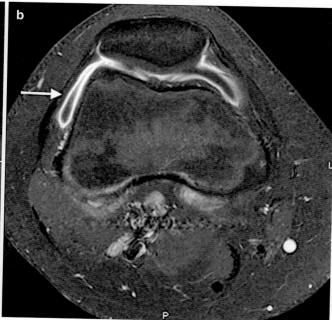

Fig. 26.16 Transient synovitis. (**a**) Axial T2-weighted fat-saturated image of the patient's right knee demonstrates normal bone marrow signal and a small suprapatellar knee effusion (*white arrow*). (**b**) Axial post-gadolinium T1-weighted image of the knee shows synovial enhancement (*arrow*), consistent with synovial inflammation

available and feasible as these patients often accumulate large radiation doses to the head over time.

- Ultrasound is an established first-line imaging modality for suspected intussusception that has an excellent sensitivity, specificity, and negative predictive value.
- When evaluating a young infant (<6 weeks) with bilious emesis, start with an abdominal radiograph to localize the obstruction.
- Pyloric ultrasound is almost 100 % sensitive and specific in confirming or excluding hypertrophic pyloric stenosis.
- Especially when physical examination of a joint is limited, ultrasound may be extremely helpful in evaluating for joint effusions.

References

1. Menge T, Hemmer B, Nessler S, Wiendl H, Neu haus O, Hartung HP, et al. Acute disseminated encephalomyelitis: an update. Arch Neurol. 2005;62:1673–80.
2. Madan S, Aneja S, Tripathi RP, Batra A, Seth A, Taluja V. Acute disseminated encephalomyelitis – a case series. Indian Pediatr. 2005;42:367–71.
3. Baum PA, Barkovich AJ, Koch TK, Berg BO. Deep gray matter involvement in children with acute disseminated encephalomyelitis. AJNR Am J Neuroradiol. 1994;15:1275–83.
4. Apak RA, Kose G, Anlar B, Turanli G, Topaloglu H, Ozdirim E. Acute disseminated encephalomyelitis in childhood: report of 10 cases. J Child Neurol. 1999;14:198–201.
5. Leach JL, Fortuna RB, Jones BV, Gaskill-Shipley MF. Imaging of cerebral venous thrombosis: current techniques, spectrum of findings, and diagnostic pitfalls. Radiographics. 2006;26 Suppl 1:S19–41; discussion S42–3.
6. Ludwig BJ, Foster BR, Saito N, Nadgir RN, Castro-Aragon I, Sakai O. Diagnostic imaging in nontraumatic pediatric head and neck emergencies. Radiographics. 2010;30:781–99.
7. Choi KH, Lee KS, Chung SO, Park JM, Kim YJ, Kim HS, et al. Idiopathic transverse myelitis: MR characteristics. AJNR Am J Neuroradiol. 1996;17:1151–60.
8. Goeser CD, McLeary MS, Young LW. Diagnostic imaging of ventriculoperitoneal shunt malfunctions and complications. Radiographics. 1998;18:635–51.
9. Eren S, Balci AE, Dikici B, Doblan M, Eren MN. Foreign body aspiration in children: experience of 1160 cases. Ann Trop Paediatr. 2003;23:31–7.
10. Denny FW, Clyde WA Jr. Acute lower respiratory tract infections in nonhospitalized children. J Pediatr. 1986;108:635–46.
11. Bramson RT, Griscom NT, Cleveland RH. Interpretation of chest radiographs in infants with cough and fever. Radiology. 2005; 236:22–9.
12. Hunter TB, Taljanovic MS. Foreign bodies. Radiographics. 2003;23:731–57.
13. Hryhorczuk AL, Strouse PJ. Validation of us as a first-line diagnostic test for assessment of pediatric ileocolic intussusception. Pediatr Radiol. 2009;39:1075–9.
14. Niramis R, Watanatittan S, Kruatrachue A, Anuntkosol M, Buranakitjaroen V, Rattanasuwan T, et al. Management of recurrent intussusception: nonoperative or operative reduction? J Pediatr Surg. 2010;45:2175–80.
15. Houston CS, Wittenborg MH. Roentgen evaluation of anomalies of rotation and fixation of the bowel in children. Radiology. 1965;84:1–18.
16. Hernanz-Schulman M, Neblett WW. Imaging of infantile hypertrophic pyloric stenosis (IHPS). In: Medina LS, Applegate K, Blackmore CC, editors. Evidence-based imaging in pediatrics: improving the quality of imaging in patient care. New York: Springer; 2009.
17. Cogley JR, O'Connor SC, Houshyar R, Dulaimy KA. Emergent pediatric us: what every radiologist should know. Radiographics. 2012;32:651–65.
18. Lee SK, Suh KJ, Kim YW, Ryeom HK, Kim YS, Lee JM, et al. Septic arthritis versus transient synovitis at mr imaging: preliminary assessment with signal intensity alterations in bone marrow. Radiology. 1999;211:459–65.

Index

A

Abdominal
    hypertrophic pyloric stenosis, 370
    ingested foreign body, 367–369
    intussusception, 369
    malrotation, midgut volvulus, 369–371
Abdominal aortic aneurysm (AAA)
    aortic dissection (*see* Aortic dissection)
    aortic rupture, 1, 2
    aorto-enteric fistula, 1, 3
    causes, 1
    draped aorta sign, 4, 5
    etiologies, 1
    hyperdense crescent sign, 4
    imaging, 4
    saccular, 1, 2
    ultrasound, 1
Acetabulum, lower extremity trauma
    anterior and posterior columns, pelvis, 280
    description, 279
    presence of abnormality, 279–280
ACF. *See* Anterior cranial fossa (ACF)
Acromioclavicular dislocation, 262
ACS. *See* Acute coronary syndrome (ACS)
Acute aortic conditions
    AAA (*see* Abdominal aortic aneurysm (AAA))
    description, 1
Acute cholecystitis
    chronic calculous cholecystitis, 175, 179
    complete common bile duct obstruction, 175, 180
    false-positives and false-negatives, HBS, 175, 179
    gallstones, 174
    gangrenous, 175, 178
    HBS, 175
    normal, 175, 178
    pathophysiologic changes, 175
    typical hepatobiliary scintigraphy technical protocol, 175, 178
Acute colonic disorders
    acute diverticulitis, 65–66
    colonic ischemia, 78, 80
    epiploic appendagitis (*see* Acute epiploic appendagitis)
    GI bleeding, 80–81
    inflammatory bowel disease, 70–72
    pseudomembranous colitis, 72, 73
    segmental omental infarction, 66, 69
    typhlitis, 72, 73–74
    volvulus, 73–79
Acute coronary syndrome (ACS)
    abnormal rest MPI, 172, 177
    clinical presentation, ECG and cardiac biomarkers, 169
    ERASE trial, 173
    high NPV, 172

medical emergencies, 169
    MPI, 172, 174
    normal rest MPI, 172, 176
    risk groups, patients, 170
    typical rest with chest pain, 172, 175
Acute disseminated encephalomyelitis (ADEM), 361, 362
Acute diverticulitis
    colovesical fistula, 65, 68
    giant sigmoid diverticulum, 65, 67
    imaging, 65
    treatment, 65
Acute epiploic appendagitis
    imaging, 70
    torsion, 66, 67
Acute gynecologic disorders
    functional ovarian cysts, 155–157
    pelvic pain, 155
    PID, 156–158
Acute head emergencies imaging
    acute hypertensive encephalopathy, 212
    brain death (*see* Brain death)
    carbon monoxide poisoning, 199, 200
    central nervous system infections, 199–202
    cerebral arterial air embolism, 209–211
    cerebral contusions, 206, 208–209
    cortical laminar necrosis, 209, 210
    CSF leak (*see* Cerebrospinal fluid (CSF) leak)
    description, 199
    extra-axial hemorrhages (*see* Extra-axial hemorrhages)
    giant MCA aneurysm, 203, 205
    herniation syndromes, 204, 206, 208
    herpes encephalitis, 202–203
    obstructive hydrocephalus, 210–212
    pseudo-subarachnoid hemorrhage (*see* Pseudo-subarachnoid hemorrhage)
    spontaneous intracranial hypotension, 204, 206
    tension pneumocephalus, 203, 204
Acute hepatitis
    diagnosis, 125
    fulminant hepatitis, 125
    pyogenic hepatic abscess, 125, 127
    ultrasound, 125–126
Acute hypertensive encephalopathy, 212
Acute ischemic stroke
    CTA (*see* Computed tomography angiography (CTA))
    CTP (*see* CT perfusion (CTP))
    goals, 4 "Ps", 230
    hemorrhage and surgically amenable lesions, 230
    hemorrhagic transformation, 232, 234
    infarct evolution, 235–236
    infarction, septic emboli, 235
    MR imaging, 232, 233

A. Singh (ed.), *Emergency Radiology*,
DOI 10.1007/978-1-4419-9592-6, © Springer Science+Business Media New York 2013

Printed by Printforce, the Netherlands